Frontiers in Human Brain Topography

Frontiers in Human Brain Topography

Proceedings of the 15th World Congress of the International Society for Brain Electromagnetic Topography (ISBET 2004) held in Urayasu, Japan between 11 and 14 April 2004

Editors:

Masafumi Nakagawa
Department of Otorhinolaryngology
Juntendo University School of Medicine
Tokyo
JAPAN
&
Vice Hospital Director
Mitsuwadai General Hospital
Chiba
JAPAN

Koichi Hirata
Department of Neurology
Dokkyo University School of Medicine
Mibu, Tochigi
JAPAN

Yoshihiko Koga
Department of Neuropsychiatry
Kyorin University School of Medicine
Mitaka, Tokyo
JAPAN

Ken Nagata
Department of Neurology
Research Institute for Brain and Blood Vessels
Senshu-Kubota Akita
JAPAN

ELSEVIER

2004

ELSEVIER B.V.
Sara Burgerhartstraat 25
P.O. Box 211, 1000 AE Amsterdam
The Netherlands

ELSEVIER Inc.
525 B Street, Suite 1900
San Diego, CA 92101-4495
USA

ELSEVIER Ltd
The Boulevard, Langford Lane
Kidlington, Oxford OX5 1GB
UK

ELSEVIER Ltd
84 Theobalds Road
London WC1X 8RR
UK

First edition 2004

Library of Congress Cataloging in Publication Data
A catalog record is available from the Library of Congress.

British Library Cataloguing in Publication Data
A catalogue record is available from the British Library.

International Congress Series No. 1270
ISBN: 0-444-51655-7
ISSN: 0531-5131

⊗ The paper used in this publication meets the requirements of ANSI/NISO Z39.48-1992 (Permanence of Paper).
Printed in The Netherlands.

ELSEVIER

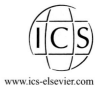

www.ics-elsevier.com

Preface

This volume contains the proceedings of the 15th Congress of the International Society for Brain Electromagnetic Topography (ISBET2004) held in the Tokyo Disney Sea, Chiba, Japan. Over 70 papers were selected for presentation among the submitted papers, 20 invited talks were given and five symposium papers were presented. We experimented this year with poster sessions and selected 10 Young Scientist Awards, including one Best Paper Award among them. Also this year, the 21st Annual Meeting of the Japanese Society for Brain Electromagnetic Topography (JASBET) was held in conjunction with ISBET2004 at the same venue.

The papers in this volume give an indication of new trends in this field. The successive meeting covered a wide aspect of topics for brain topography and brain mappings from basic neuroscience to clinical applications using EEG, ERP, SPECT, PET, MEG, f-MRI, NIRS, Transcranial Magnetic Stimulation (TMS), etc. These focused especially on multimodal integration, hearing and language, oral and masticatory science, plasticity and deprivation and new methods, including NIRS and event-related f-MRI.

The technical program comprised of paper sessions, invited talks and symposiums. The invited speakers are internationally distinguished researchers. We thank them for preparing papers on their talks. These papers are included in these proceedings.

The success of the conference depends on support and cooperation from many individuals and organizations; ISBET2004 was no exception. We would like to take this opportunity to thank the authors, and the organizing and program committee members of the conference for their time and effort spent on making ISBET2004 a successful and enjoyable conference.

Last but not least, we would like to thank everyone who was involved with this conference for his/her cooperation.

Masafumi Nakagawa
Yoshihiko Koga
Ken Nagata
Koichi Hirata

0531-5131/ © 2004 Elsevier B.V. All rights reserved.
doi:10.1016/j.ics.2004.05.154

International Congress Series 1270 (2004) vi

ELSEVIER

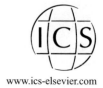

www.ics-elsevier.com

Address

As a symposium organizer, I am very glad to address the keystone of planning this symposium of the ISBET2004 Congress.

The 20th century was filled with major advances in science and technology. At the beginning of the century, the first Nobel Prize in physics was presented in 1901 to Wilhelm Conrad Roentgen, the discoverer of the X-ray. The invention of radiography contributed greatly to medical diagnostics. However, there was a long wait until the appearance of a new modality for the noninvasive observation of the structure and function of a vital brain.

Last year, the Nobel Prize in physiology or medicine was presented to two inventors of Magnetic Resonance Imaging (MRI), which came 100 years after the discovery of the X-ray. Although MRI is an integration of various advanced technologies, obviously this technology has not been utilized without the application of superconductivity. Another remarkable contribution of superconductivity for brain research is Magneto-encephalography (MEG). These new modalities have improved spatial and temporal resolution for brain imaging and functional examination, which rapidly replaced legacy techniques.

Numerous corroborations have been demonstrated that oral function may relate closely to brain function or that oral function is regulated by the central nervous system. We have investigated the relationship between oral and brain function by means of magneto-encephalography (MEG). Only a few studies on oral function have been carried out using fMRI or MEG, and there was no other place to meet and exchange information on this matter.

I am more than happy that all of us are gathered in this symposium today to exchange the successful outcomes of studies on brain and oral function. Sincere gratitude is expressed to the Congress President, Dr. Nakagawa, who provided the opportunity to have this symposium.

I would like to encourage your further interest in and attention to the topics.

Tatsuya Ishikawa

0531-5131/ © 2004 Published by Elsevier B.V.
doi:10.1016/j.ics.2004.05.153

Young Scientist Award Winners

These papers were awarded in the poster competition for young scientists

Sayaka Imaeda, Himeji Institute of Technology, Japan
Wavelet-based hemodynamic analyzing method in event-related fMRI with statistical parocessing

Yohei Tamura, National Institute for Physiological Sciences, Japan
Effects of repetitive transcranial magnetic stimulation on acute pain

Kotoe Sakihara, Osaka University Graduate School of Medicine, Japan
The late response in the soleus muscle evoked by transcranial magnetic stimulation at the foramen magnum level

Noriko Yazawa, Ibaraki University, Japan
Event related potential due to vocalization of a single syllable in Down syndrome

Takashi Abe, Hiroshima University, Japan
Current sources of the brain potentials before rapid eye movements in human REM sleep

Keiichi Onoda, Hiroshima University, Japan
LORETA analysis of CNV in time perception

Megumi Masuzawa, Ibaraki University, Japan
SERPs due to vibration presented at index fingers and selective-attention in the blind

Mai Fukumoto, Graduate School of Tokyo Medical and Dental University Japan
Functional MRI study on neural network dysfunction in schizophrenia and epileptic psychosis

ISBET 2004 Organizing Committee

Honorary Conference Chair
Ginichiro Ichikawa Juntendo University, Japan

Conference Chair
Masafumi Nakagawa Mitsuwadai General Hospital, Japan

Vice Conference Chairs
Ken Nagata Research Institute for Brain and Blood Vessels Akita, Japan
Yoshihiko Koga Kyorin University, Japan

Program Chair
Koichi Hirata, Dokkyo University School of Medicine, Japan

Advisors:
Shigeaki Matsuoka, University of Occupational and Environmental Health, Japan
Tada Tomio University of Tokyo, Japan
Hisamasa Imai Tokyo Rinkai Hospital, Japan

Organizing Committee
Keiichiro Kasai Tokyo Rinkai Hospital, Japan
Toshiaki Masumura Tokyo Rinkai Hospital, Japan
Tsuneya Nakajima Tokyo Dental College, Japan
Yoshinori Matsuwaki Tokyo Dental College, Japan
Yasutomo Yoshida Juntendo University, Japan
Shotaro Nakamura Mitsuwadai General Hospital, Japan
Yoshiyuki Iida Koshigawa Municipal Hospital, Japan
Ryuta Tokumaru Juntendo University, Japan
Takafumi Yuasa Toho University, Japan
Shin-ya Inami Tokyo Rinkai Hospital, Japan
Eiji Kirino Juntendo University, Japan

Under the auspices of
ISBET Executive Committee
Chairman
Wolfgang Skrandies, Giessen, Germany

Co-Chairman
Frank Duffy, Boston, USA

Treasurer
Thomas Dierkes, Bern, Switzerland

Secretary
Koichi Hirata, Mibu, Tochigi, Japan

Members at large
Alan Gevins, San Francisco, USA
Ken Nagata, Akita, Japan
Yoshio Okada, Albuquerque, USA
Richard Silberstein, Melbourne, Australia
Fernando Lopes da Silva, Amsterdam
Peter K.H. Wong, Vancouver, Canada

Honorary Emeritus Chairman
Dietrich Lehmann, Zurich, Switzerland

Honorary Founding member
Konrad Maurer, Frankfurt, German

Honorary Emeritus member
Shigeaki Matsuoka, Kitakyushu, Japan

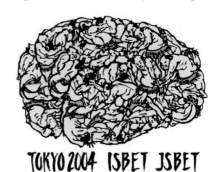

TOKYO 2004 ISBET JSBET

Contents

Keynote contributions

International Congress Series 1270 (2004) 3–8

ELSEVIER

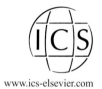

www.ics-elsevier.com

From high-resolution EEG to electrophysiological neuroimaging

Bin He*, Lei Ding

Department of Biomedical Engineering, University of Minnesota, 7-105 BSBE, 312 Church Street, Minneapolis, MN 55455, USA

Abstract. This article provides a brief review of the state-of-the-art of EEG inverse problem in several important areas. Developments in Laplacian mapping, cortical imaging, dipole source localization, and distributed source estimation are covered. It is our intent to provide an overall introduction instead of exhaustive review of this fascinating field in this short article. © 2004 Elsevier B.V. All rights reserved.

Keywords: High-resolution EEG; Electrophysiological neuroimaging; Inverse problem; Neuroimaging

1. Introduction

Advanced functional brain imaging techniques have greatly enhanced our understanding of the human brain through noninvasive imaging of the electrophysiological, metabolic, and hemodynamic processes underlying normal or pathological brain activity. Among these modalities, the EEG has an unsurpassed millisecond-scale temporal resolution, but has limited spatial resolution due to the smearing effect of the low-conductivity skull. Over the past few decades, a significant effort has been made by a number of investigators to enhance the spatial resolution of EEG by increasing substantially the number of recording channels, developing numerical algorithms to restore the lost high-frequency components in the scalp EEG signals. Such approach has been usually called High-Resolution EEG (HR-EEG), which has achieved a great deal in the past decade.

An important advancement in the history of science is the development of magnetic resonance imaging (MRI). Numerous studies have shown that structure and functional MRI have changed the state-of-the-art of neuroimaging. A great effort has been made in the past several years to develop electrophysiological neuroimaging modalities, which incorporate anatomic details, as obtained from MRI, into HR-EEG, such that electrophysiological information can be coded over the anatomically realistic brain [1].

This article provides a brief review of several selected areas of research activity in the field of electrophysiological neuroimaging.

* Corresponding author. Tel.: +1-612-626-1115; fax: +1-612-626-6583.
E-mail address: binhe@umn.edu (B. He).

0531-5131/ © 2004 Elsevier B.V. All rights reserved.
doi:10.1016/j.ics.2004.06.015

2. Surface source imaging

Two important surface source imaging techniques have been developed to restore high-frequency spatial information regarding brain electrical activity over different surfaces, i.e. the scalp or the cortical surface. The first approach is the so-called surface Laplacian (SL), which employs a Laplacian filter to enhance the high-frequency components of brain electrical activity that are smeared and distorted by the low-conductivity skull and achieve high-resolution imaging over the scalp surface [2–7]. The SL can be interpreted as an equivalent charge density or equivalent current density over the scalp surface [8,9]. Implementations of Laplacian operator have been realised by local-based methods [2–4], global-based methods [5–7], or application of the spline algorithm to regional potential recordings [4]. Among the reported SL methods, spline SL algorithms [5–7], have been shown to provide the best performance and robustness against measurement noise.

Another approach is cortical potential imaging technique (CIT) which uses an explicit biophysical model of the passive conducting properties of a head to deconvolve the smeared scalp potential (SP) into the epicortical potential distributions [10–18]. Taking advantage of numerical computational methods, such as boundary element method (BEM) and finite element method (FEM), the realistic geometry (RG) CIT algorithms avoid the co-registration error when using approximated spherical head models and offer much-enhanced spatial resolution as compared with the blurred scalp potentials. FEM-based CIT demonstrates great flexibilities to incorporate the detailed three-dimensional (3D) conductivity distribution [11]. Recently, BEM-based CIT has been shown to provide excellent performance in directly estimating cortical potentials from SPs in humans [17]. Compared with SL estimate over the scalp, RG CIT techniques allow reconstruction of electrical potential fields directly over the brain surface and with anatomic details [11,13,17]. Due to the anatomic details provided by structure imaging such as MRI, RG CIT techniques offer important capabilities of imaging electrocorticograms from noninvasive SPs.

3. Dipole source localization

The basic dipole source localization (DSL) method is the least-squares source estimation which estimates the dipole parameters [19–23] that can best explain the observed SP measurements in the least-squares sense. Due to the nonlinear characteristic of parameter space, nonlinear multidimensional minimization procedures should be employed with the expense of computation time. Minimization methods range from Levenberg–Marquardt and Nelder–Meade downhill simplex searches to global optimization schemes, genetic algorithms and simulated annealing [24]. Simulation and experimental studies have demonstrated that incorporating the anatomic details, as obtained from MRI, allows DSL to localize neural sources with greater accuracy [22,23,25].

A key problem with the least-squares source estimation is that the number of sources has to be decided a priori. Furthermore, the nonconvexity of the least-squares cost function becomes much more severe and nonlinear multidimensional search becomes unpractical as the number of sources increases. The alternatives described below avoid such difficulties by scanning a region of interest.

Beamforming approaches perform spatial filtering on data from sensory array to separate signals between those arriving from a location of interest and those originating somewhere else. Linearly constrained minimum variance (LCMV) beamforming [26] provides an adaptive version in which the limited degrees of freedom are used to place nulls in the response at positions corresponding to interfering sources. Another alternative is a group of methods termed subspace source localization methods, e.g. multiple signal classification (MUSIC) algorithm [27], which give estimates for multiple dipole locations using a 3D search. The procedure of subspace source localization methods can be divided into two steps. The first step is to estimate the signal and the noise-only subspace from the measured EEG data, and then apply a projection, as the second step, onto the estimated noise-only subspace to get their cost functions' extrema. After MUSIC, Mosher and Leahy [28] further introduced recursively applied and projected MUSIC (RAP-MUSIC), which had better source resolvability in highly correlated source localization problems. Sekihara et al. [29] incorporated estimated noise covariance into classic MUSIC algorithm to reduce the influence from background activity. We have recently introduced another subspace method, *first principle vectors* (FINES) [30] to EEG source localization, which demonstrates smaller estimation bias and better spatial resolution for closely spaced sources by employing projections onto a particular set of vectors in the noise-only subspace instead of entire noise-only subspace.

4. Distributed source estimation

The distributed source model assumes brain electrical sources continuously distribute over all specified surface or volume and does not require the ad hoc assumption about the number of sources. Because nonlinear parameters, such as source locations, can be incorporated into the lead field matrix, the distributed source estimation problems, in most cases, can be expressed as a linear formulation which is a highly underdetermined system. In order to achieve the unique solution, additional constraint, e.g. minimum norm [31], must be applied. Furthermore, regularization methods [32,33] need to be employed to suppress the noise effect on the underdetermined linear problem.

The cortical current source imaging is a two-dimensional surface current source imaging technique and is developed to estimate the strength of the equivalent cortical current dipole layer from the scalp potentials [31,34–37]. There are two ways to reconstruct the equivalent cortical current dipole layer. One is to model the cortex as a flattened surface without the detailed sulci and gyri information and equivalent cortical current dipole layer defined on a surface which is very close to the flattened cortex [35,38]. Another is to model the cortex as a folded surface where sulci and gyri are preserved [39,40,36,37]. The anatomical constraint applied in such model is based on the observation that the cortical generators of EEG signals are localized to the grey matter and oriented perpendicularly to the cortical sheet [8].

The abovementioned approaches are mainly achieved using BEM and FEM because detailed anatomical information is required. Furthermore, integration with fMRI are available in the constrained cortical current imaging techniques. Dale and Sereno [34] proposed a framework to integrate EEG, MEG, MRI, and fMRI based on the Wiener linear inverse filter. Liu et al. [41] investigated the proposed framework and demonstrated that using fMRI as constraint with proper weighting showed much improved source estimation performance by means of so-called "crosstalk" metric and spatial point spread function.

The well-known 3D estimation is minimum norm (MN) solution [31]. Unfortunately, the MN solution exhibits an undesired depth dependency which favors superficial sources.

Then, two other well-known weighting solutions, i.e. diagonal matrix weighted minimum norm (WMN) solution [42,43] and the Laplacian weighted minimum norm (LWMN) solution, also known as LORETA [44], were introduced to compensate such bias. Furthermore, these variants of MN solutions can be represented in the Bayesian framework [45]. Another kind of nonlinear approach can be achieved using L1-norm instead of L2-norm which is commonly used in the abovementioned solutions to partially overcome the smeared effect due to the regularization procedure. Iterative methods, such as FOCUSS [43], using MN as initial estimate, and SCEA, using LORETA or others as initial estimate [46], are also available to find the localized sparse solutions.

Alternative approaches which are not based on the equivalent dipole source model are also worthy of inclusion here because they belong to the category of 3D estimation problem. ELECTRA [47] reconstructed the 3D electric potential distribution over the brain volume. Meanwhile, 3D distribution of equivalent current source (monopole) was estimated by means of LWMN algorithm [48].

Statistical inference over the distributed source estimation has been taken into consideration on the cortical current source imaging and 3D estimation. The cortical current source imaging was normalized in terms of noise sensitivity at each spatial location to obtain statistical parametric maps of brain activity [49] and standardized LORETA method using similar procedure in 3D estimation were proposed [50].

5. Discussion

This article briefly reviews important techniques which have been developed for electrophysiologic neuroimaging, including surface source imaging, dipole source localization, and distributed source estimation. As discussed above, it is clear that there has been no unified solution in the functional brain imaging problem. Each method has its own advantage and bears its own limitations. While surface source imaging, dipole source localization, and cortical current density estimation have been well developed, explored, and analyzed, 3D source estimation is still developing and exhibits the potential to achieve full knowledge of 3D distributed brain activity.

Integration with other imaging modalities in electrophysiological neuroimaging has attracted increasing attention because of its potential benefits of both higher spatial resolvability and higher dynamic resolution on time courses. This ability has been partially demonstrated in the dipole source localization and the cortical current imaging. In addition to the integration of fMRI prior to the cortical current source imaging [34,36,37,41], integration with other functional imaging modalities in dipole source localization has also been developed and implemented (see Ref. [51] for review). The challenge of integration will be how to unify the experimental design and stimulus protocol and how to carry out co-registration between the measurements from different modalities.

In summary, tremendous efforts have been made in the field of HR-EEG and electrophysiological neuroimaging. The electrophysiological neuroimaging shall further advance the field, as the HR-EEG has, towards our ultimate goal of achieving high-resolution spatiotemporal imaging of brain functions, and would have an important impact on the fields of clinical neurosurgery, neural pathophysiology, cognitive neuroscience and neurophysiology.

Acknowledgements

This work was supported in part by NIH R01 EB00178, NSF BES-0218736 and NSF-9875344.

References

[1] B. He (Ed). Modeling and Imaging of Bioelectric Activity—Principles and Applications, Kluwer Academic/ Plenum Publishers, 2004.

[2] B. Hjorth, An on-line transformation of EEG scalp potentials into orthogonal source derivations, Electroencephalogr. Clin. Neurophysiol. 39 (1975) 526–530.

[3] A.S. Gevins, Dynamic functional topography of cognitive tasks, Brain Topogr. 2 (1989) 37–56.

[4] F. Zhao, B. He, A new algorithm to estimate surface Laplacian and its applications to visual evoked potentials, Electromagnetics 21 (2001) 633–640.

[5] F. Perrin, O. Bertrand, J. Pernier, Scalp current density mapping: value and estimation from potential data, IEEE Trans. Biomed. Eng. 34 (1987) 283–288.

[6] F. Babiloni, et al., Spline Laplacian estimate of EEG potentials over a realistic magnetic resonance-constructed scalp surface model, Electroencephalogr. Clin. Neurophysiol. 98 (1996) 363–373.

[7] B. He, J. Lian, G. Li, High-resolution EEG: a new realistic geometry spline Laplacian estimation technique, Clin. Neurophysiol. 112 (2001) 845–852.

[8] P.L. Nunez, Electric Field of the Brain, Oxford Univ. Press, London, 1981.

[9] B. He, R.J. Cohen, Body surface Laplacian ECG mapping, IEEE Trans. BME 39 (1992) 1179–1191.

[10] R. Sidman, et al., Age-related features of the resting and P300 auditory evoked responses using the dipole localization method and cortical imaging technique, J. Neurosci. Methods 33 (1990) 22–32.

[11] A. Gevins, et al., High resolution EEG: 124-channel recording, spatial deblurring and MRI integration methods, Electroencephalogr. Clin. Neurophysiol. 90 (1994) 337–358.

[12] B. He, et al., Cortical source imaging from scalp electroencephalograms, Med. Biol. Eng. Comput. 34 (1996) 257–258.

[13] F. Babiloni, et al., High resolution EEG: a new model-dependent spatial deblurring method using a realistically-shaped MR-constructed subject's head model, Electroencephalogr. Clin. Neurophysiol. 102 (1997) 69–80.

[14] B. He, Y. Wang, D. Wu, Estimating cortical potentials from scalp EEG's in a realistically shaped inhomogeneous head model, IEEE Trans. Biomed. Eng. 46 (1999) 1264–1268.

[15] B. He, et al., A cortical potential imaging analysis of the P300 and novelty P3 components, Hum. Brain Mapp. 12 (2001) 120–130.

[16] J.O. Ollikainen, et al., A new computational approach for cortical imaging, IEEE Trans. Med. Imag. 20 (2001) 325–332.

[17] B. He, et al., Boundary element method based cortical potential imaging of somatosensory evoked potentials using subjects' magnetic resonance images, NeuroImage 16 (2002) 564–576.

[18] X. Zhang, et al., High resolution EEG: cortical potential imaging of interictal spikes, Clin. Neurophysiol. 114 (2003) 1963–1973.

[19] R.N. Kavanagh, et al., Evaluation of methods for three-dimensional localization of electrical sources in the human brain, IEEE Trans. BME 25 (1978) 421–429.

[20] M. Scherg, D. Von Cramon, Two bilateral sources of the AEP as identified by a spatio-temporal dipole model, Electroencephalogr. Clin. Neurophysiol. 62 (1985) 32–44.

[21] B. He, et al., Electrical dipole tracing in the brain by means of the boundary element method and its accuracy, IEEE Trans. BME 34 (1987) 406–414.

[22] B.N. Cuffin, A method for localizing EEG sources in realistic head models, IEEE Trans. BME 42 (1995) 68–71.

[23] T. Musha, Y. Okamoto, Forward and inverse problems of EEG dipole localization, Crit. Rev. Biomed. Eng. 27 (1999) 189–239.

[24] K. Uutela, M. Hamalainen, R. Salmelin, Global optimization in the localization of neuromagnetic sources, IEEE Trans. Biomed. Eng. 45 (1998) 716–723.

[25] B.J. Roth, et al., Dipole localization in patients with epilepsy using the realistically shaped head model, Electroencephalogr. Clin. Neurophysiol. 102 (1997) 159–166.

[26] B.D. Van Veen, et al., Localization of brain electrical activity via linearly constrained minimum variance spatial filtering. 44 (1997) 867–880.

[27] J.C. Mosher, P.S. Lewis, R.M. Leahy, Multiple dipole modeling and localization from spatio-temporal MEG data IEEE, Trans. Biomed. Eng. 39 (1992) 541–557.

[28] J.C. Mosher, R.M. Leahy, Source localization using recursively applied and projected (RAP) MUSIC, IEEE Trans. Signal Process. 47 (1999) 332–340.

[29] K. Sekihara, et al., Noise covariance incorporated MEG-MUSIC algorithm: a method for multiple–dipole estimation tolerant of the influence of background brain activity, IEEE Trans. Biomed. Eng. 44 (1997) 839–849.

[30] X.L. Xu, B. Xu, B. He, An alternative subspace approach to EEG dipole source localization, Phys. Med. Biol. 49 (2004) 327–343.

[31] M. Hamalainen, R. Ilmoniemi, Interpreting measured magnetic fields of the brain: estimates of current distributions, Tech. Rep. TKF-F-A559, Helsinki Uni. of Tech., 1984.

[32] A.N. Tikhonov, V.Y. Arsenin, Solutions of Ill-Posed Problems, Wiley, New York, 1977.

[33] Y.S. Shim, Z.H. Cho, SVD pseudoinversion image reconstruction, IEEE Trans. Acoust. Speech Process. 29 (1981) 904–909.

[34] A.M. Dale, M.I. Sereno, Improved localization of cortical activity by combining EEG and MEG with MRI cortical surface reconstruction: a linear approach, J. Cogn. Neurosci. 5 (1993) 162–176.

[35] B. He, D. Yao, J. Lian, High resolution EEG: on the cortical equivalent dipole layer imaging, Clin. Neurophysiol. 113 (2002) 227–235.

[36] F. Babiloni, et al., Multimodal integration of high-resolution EEG and functional magnetic resonance imaging data: a simulation study, NeuroImage 19 (1) (2003 May) 1–15.

[37] F. Babiloni, et al., Assessing time-varying cortical functional connectivity with the multimodal integration of high resolution EEG and fMRI data by Directed Transfer Function, NeuroImage, submitted for publication.

[38] J. Hori, M. Aiba, B. He, Spatio-temporal cortical source imaging of brain electrical activity by means of time-varying parametric projection filter, IEEE Trans. Biomed. Eng. (2004) 768–777.

[39] M. Fuchs, et al., Linear and nonlinear current density reconstructions, J. Clin. Neurophysiol. 16 (1999) 267–295.

[40] A.M. Dale, B. Fischl, M.I. Sereno, Cortical surface-based analysis: I. Segmentation and surface reconstruction, NeuroImage 9 (1999) 179–194.

[41] A.K. Liu, J.W. Belliveau, A.M. Dale, Spatiotemporal imaging of human brain activity using fMRI constrained MEG data: Monte Carlo simulations, Proc. Natl. Acad. Sci. U. S. A. 95 (1998) 8945–8950.

[42] B. Jeffs, R. Leahy, M. Singh, An evaluation of methods for neuromagnetic image reconstruction, IEEE Trans. Biomed. Eng. 34 (1987) 713–723.

[43] I.F. Gorodnitsky, J.S. George, B.D. Rao, Neuromagnetic source imaging with FOCUSS: a recursive weighted minimum norm algorithm, Electroencephalogr. Clin Neurophysiol. 95 (1995) 231–251.

[44] R.D. Pascual-Marqui, C.M. Michel, D. Lehmann, Low resolution electromagnetic tomography: a new method for localizating electrical activity in the brain, Int. J. Psychophysiol. 18 (1994) 49–65.

[45] S. Baillet, L. Garnero, A Bayesian approach to introducing anatomo-functional priors in the EEG/MEG inverse problem, IEEE Trans. Biomed. Eng. 44 (1997) 374–385.

[46] D. Yao, B. He, A self-coherence enhancement algorithm and its application to enhancing three-dimensional source estimation from EEGs, Ann. Biomed. Eng. 29 (2001) 1019–1027.

[47] R. Grave de Peralta-Menendez, et al., Imaging the electrical activity of the brain: ELECTRA, Hum. Brain Mapp. 9 (2000) 1–12.

[48] B. He, et al., An equivalent current source model and Laplacian weighted minimum norm current estimates of brain electrical activity, IEEE Trans. BME 49 (2002) 277–288.

[49] A.M. Dale, et al., Dynamic statistical parametric mapping: combining fMRI and MEG for high-resolution imaging of cortical activity, Neuron 26 (2000) 55–67.

[50] R.D. Pascual-Marqui, Standardized low resolution brain electromagnetic tomography (sLORETA): technical detail, Methods Find. Exp. Clin. Pharmacol. 24D (2002) 5–12.

[51] B. He, J. Lian, Spatio-temporal functional neuroimaging of brain electric activity, Crit. Rev. Biomed. Eng. 30 (2002) 283–306.

International Congress Series 1270 (2004) 9–14

www.ics-elsevier.com

Transcranial magnetic stimulation and magnetic resonance imaging of currents and conductivity tomography of the brain

Shoogo Ueno*, Masaki Sekino

Department of Biomedical Engineering, Graduate School of Medicine, University of Tokyo, 7-3-1 Hongo, Bunkyo, Tokyo 113-0033, Japan

Abstract. This paper focuses on two topics in biomagnetics: transcranial magnetic stimulation (TMS) and conductivity magnetic resonance imaging (MRI). We studied an associative memory task involving pairs of Kanji (Chinese) pictographs and unfamiliar abstract patterns. During memory encoding, TMS was applied over the left and right dorsolateral prefrontal cortex (DLPFC). A significant ($P < 0.05$) reduction in subsequent recall of new associations was seen only with TMS over the right DLPFC. Eddy current distribution in the brain during TMS was calculated using the finite element method. In addition, current distribution in electroconvulsive therapy (ECT) was calculated and compared with the current distribution in TMS. TMS could generate eddy currents of comparable intensity with ECT. Conductivity MRI is a method for imaging conductivity distributions in tissues using diffusion tensor MRI. Conductivity images of the rat brain were acquired by a 4.7-T MRI system with motion probing gradients (MPGs) applied in three directions. The mean conductivity in the cortex and the corpus callosum were 0.014 and 0.018 S/m, respectively. © 2004 Elsevier B.V. All rights reserved.

Keywords: Transcranial magnetic stimulation; Conductivity; Magnetic resonance imaging

1. Introduction

Bioelectromagnetic approaches to understanding the functional organization of the human brain include transcranial magnetic stimulation (TMS) [1–8], electroencephalography (EEG), magnetoencephalography (MEG), and new types of magnetic resonance imaging (MRI) techniques such as functional MRI, electrical current MRI and impedance or conductivity MRI [9–15]. This paper focuses on the TMS and conductivity MRI. We developed a method of localized and vectorial TMS using a figure eight coil [2,3]. This method facilitates stimulation of the brain within a 5-mm resolution. TMS is a useful method to examine dynamic brain function without causing any pain, producing so-called "virtual lesions" for a short period of time. We were able to non-invasively evaluate the cortical reactivity and functional connections between different brain areas. We used TMS

* Corresponding author. Tel.: +81-3-5841-3563; fax: +81-3-5689-7215.
E-mail address: ueno@medes.m.u-tokyo.ac.jp (S. Ueno).

0531-5131/ © 2004 Elsevier B.V. All rights reserved.
doi:10.1016/j.ics.2004.04.057

to investigate memory encoding and retrieval, particularly the role of dorsolateral prefrontal cortex in associative memory for visual patterns [4]. TMS disrupts associative learning for abstract patterns over the right frontal area, which suggests that the participating cortical networks may be lateralized in accordance with classic concepts of hemispheric specialization. We also investigated the effects of repetitive TMS (rTMS) with 25 pulses/s on the rat hippocampus by focusing on long-term potentiation (LTP), and we obtained the results that the effects of rTMS depend on the stimulus intensity, and rTMS administered at the appropriate stimulus intensity may potentially activate hippocampal function [5,6].

Although MEG allows us to follow changes in brain activity millisecond by millisecond, there are still many limitations in solving the inverse problem, that is in accurately inferring the source of activity inside the brain based on current distribution within the head as observed by MEG. We proposed new methods to visualize electrical current distributions [9–12] and impedance distributions [13–15] in the head based on new principles of MRI. We developed two methods of impedance MRI; eddy current method [13,14] and diffusion tensor method [15]. The basic idea of the eddy current method is to use shielding effects of induced eddy currents in the body on spin precession. The degree of disturbance of MRI signals due to the eddy currents varies with the tissue conductivity or impedance. We were able to obtain impedance-enhanced MRI of rat brain. We also obtained conductivity tensor images of rat brain and the brain of human subjects by a method using diffusion-weighted MRI. The basic idea is to use an assumption that the tissue conductivity is proportional to the diffusion coefficient of water molecules at low frequencies. The conductivity MR images showed that the tissues with highly anisotropic cellular structures, such as corpus callosum, internal capsule, and trigeminal nerves, exhibited high anisotropy in conductivity.

2. Transcranial magnetic stimulation

Our newly devised method of applying magnetic stimulation locally to the brain from outside uses a figure-eight coil. When a strong electric current is applied to a figure-eight coil over the head for 0.1 ms, a pulse magnetic field of 1 T is produced. This pulse magnetic field generates eddy currents in the brain, which stimulate the nervous system. For example, by electrically stimulating the motor area of the brain, which is responsible for movement control, a person's fingers can be induced to move involuntarily. We have succeeded in selectively stimulating the human cerebral cortex with a spatial resolution of 3–5 mm. TMS is a useful method to examine brain function and structure without causing any pain. In recent years, an increasing number of studies on the clinical applications of magnetic stimulation have been performed. There are high expectations for magnetic stimulation to regulate paralysed muscles, promote regeneration of a damaged nervous system, regulate gene expression, and compensate for the loss of sensory functions. TMS may also provide beneficial therapeutic applications in treating patients with pain and psychoneurotic disorders. Results obtained in recent studies concerning TMS have provided a basic understanding of its clinical application in the treatment of depression and Parkinson's disease, as well as its clinical usefulness in protecting or repairing neurons damaged by cerebral infarction or other brain injury.

Medical applications of transcranial magnetic stimulation include estimation of localized brain function, creating virtual lesions to disturb dynamic neuronal connectivities, damage prevention and regeneration of neurons, modulation of neuronal plasticity, and therapeutic and diagnostic applications for the treatment of central nervous system (CNS) diseases and mental illnesses.

Functional neuroimaging suggests asymmetries of memory encoding and retrieval in the prefrontal lobes, but different hypotheses have been presented concerning the nature of prefrontal hemispheric specialization. We studied an associative memory task involving pairs of Kanji (Chinese) pictographs and unfamiliar abstract patterns [4]. Subjects were 10 Japanese adults fluent in Kanji, so only the abstract patterns represented novel material. During encoding, TMS was applied over the left and right dorsolateral prefrontal cortex (DLPFC). A significant ($P < 0.05$) reduction in subsequent recall of new associations was seen only with TMS over the right DLPFC. This result suggests that the right DLPFC contributes to encoding of visual-object associations, and is consistent with a material-specific rather than a process-specific model of mnemonic function in DLPFC.

Electroconvulsive therapy (ECT), in which electric currents are applied to the brain, improves severe mental illnesses such as depression (Fig. 1). Because TMS has a potential to give a comparable therapeutic effect to ECT with less invasiveness, TMS has been used for treatment of depression in numerous studies. However, these trials have not necessarily given beneficial results. We compared current density distributions in ECT and TMS by numerical calculations [7,8]. The model consisted of an air region and three types of tissues with different conductivities representing the brain, the skull, and the scalp. In the ECT model, electric currents were applied through electrodes with a voltage of 100 V. In the TMS model, a figure-eight coil (6 cm diameter per coil) was placed on the vertex of the head model. An alternating current with a peak intensity of 3.0 kA and a frequency of 4.2 kHz was applied to the coil. The maximum current densities inside the brain in ECT (bilateral electrode position) and TMS were 234 and 322 A/m², respectively. The results indicate that magnetic stimulators can generate current densities comparable with ECT. While the skull significantly affected current distributions in ECT, TMS efficiently induced eddy currents in the brain. In addition, TMS is more beneficial than ECT because the localized current distribution reduces the risk of adverse side effects (Fig. 2).

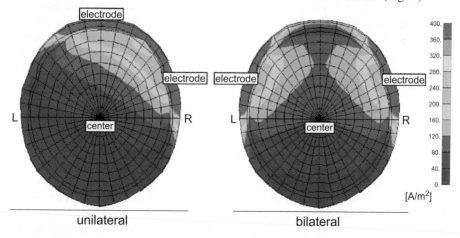

Fig. 1. Current density distributions in ECT.

3. Conductivity magnetic resonance imaging

The estimation of conductivity distributions in the brain is essential for various biomedical engineering analyses. Though tissue conductivity has anisotropy and can be expressed by tensor, it is difficult to investigate distributions of conductivity anisotropy by conventional methods in which currents are applied via surface electrodes. We introduce a method of conductivity tensor imaging based on diffusion MRI [15].

The effective conductivity σ of tissue is obtained using the following equation [16]:

$$\sigma = \frac{2v_{ext}\sigma_{ext}}{3 - v_{ext}} \tag{1}$$

where v_{ext} is the fractional volume of extracellular space, σ_{ext} is the conductivity of the extracellular fluid. The relationship between the conductivity σ_{ext} and the diffusion coefficient D_{ext} of the extracellular fluid is obtained from the Stokes–Einstein equation and the balance between the electrostatic force and viscous drag as

$$\sigma_{ext} = \frac{j}{E} = \frac{q^2 N}{6\pi r_i \eta} = \frac{r_w q^2 N}{r_i kT} D_{ext} \tag{2}$$

where r_w and r_i are the Stokes radius of water molecules and ions, q is the charge of the ions, N is the density of the ions, k is the Boltzmann constant, and T is the temperature. Based on the assumption that the composition of extracellular fluid is equal to that of saline solution (0.15 mol/l NaCl), the constants in Eq. (2) are $r_w/r_i = 0.76$, $q = 1.6 \times 10^{-19}$ C, $N = 2.0 \times 10^{25}$ m^{-3}, and $kT = 4.1 \times 10^{-21}$ J. Diffusion studies using high b values in the brain indicate that the diffusional signal decay is described in terms of a biexponential function

$$\frac{S(b)}{S(0)} = f_{fast}\exp(-bD_{fast}) + f_{slow}\exp(-bD_{slow}) \tag{3}$$

where D_{fast} and D_{slow} are called the fast component and the slow component of the apparent diffusion coefficient (ADC), respectively. Though interpretation of the origins of the two components has not yet been established, the fast component and the slow component have been attributed to extracellular fluid and intracellular fluid, respectively [17]. We assume that the diffusion coefficient and the fractional volume of extracellular fluid are equal to the fast component of the ADC and the fraction of the fast component. Based on the models described above, tissue conductivity is obtained from the fast component of the ADC and the fraction of the fast component as

$$\sigma = \frac{2f_{fast} \times 9.5 \times 10^{-7} \times D_{fast}}{3 - f_{fast}} \tag{4}$$

Images of the rat brain were obtained using a 4.7-T MRI system. Motion probing gradients (MPGs) were applied with four arrayed b factors of $b = 0, 1200, 2400, 3600$ s/mm^2, in the following three directions: $G_1 = G(1\ 0)^T$, $G_2 = G(0\ 1)^T$, $G_3 = G(-1/\sqrt{2}\ 1/\sqrt{2})^T$. A linearized version of function (3) was used to calculate the components of ADC [18]. The conductivity tensor elements were calculated as $\sigma_{xx} = \sigma_1$, $\sigma_{yy} = \sigma_2$, and $\sigma_{xy} = (2\sigma_3 - \sigma_1 - \sigma_2)/2$. The mean conductivity was defined as MC$(\sigma) = (\sigma_{xx} + \sigma_{yy})/2$.

Fig. 3a,b shows the relationships between the b factor and the logarithm of the signal intensity in the cortex and the corpus callosum. Linear relations were not observed between the logarithm of the signal intensity and the b factor at high b values. In the

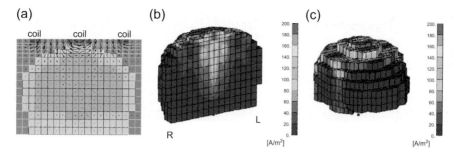

Fig. 2. (a) Vector maps of magnetic field distributions in TMS. Eddy current distributions on (b) the coronal slice and (c) the brain surface.

cortex, as shown in Fig. 3a, the fast components of the ADC obtained for each MPG direction were as follows: $D_{fast}=6.1\times10^{-10}$ m^2/s, $f_{fast}=0.39$ in the direction G_1, $D_{fast}=5.2\times10^{-10}$ m^2/s, $f_{fast}=0.30$ in the direction G_2, and $D_{fast}=5.9\times10^{-10}$ m^2/s, $f_{fast}=0.32$ in the direction G_3. Conductivities calculated by Eq. (4) in each direction were $\sigma_1=0.017$ S/m, $\sigma_2=0.011$ S/m, $\sigma_3=0.013$ S/m. The mean conductivity was 0.014 S/m. In the corpus callosum, as shown in Fig. 3b, the fast components of the ADC obtained with each MPG direction were as follows: $D_{fast}=8.1\times10^{-10}$ m^2/s, $f_{fast}=0.39$ in the direction G_1, $D_{fast}=4.8\times10^{-10}$ m^2/s, $f_{fast}=0.32$ in the direction G_2, and $D_{fast}=6.3\times10^{-10}$ m^2/s, $f_{fast}=0.42$ in the direction G_3. Conductivities in each direction, $\sigma_1=0.023$ S/m, $\sigma_2=0.011$ S/m, $\sigma_3=0.019$ S/m, exhibited higher anisotropy than the values in the cortex. The eigenvalues of the conductivity tensor were $\lambda_1=0.023$ S/m and $\lambda_2=0.011$ S/m indicating that conductivity varies by approximately $2(\lambda_1-\lambda_2)/(\lambda_1+\lambda_2)=75\%$ depending on the direction of the electric field. The mean conductivity was 0.018 S/m.

Fig. 4a,b,c shows distributions of the components of the conductivity tensor, σ_{xx}, σ_{yy}, and σ_{xy}. Measurement of conductivity distribution in the brain is important for the investigation of brain function and various biomedical engineering analyses. Conventional methods to obtain conductivity distributions using currents that are applied via surface electrodes provide less accurate tissue measurements when the surrounding tissues such as bone exhibit extremely low conductivity. In addition, it has been difficult to investigate the anisotropy by conventional methods even though highly anisotropic conductivity is expected in the brain due to the fibrous nature of neurons. This new method based on

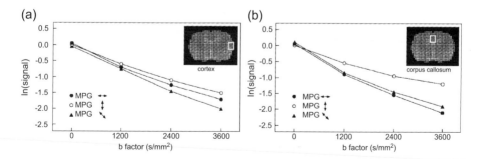

Fig. 3. Diffusional signal attenuations in (a) the cortex and (b) the corpus callosum.

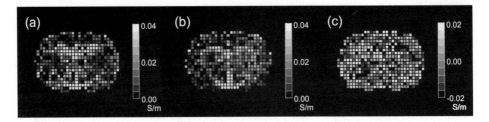

Fig. 4. Images of the conductivity tensor elements (a) σ_{xx}, (b) σ_{yy}, and (c) σ_{xy}.

MRI has high spatial resolution compared with conventional methods such as electrical impedance tomography, and the surrounding tissues do not affect measurement. Moreover, this new method to obtain conductivity distributions from the ADC can easily visualize the distribution of conductivity anisotropy.

Acknowledgement

This study was supported by a Grant-in-Aid for Specially Promoted Research (No. 12002002) from the Ministry of Education, Culture, Sports, Science and Technology, Japan.

References

[1] A.T. Barker, R. Jalinous, I.L. Freeston, Lancet 1 (8437) (1985) 1106–1107.
[2] S. Ueno, T. Matsuda, M. Fujiki, IEEE Trans. Magn. 26 (5) (1990) 1539–1544.
[3] S. Ueno, T. Tashiro, K. Harada, J. Appl. Phys. 64 (10) (1988) 5862–5864.
[4] C.M. Epstein, et al., Neurosci. Lett 320 (1–2) (2002) 5–8.
[5] M. Ogiue-Ikeda, S. Kawato, S. Ueno, IEEE Trans. Magn. 39 (5) (2003) 3390–3392.
[6] M. Ogiue-Ikeda, S. Kawato, S. Ueno, Brain Res. 993 (1–2) (2003) 222–226.
[7] M. Sekino, S. Ueno, J. Appl. Phys. 91 (10) (2002) 8730–8732.
[8] M. Sekino, S. Ueno, IEEE Trans. Magn. (in press).
[9] K. Yamaguchi, et al., J. Appl. Phys. 93 (10) (2003) 6739–6741.
[10] M. Sekino, et al., J. Appl. Phys. 94 (8) (2003) 5359–5366.
[11] H. Kamei, et al., IEEE Trans. Magn. 35 (5) (1999) 4109–4111.
[12] M. Sekino, et al., IEEE Trans. Magn. (in press).
[13] S. Ueno, N. Iriguchi, J. Appl. Phys. 83 (11) (1998) 6450–6452.
[14] Y. Yukawa, N. Iriguchi, S. Ueno, IEEE Trans. Magn. 35 (5) (1999) 4121–4123.
[15] M. Sekino, et al., J. Appl. Phys. 93 (10) (2003) 6730–6732.
[16] K.S. Cole, C.L. Li, A.F. Bak, Exp. Neurol. 24 (3) (1969) 459–473.
[17] T. Niendorf, et al., Magn. Reson. Med. 36 (6) (1996) 847–857.
[18] C.A. Clark, M. Hedehus, M.E. Moseley, Magn. Reson. Med. 47 (4) (2002) 623–628.

International Congress Series 1270 (2004) 15–19

www.ics-elsevier.com

Brain source montages improve the non-invasive diagnosis in epilepsy

M. Scherg[a,b,*], T. Bast[c], K. Hoechstetter[a], N. Ille[a,b], D. Weckesser[a],
H. Bornfleth[a], P. Berg[d]

[a] MEGIS Software GmbH, Bahnhofstr. 95, 82166 Gräfelfing/Munich, Germany
[b] Department of Neurology, University Hospital Heidelberg, Heidelberg, Germany
[c] Department of Pediatric Neurology, University Hospital Heidelberg, Heidelberg, Germany
[d] Department of Psychology, University of Konstanz, Konstanz, Germany

Abstract. Using multiple regional source models, brain source montages can be defined to compute continuous, single trial or averaged brain source activity by applying a fixed or adaptive source transformation to the raw or averaged EEG or MEG data. Brain source montages can dissociate the activities of the different lobes, hemispheres and sublobar areas, e.g. the different surfaces of the right and left temporal lobes. Epileptiform spike and seizure activities in EEG and MEG can be made more conspicuous by using brain source montages as compared with conventional montages or raw surface signals. By using mirror sources in both hemispheres, lateralized focal activity can be immediately recognized from the on-going EEG and MEG data. © 2004 Elsevier B.V. All rights reserved.

Keywords: Dipole source; Source analysis; Source montages; EEG deblurring; Epilepsy diagnosis

1. Introduction

EEG electrodes and MEG sensors record overlapping signals from all active brain regions. The overlap depends on sensor location, volume conduction properties and the distance and orientation of the different brain activities from the recording electrode or magnetic coil. Discrete multiple source analysis is capable of separating these spatially and temporally overlapping surface signals provided that each region contributing significantly to the recorded signals is modeled by an equivalent source [1]. The time courses of the activities in the different brain regions can be represented by source waveforms, i.e. the time-varying regional dipole moments that are calculated by a spatial transformation of all surface signals. This transformation of scalp into brain source waveforms [2] was first applied to continuous epileptiform EEG data using a set of 16–19 single dipoles to

* Corresponding author. MEGIS Software GmbH, Bahnhofstr. 95, 82166 Gräfelfing/Munich, Germany.
Tel.: +49-89-89809966; fax: +49-89-89809967.
 E-mail address: mscherg@besa.de (M. Scherg).

separate the activities at the different aspects of the temporal lobe from those at other cortical surfaces [3,4].

Better separation of the different brain activities is obtained using regional sources. A regional source models the compound current flow of a brain region in any direction by three orthogonal current dipoles. They can be oriented according to the main superficial and fissural cortical surfaces of the modeled region [2,5]. Brain source montages can dissociate the activities of the different lobes, hemispheres and sublobar areas, e.g. the different surfaces of the right and left temporal lobes [3,4,6].

The goal of this paper was to apply regional brain source montages to brain areas other than the temporal lobes, and to demonstrate the usefulness of brain source montages in the non-invasive EEG diagnosis of extra-temporal lobe epilepsies.

2. Materials and methods

EEGs recorded during epilepsy monitoring were reviewed with standard scalp and source montages using the EEGFOCUS 3.0 software. Multiple source models and source montages were generated using the BESA 5.0 software. A regional source model was created with 15 sources to cover the lateral frontal, central and parietal regions, and the anterior and posterior temporal lobes bilaterally, and 5 midline sources to cover the parasagittal brain regions. Specific montages were created for the frontal, central and parietal regions by separating the source in the region of interest into a radial inward and two tangential dipoles. For the specific temporal regional montage, four dipoles were used on each side. The signals of the other regional sources were displayed either using one trace oriented along maximum amplitude, rectified magnitude or split into three orthog-

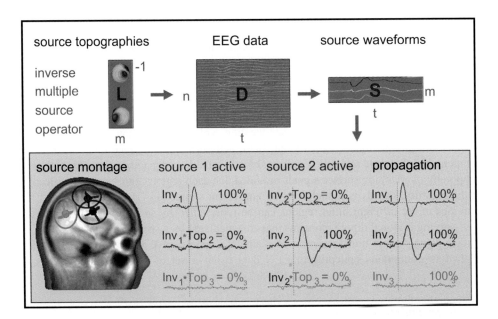

Fig. 1. Illustration of the separation capability of an inverse regional source operator using simulated data.

onal signals. The inverse linear operator was calculated using 81 standard 10–10 electrode locations and applied to the individual EEG interpolated onto these electrodes using spherical splines [6].

An important property of the inverse linear operator is illustrated in Fig. 1. The operator picks up 100% of the activity at the center location of the source of interest, but rejects all overlap from the centers of the other modeled regions (0%). If spike activity is spreading, for example by fibres connecting areas 1 and 2, the activities of the two regions are separated and their sequential spike–wave patterns become apparent. The third source does not pick up any activity although the overlying scalp electrode might show large signals due to volume conduction. Thus, a significant contribution of the third source region to the generation of the spike can be excluded. However, the centers of activation are not precisely coinciding with the source locations, and the inverse operator must be modestly smoothed by regularization (1%) to reduce noise enhancement. This results in cross-talk, or sharing of activity with the nearby sources. In practice, the cross-talk is in the order of 5–20%, i.e. considerably less than in scalp montages.

3. Results

The comparison of spikes in continuous EEG recordings using a standard longitudinal bipolar montage with standard and individual brain source montages is depicted for two children (ages 10 and 12) with rolandic and frontal lesional epilepsy, respectively, in Figs. 2 and 3. In most cases, spikes became more apparent and emerged better from the on-going EEG in the source channels as compared with conventional bipolar scalp or average referenced scalp channels. When using spike pattern search in the case of left frontal cortical dysplasia (Fig. 3), the overlap with the widespread concurrent alpha rhythm resulted in phase shifts of the apparent spike in the bipolar channels. Thus, the alpha activity was not sufficiently suppressed by averaging and needed to be modeled using an additional source [7]. Using the standard frontal source montage, spikes were much better separated from the posterior alpha activity and the average was not biased.

4. Discussion

As shown also in previous publications on temporal lobe epilepsy [3,4,6], brain source montages provide a better separation of the activities of both hemispheres and the different brain regions as compared with routine bipolar and average reference montages. Thus, focal activities can be recognized more easily as they emerge better above the on-going EEG of the brain region they model. Source montages based on multiple discrete sources can be optimized individually to provide for strong contrast and separation of specific regions of interest. But, also standard regional source montages separated the activities sufficiently well at a sublobar level. Other methods, e.g. beamformers [8], principally can create comparable source montages for the different brain regions. However, they are less capable of dissociating correlated activities from different areas.

In conclusion, brain source montages can considerably improve the non-invasive diagnosis in epilepsy when applied to the review of spike and seizure onset activities.

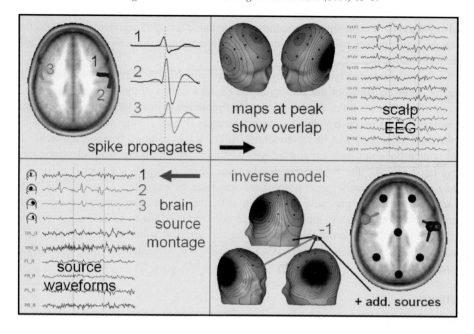

Fig. 2.

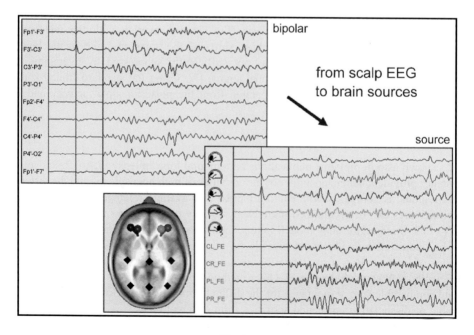

Fig. 3.

Acknowledgements

The authors are grateful to R. Boor and J. Ebersole for providing valuable data and advice. Some of the material used in this paper has been presented on www.besa.de.

References

[1] M. Scherg, D. von Cramon, Two bilateral sources of the late AEP as identified by a spatio-temporal dipole model, Electroencephalogr. Clin. Neurophysiol. 62 (1985) 32–44.

[2] M. Scherg, D. von Cramon, Evoked dipole source potentials of the human auditory cortex, Electroencephalogr. Clin. Neurophysiol. 65 (1986) 344–360.

[3] M. Scherg, J.S. Ebersole, Brain source imaging of focal and multifocal epileptiform EEG activity, Neurophysiol. Clin. 24 (1994) 51–60.

[4] B.A. Assaf, J.S. Ebersole, Visual and quantitative ictal EEG predictors of outcome after temporal lobectomy, Epilepsia 40 (1999) 52–61.

[5] M. Scherg, P. Berg, New concepts of brain source imaging and localization, in: C. Barber, et al (Ed.), Functional neuroscience, Electroencephalogr. Clin. Neurophysiol., Suppl. 46, (1996) 127–137.

[6] M. Scherg, et al, Advanced tools for digital EEG review: virtual source montages, whole-head mapping, correlation, and phase analysis, J. Clin. Neurophysiol. 19 (2002) 91–112.

[7] M. Scherg, T. Bast, P. Berg, Multiple source analysis of interictal spikes: goals, requirements, and clinical value, J. Clin. Neurophysiol. 16 (1999) 214–222.

[8] K. Sekihara, et al, Reconstructing spatio-temporal activities of neural sources using an MEG vector beamformer technique, IEEE Trans. Biomed. Eng. 48 (2001) 760–771.

Fig. 2. Individual source montage applied to rolandic spikes. Upper left: source regions and source waveforms identified by multiple source modeling (average of 637 spikes, ± 200 ms). Upper right: longitudinal bipolar montage shows polarity reversal at T7, but no clear evidence of propagation. Map at spike peak shows bilateral negativities. Lower right: a source montage is constructed using the 3 dipoles and 11 regional sources to cover the other brain regions. Lower left: consistent spike propagation is revealed for the single spike discharges.

Fig. 3. Comparison of standard and individual frontal source montage in a case of left frontal cortical dysplasia [7]. The small spikes were hard to recognize in the bipolar montage due to considerable overlap with alpha rhythm. The standard left frontal radial source channel (trace 1) showed a clear emergence of individual spikes allowing for spike detection using pattern search. Traces 2 and 3 showed the propagation within the left frontal regions, modeled individually by a near-radial (red) and near-tangential (blue) source. Propagation was consistent across single spikes, as can be seen from the two spikes of the displayed source segment.

International Congress Series 1270 (2004) 20–25

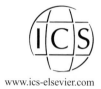

www.ics-elsevier.com

Localization of impaired cortical neurons by EEG power fluctuation analysis

Toshimitsu Musha[a,*], Yuusuke Mochiduki[b], Takayoshi Kurachi[a], Hiroshi Matsuda[c], Takashi Asada[d]

[a]*Brain Functions Laboratory, Inc., Head of the Company, KSP E-211, Sakado, Takatsu, Kawasaki-shi 213-0012, Kanagawa-pref., Japan*
[b]*Tokyo Institute of Technology, Japan*
[c]*National Center of Neurology and Psychiatry, Japan*
[d]*Tsukuba University, Japan*

Abstract. Electrical activities of cortical neurons produce a scalp potential distribution. It was already found that this potential distribution for the alpha rhythm is smooth and stable in normal subjects, whereas it loses smoothness and is unstable in AD patients. We investigated a histogram of the normalized power variance (NPV) evaluated for 100 ms of the beta component (13–30 Hz), recorded with 21 electrodes placed according to the 10–20 method. It was evaluated in 56 normal subjects for each electroencephalogram (EEG) channel, and its mean $\langle NPV \rangle$ and standard deviation σ were calculated. When an NPV of a patient with Alzheimer's disease (AD) lies outside of a range $\langle NPV \rangle \pm \sigma$, cortical neurons related to that channel are regarded as partly impaired, where impairment is classified as being more unstable (over-active) and more inactive (under-active) than averaged normal neurons. The neuronal impairment map (NIM) was defined based on such evaluations of the 21 channels, where the NIP is characterised in red and blue regions correspond to over- and under-activity. The NIM pattern is similar to the regional cerebral blood flow (rCBF) reduction pattern measured by SPECT. The NIM is a simple tool to see local, cortical, neuronal impairment. © 2004 Elsevier B.V. All rights reserved.

Keywords: Alzheimer; EEG; Neuronal impairment; SPECT; Diagnosis

1. Introduction

The electroencephalogram (EEG) is rich in information on cortical, neuronal activity in the brain, and an appropriate signal processing will give us valuable information on the brain activity, which could not be obtained by other imaging tools. The band-limited alpha rhythm in a normal subject generates a smooth scalp potential distribution, which is well approximated by a single current dipole. Partial impairment of cortical neuronal activity

* Corresponding author. Tel.: +81-44-819-2454; fax. +81-44-813-7252.
E-mail address: musha@bfl.co.jp (T. Musha).

0531-5131/ © 2004 Elsevier B.V. All rights reserved.
doi:10.1016/j.ics.2004.04.051

results in non-uniform electric current density on the cortical surface of sulci, and electric currents no longer cancel each other anymore. As a result, random electric current sources appear in the brain and disturb the smoothness of the scalp potential distribution. This effect is well expressed in terms of dipolarity [1]. The dipolarity of the alpha rhythm varies periodically, and peak dipolarity can be a measure of neuronal impairment, which is actually fluctuating from peak to peak. Musha et al. [2] already reported that the degree of cortical neuronal impairment is characterised in terms of standard deviation D_σ of the peak dipolarity values of the alpha rhythm and its mean D_α. As Alzheimer's disease (AD) progresses, D_α decreases and D_σ increases.

Based on this finding, we made use of fluctuations of local EEG power to estimate how much local, cortical, neuronal activity is impaired. With 21 electrodes, the neuronal impairment map (NIM) was made on the standard brain surface. NIMs of AD patients look similar to the corresponding regional cerebral blood flow (rCBF) reduction maps measured by SPECT.

2. Method

2.1. Neuroactivity diagram

The alpha rhythm with 3 Hz bandwidth has a smooth scalp potential distribution so that it can be well approximated by a single dipole potential, and its goodness of fit (dipolarity), D, is defined as $D = \sqrt{1 - \langle (u_{obs} - u_{dip})^2 \rangle_{channel} / \langle (u_{obs})^2 \rangle_{channel}}$, where u_{obs} and u_{dip} are observed and dipole potentials, respectively, at an electrode site, and $\langle \ldots \rangle$ denotes averaging over all the electrode sites. EEGs were recorded in a rest state with closed eyes for 5 min with 21 scalp electrodes placed according to the international 10–20 standard and digitized at every 5 ms. The reference electrode was on the right earlobe.

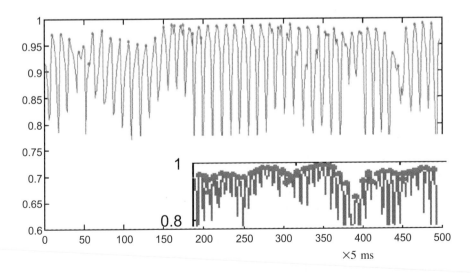

Fig. 1. Dipolarity of the alpha rhythm in a normal subject. Insert is in an AD patient.

Dipolarity was computed at every sample point. An example of calculated D values for a normal control subject is shown in Fig. 1. The D value varies almost periodically at twice the alpha frequency, and peaks are observed at positive and negative potential maxima of the alpha rhythm. In the case of a normal subject, the peak value mostly stays close to unity for relatively long periods, sometimes going below unity. An example of an AD patient is inserted in this figure; the peak value fluctuates more and mostly stays way below unity. This up-and-down process of the peak value is repeated rapidly in AD patients. The mean and standard deviation of peak dipolarity are denoted as D_α and D_σ, which form the *Neuroactivity Diagram* as shown in Fig. 2. According to the result, which is based on examinations of 56 normal subjects (MMSE 28.5 ± 1.6), 25 very mild (MMSE 26 ± 1.8) and 33 moderately severe (MMSE 15.3 ± 6.4) AD patients, points of (D_α and D_σ) were distributed within a fan-beam area [1]. This area is divided into the following three regions: (1) normal region: the mean peak dipolarity is close to unity and is relatively stable, and the subject tested is diagnosed as normal, at the risk of including 10% of AD patients; (2) the impaired region: the mean peak dipolarity is low and unstable and the subject is diagnosed as AD, at the risk of including 10% of normal subjects; and (3) the sub-normal region: the subject should be examined again several months later; when, in the second examination, the subject is almost in the same state, he/she will be normal.

This diagnosis method in reference to the *Neuroactivity Diagram* is named DIMEN-SION for *Diagnosis Method of Neuronal Dysfunction*. This method is now used for

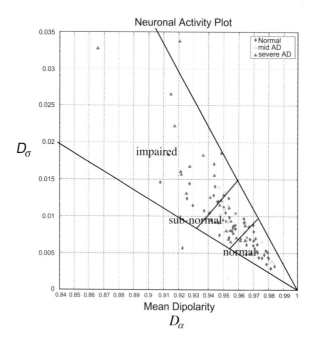

Fig. 2. Neuroactivity diagram. D_α and D_σ denote the mean alpha peak dipolarity and the standard deviation of peak dipolarity. Data of normal and AD patients are in a fan-beam area.

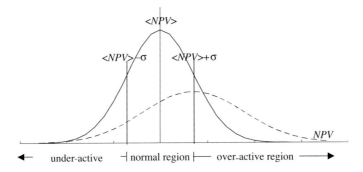

Fig. 3. Distributions of NPV values in normal subjects (solid line). It has a mean $\langle$NPV$\rangle$ and a standard deviation σ. When an NPV value of a subject to be tested is in the overactive region, the neuronal activity is regarded as unstable. When, on the other hand, it is in the under-active region, the neuronal activity is regarded as more inactive than normal.

monitoring the progress of AD and the efficacy of various kinds of therapy for rehabilitation.

2.2. Regional impairment of neurons

In the previous study [1], we found that D_α and D_σ are closely related to each other as shown in Fig. 2, and this fact suggests that variance of EEG power in a limited frequency band can be a marker of regional impairment of cortical neurons. Since the magnitude of EEG amplitude or power itself is not what we want, the power variance is normalized by a square of the mean power. This normalized power variance, NPV, is defined as NPV = PV/$\langle(u_{\text{obs}})^2\rangle^2$ where power variance PV is defined as PV = $\langle(u_{\text{obs}})^4\rangle - \langle(u_{\text{obs}})^2\rangle^2$. Here, u_{obs} is a potential observed with a specified electrode and averaging is taken over a specified time period, say 100 s. Now the beta band of 13–40 Hz was used instead of the alpha rhythm because the alpha rhythm is sensitive to an emotional state of a subject and, moreover, it is sometimes unobservable.

The NPV value of a normal subject depends on individuals, and a distribution of NPV values of normal control subjects is schematically shown by a solid line in Fig. 3. The mean of NPV in normal control subjects is written as $\langle$NPV$\rangle$ and the related standard deviation is σ. If a measured NPV on a specified electrode site is between $\langle$NPV$\rangle - \sigma$ and $\langle$NPV$\rangle + \sigma$, the neuronal activity related to that electrode site is regarded as normal. If it is out of this range, the fluctuations are regarded as abnormal and the related neuronal activity is regarded as abnormal, such that it is more unstable or more inactive than the normal neurons. Therefore, the degree of neuronal activity or inactivity is numerically represented by

Degree of neuronal instability $= \text{NPV} - \langle\text{NPV}\rangle - \sigma$

Degree of neuronal inactivity $= \langle\text{NPV}\rangle - \sigma - \text{NPV}.$

3. Result

By repeating this process with the 21 channels, the degree of over- and under-activity of cortical neurons is allotted to each of the 21 electrode sites, and mapped on the standard brain surface after interpolation. The map is coloured in the following way. The overactive regions are in red and brightness increases in three steps: $\langle NPV \rangle +$ $\sigma \sim \langle NPV \rangle + 2\sigma$; $\langle NPV \rangle + 2\sigma \sim \langle NPV \rangle + 3\sigma$ and $\langle NPV \rangle + 3\sigma \sim$. Similarly, the under active regions are in blue and brightness of blue colour increases in three steps: $\langle NPV \rangle - \sigma \sim \langle NPV \rangle - 2\sigma$; $\langle NPV \rangle - 2\sigma \sim \langle NPV \rangle - 3\sigma$; and $\langle NPV \rangle - 3\sigma \sim$. This map

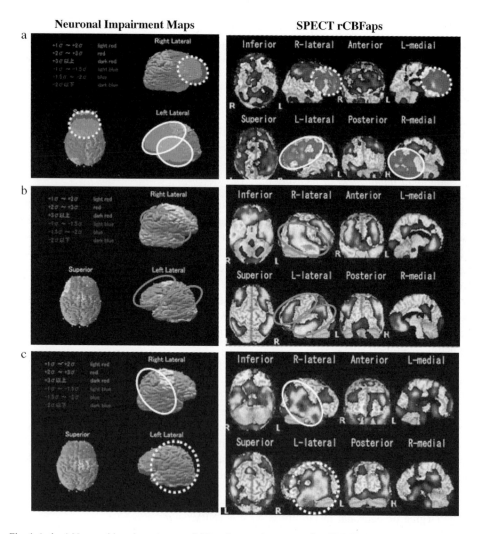

Fig. 4. (a, b, c) Neuronal impairment maps of AD patients and corresponding SPECT rCBF reduction maps. Red areas indicate more unstable neuronal activity, and blue areas indicate more quiet neuronal activity. These areas have correspondent rCBF reduction in SPECT maps.

is called the *Neuronal Impairment Map* (NIM), and some examples of the NIM of AD patients are compared with corresponding SPECT rCBF maps in Fig. 4, where a good correspondence is observed between NIM and the rCBF reduction map. In (a) of Fig. 4, rCBF reduction is related to overactive synapse-neuronal activity, which is a sign of impairment. In (b) and (c), rCBF reduction is related to under-active synapse-neuronal activity. It seems that rCBF reduction areas refer either to abnormally unstable neuronal activity or to abnormally inactive neuronal activity.

As regards SPECT measurement, each subject received a 600-MBq intravenous injection of ^{99m}Tc-ethy cysteinate dimmer (ECD) just prior to the SPECT scan. The global cerebral blood flow was non-invasively measured using graphical analysis [3,4] without any blood samples. Ten minutes after injection of ^{99m}Tc-ECD, brain SPECT equipped with high-resolution fan-beam collimators was performed. The linearization algorithm of a curvilinear relationship between brain activity and blood flow was applied to calculate rCBF and to correct for incomplete retention of ^{99m}Tc-ECD in the brain [5]. Using SPM99, SPECT images were spatially normalized to a standardized stereotactic space based on the Talairach and Tournoux Atlas [6]. Each subject's SPECT image data were standardized using 12-parameter linear affine normalizations and 8 nonlinear iteration algorithms to provide the best fit to a brain image template [7].

4. Discussion

The NIM is made by averaging neuronal activity for, say, 100 s. A high time-resolution investigation showed that impaired regions are very dynamic. So far, we have attributed impairment of electrical activity of the cortex to neuronal impairment. A rapid change of impairment seems to show that not only neurons, but also synapses are responsible for such dynamic behaviour of impairment. The rCBF map refers to averaged impairment. Therefore, we should say that what we have analysed is a *synapse-neuronal impairment map* (SNIM).

Through the present analysis, we have found rCBF is related to two different states of synapse-neuronal impairment; one is enhanced fluctuation of synapse-neuronal activity as compared with the normal one, which is caused by their functional impairment. Another is more inactive neuronal activity than the normal one.

References

[1] T. Musha, Y. Okamoto, Forward and inverse problems of EEG dipole localization, Crit. Rev. Biol. Eng. 27 (1999) 189–239.
[2] T. Musha, et al., A new EEG method for estimating cortical neuronal impairment that is sensitive to early stage Alzheimer's disease, Clin. Neurophysiol. 113 (2002) 1052–1058.
[3] H. Matsuda, et al., Quantitative approach to technetium-9m ethyl cysteinate dimmer: a comparison with technetium-99m hexametyl propylene amine, Eur. J. Nucl. Med. 22 (1995) 633–637.
[4] R. Takeuchi, et al., Noninvasive quantitative measurements of regional cerebral blood flow using technetium-99m-L,L-ECD SPECT activated with acetazolamide: quantification analysis by equal-volume-split 99mTc-ECD consecutive SPECT method, J. Cereb. Blood Flow Metab. 17 (1997) 1020–1032.
[5] D. Kogure, et al., Longitudinal evaluation of early Alzheimer's disease using brain perfusion SPECT, J. Nucl. Med. 41 (2000) 1152–1162.
[6] J. Talairach, P. Tournoux, Co-planar Stereotactic Atlas of the Human Brain, 1st ed., Tieme, Stuttgart, 1988.
[7] T. Ohnishi, et al., Abnormal cerebral blood flow in autism, Brain 123 (2000) 1838–1844.

International Congress Series 1270 (2004) 26–31

ELSEVIER

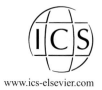

www.ics-elsevier.com

The action-perception paradigm: a new perspective in cognitive neuroscience

Hiroshi Nittono*

Faculty of Integrated Arts and Sciences, Hiroshima University, 1-7-1 Kagamiyama, Higashi-Hiroshima 739-8521, Japan

Abstract. The traditional research approach in cognitive neuroscience uses passive participants who keep still and wait for stimuli presented by the experimenter. Although this monitoring or vigilance paradigm has effectively revealed various aspects of cognitive processes, it does not cover the full range of human cognitive activity. The present article introduces a new experimental paradigm to examine another mode of stimulus information processing in which participants process stimuli produced by their voluntary actions. Three event-related brain potential experiments using oddball tasks showed consistently that a fronto-central P3 (P3a) component was larger in amplitude when the eliciting stimulus was triggered by a voluntary button press than when the same stimulus was presented automatically. This effect was obtained in both auditory and visual modalities. The findings suggest that voluntary stimulus presentation boosts the process of attention switching to deviant events, possibly because the planning of action activates the representation of its most frequent perceivable outcome. © 2004 Elsevier B.V. All rights reserved.

Keywords: Event-related potential; Voluntary action; P3; Methodology

1. Introduction

In cognitive neuroscience research, participants are typically asked to keep still and wait for stimuli presented by the experimenter. This experimental protocol, sometimes called a monitoring or vigilance paradigm, is useful for examining brain activities related to stimulus information processing, since it minimizes artifactual effects of movement-related processes. However, this is not the only mode of human cognitive processing. In daily life, we often process stimuli produced by voluntary actions. For example, when we want to watch television we normally turn on the switch instead of waiting for someone else to do so. Although many studies have examined the preparation and execution processes of voluntary actions [1], little is known about how the outcomes of these actions are processed in the brain. Despite a few preliminary reports on this subject [2–4], it remains unclear whether the processing of stimuli produced by voluntary action is the same as that of stimuli presented by an experimenter. This issue can be resolved by

* Tel.: +81-82-424-6565; fax: +81-82-424-0759.
E-mail address: nittono@hiroshima-u.ac.jp (H. Nittono).

0531-5131/ © 2004 Elsevier B.V. All rights reserved.
doi:10.1016/j.ics.2004.04.093

measuring brain activity during tasks in which stimuli are produced by a participant's voluntary action. I refer to this methodology as the "action-perception" paradigm.

In two previous studies, event-related potentials (ERPs) were recorded in the action-perception paradigm using auditory and visual "oddball" tasks. In the first study [5], 14 healthy adults performed an auditory novelty oddball task with three different methods of stimulus presentation. The stimuli consisted of standard (1000 Hz, $p=0.8$), target (2000 Hz, $p=0.1$), and novel stimuli (various computer-edited sounds, $p=0.1$). In the first block, these stimuli were presented with a fixed onset-to-onset interval of 2 s (fixed condition). In the second block, each stimulus was presented immediately after the participant's voluntary button press (self condition). In the third block, the same stimuli were presented automatically by a computer with the same interstimulus intervals as those produced by the participant in the previous self condition (auto condition). The task was pressing another button when the target stimulus was presented. The effect of voluntary stimulus presentation manifested itself particularly on the P3 waves elicited by the target and novel stimuli. The amplitudes of both P3s were larger in the self condition than in the fixed and auto conditions. Interestingly, the amplitude increase was prominent at fronto-central sites for both target and novelty P3s. The ERPs to standard stimuli showed little difference between conditions except for post-motor somatosensory potentials [6].

The second study replicated these findings in the visual modality [7]. Twelve university students performed a three-stimulus oddball task with three conditions similar to the above experiment. The stimuli consisted of three alphabetic letters (S, H, and O) assigned to target ($p=0.125$), nontarget ($p=0.125$), and standard stimuli ($p=0.750$). Participants were asked to count silently the number of target stimuli. Again, in the self condition, the amplitudes of the P3s to target and nontarget stimuli were larger particularly at fronto-central sites than in the other conditions where the stimuli were presented automatically. These results suggest that part of the processing of infrequent events, which is reflected in the fronto-central component of the P3, is modulated by voluntary presentation of stimuli.

The present article describes the results of a supplementary experiment conducted to examine whether the effect of voluntary stimulus presentation on the P3 was replicated in typical two-stimulus auditory and visual oddball tasks. It was predicted that in both sensory modalities the amplitude of the P3 to target stimuli would be increased particularly at fronto-central sites when the stimuli were produced by voluntary button presses.

2. Methods

2.1. Participants

Sixteen right-handed student volunteers at Hiroshima University participated in the study (8 men and 8 women, 21–24 years old, mean age 22.3 years). All of them had normal or corrected-to-normal vision and normal hearing assessed by standard audiometry. They gave written informed consent.

2.2. Stimuli

In the auditory task, 2000 and 1000 Hz pure tones (duration 70 ms, rise/fall 10 ms) were used as target and standard stimuli, respectively. They were presented via headphones at 60 dB/SPL. In the visual task, "X" and "O" were used as target and standard stimuli, respectively. They were presented in white on a black CRT display for 70 ms with a visual angle of 1°. The target stimulus probability was 0.25.

2.3. Procedure

In the self condition, the stimuli were triggered by voluntary mouse clicks. Participants were asked to press a computer mouse button at a pace of once per 1–2 s with the index finger of either the right or left hand. Each button press triggered one of the two stimuli immediately after the microswitch closure (<10 ms). In the auto condition, the same stimuli were presented automatically (without button presses) with the same interstimulus intervals as those produced in the self condition. Participants were instructed to respond to target stimuli by pressing a space key on the keyboard with the index finger of the opposite hand. Three pairs of the self and auto conditions were performed (120 trials × self/auto × 3 blocks). The order of the auditory and visual tasks and the hands for triggering and response were counterbalanced across participants. At the end of the experiment, participants were asked to click a mouse button in the same way as in the self condition, but this time no stimulus followed (motor control condition, 120 trials).

2.4. Recording and data reduction

Electroencephalogram (EEG) was recorded from 23 scalp electrode sites referenced to the nose tip. The bandpass filter was set at 0.016 Hz (time constant 10 s) to 60 Hz. The sampling rate was 200 Hz. After rejecting the trials contaminated by ocular or muscular artifacts, the epoch between 200 ms before and 800 ms after stimulus onset was averaged separately for modalities, conditions, stimuli, and sites. The baseline was aligned to the mean amplitude of the 200-ms prestimulus period. To examine the ERPs to infrequent events without contamination of movement-related potentials, difference waveforms were calculated by subtracting the ERPs to standard stimuli from the ERPs to target stimuli recorded in each of the self and auto conditions. The P3 was identified in the difference waveforms. The amplitude was measured at each of the five midline sites (Fpz, Fz, Cz, Pz, and Oz) as the mean amplitude of the five data points ($\pm$ 10 ms) around the peak latency determined at the most dominant site, Pz.

3. Results

The means $\pm$ standard deviations of button press intervals were 1232 ± 173 and 1266 ± 187 ms in the auditory and visual tasks, respectively (1299 ± 219 ms in the

Table 1
Means $\pm$ standard errors of performance measures ($N = 16$)

	Auditory		Visual	
	Self	Auto	Self	Auto
Reaction time (ms)	$432 \pm 16^*$	409 ± 20	$460 \pm 14^*$	426 ± 12
Miss (%)	0.52 ± 0.28	1.04 ± 0.48	0.35 ± 0.16	0.52 ± 0.25
False alarm (%)	0.35 ± 0.11	0.21 ± 0.07	0.06 ± 0.04	0.18 ± 0.09

*Significantly different from the value in the auto condition, $p < 0.05$.

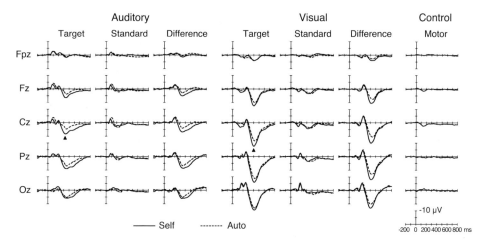

Fig. 1. Grand mean ERP waveforms in the self and auto conditions ($N = 16$). Solid triangles indicate the P3s elicited by target stimuli in the auditory and visual tasks. Difference waveforms are obtained by subtracting the ERPs to standard stimuli from the ERPs to target stimuli. P3 amplitude was larger in the self than in the auto condition and the difference was prominent at central sites. The ERP waveforms in the motor control condition in which no stimulus appeared after button press are also shown for reference.

motor control condition). Table 1 summarizes the performance measures. A repeated-measures analysis of variance (ANOVA) with factors of modality and condition showed that the mean reaction time to target stimuli was longer in the self than in the auto condition, $F(1, 15) = 22.31$, $p = 0.0003$, and was longer in the visual than in the auditory task, $F(1, 15) = 5.39$, $p = 0.0347$. The interaction was not significant. Error rates were uniformly low and did not differ significantly between conditions.

Fig. 1 shows the grand mean ERP waveforms. A large P3 wave was elicited by target stimuli in both modalities, the amplitude of which was larger in the self than in the auto condition. In the motor control condition, low-amplitude post-motor potentials appeared at fronto-central sites. Table 2 shows the mean amplitudes of the P3 in the difference waveforms. A repeated-measures ANOVA with factors of modality, condition, stimulus, and site showed significant main effects of modality and condition, $Fs(1, 15) = 60.96$ and 29.68, $ps < 0.0001$, respectively. The Condition $\times$ Site interaction was significant, $F(4, 60) = 9.74$, $p = 0.0008$, H-F epsilon $= 0.47$, suggesting that the effect of condition differed

Table 2
Means $\pm$ standard errors of P3 amplitudes (μV) at midline sites in the difference waveforms ($N = 16$)

	Fpz	Fz	Cz	Pz	Oz
Auditory					
Self	1.80 ± 0.59	6.28 ± 0.81*	8.84 ± 0.94*	10.88 ± 0.94	8.03 ± 1.06
Auto	0.81 ± 0.66	3.51 ± 0.81	5.25 ± 0.99	8.31 ± 1.11	6.39 ± 1.05
Visual					
Self	4.25 ± 0.72*	11.09 ± 0.92*	15.82 ± 1.14*	18.20 ± 1.11*	13.74 ± 1.21
Auto	2.65 ± 0.65	7.71 ± 0.91	11.03 ± 1.21	14.11 ± 1.22	10.95 ± 1.14

*Significantly different from the value in the auto condition, $p < 0.05$ (comparison-wise $p < 0.01$).

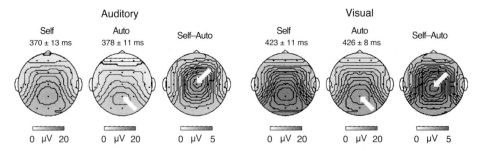

Fig. 2. Scalp topographic maps of the P3 in the difference waveforms. Means ± standard errors of peak latencies are also shown. The P3 in the auto condition is a classical, parietal dominant P3 elicited by infrequent target stimuli, whereas the effect of voluntary stimulus presentation on the P3 is prominent at more anterior sites.

across sites. Tests of simple effect showed that significant differences were found at fronto-central sites for both modalities. Fig. 2 depicts scalp topographic maps of the P3 in the difference waveforms. While the classical target P3 in the auto condition was dominant at parietal sites, the amplitude increase was dominant at more anterior sites as shown in the self-auto difference maps. P3 latency did not differ between conditions.

4. Discussion

When participants triggered auditory or visual stimuli by voluntary button presses, the P3 wave elicited by infrequent stimuli was increased in amplitude particularly at fronto-central sites. This finding is consistent with the results of the previous studies using three-stimulus oddball tasks [5,7] and confirms the robustness of the effect. The mean reaction time was longer in the self than in the auto condition. This behavioral result is similar to that of a previous study [5] and suggests that there was a motor conflict between the left and right index fingers used for triggering and response. However, the change in P3 amplitude is not attributable to this conflict since the effect was observed even when no motor responses were required [7]. The fixed order of the self and auto conditions might contribute partly to the amplitude difference between conditions, but practice or fatigue cannot explain the overall results. Previous studies showed that the amplitude of the P3 was larger in the self condition than in the preceding condition where the stimuli were presented automatically [5,7].

The effect of voluntary stimulus presentation was dominant at fronto-central sites, which was different from the parietal dominant P3 elicited by infrequent target stimuli. The scalp-recorded P3 wave has been assumed to consist of at least two different (but mutually related) components, fronto-central P3a and parietal P3b [8,9]. The scalp topography of the increased potential suggests that the P3a component was enhanced by voluntary stimulus presentation. This view is supported by a recent study showing that self-triggering of stimuli increased the amplitude of the P3 to perceptually deviant nontarget stimuli but not the P3 to less deviant target stimuli [10].

A plausible explanation of this phenomenon may be derived from the common coding theory, which holds that action and perception share a common representation and prime or interfere with each other [11]. When a participant intends to produce a stimulus by voluntary action, the perceptual representation of the forthcoming stimulus is activated before its arrival. This anticipatory representation is probably based on the most frequent outcome (i.e., frequent stimulus). The discrepancy between the activated representation and the actual event induces the attention switching, which is reflected in the P3a component. The more the representation is activated, the more salient is the discrepancy, and the larger is the amplitude of the P3a. Voluntary stimulus presentation may facilitate this anticipatory activation process and boost the deviance-induced processing.

In conclusion, the three ERP experiments using the action-perception paradigm have unambiguously shown that stimuli triggered by a participant's voluntary action are processed differently from the same stimuli presented automatically by a computer. These findings open up a new research field investigating the bidirectional link between human cognition and action in cognitive neuroscience. Besides the theoretical interest, the recording of ERPs to events following a participant's intentional action would be useful for examining cognitive processes in real-world settings such as human–computer interaction [7]. Whether the intentionality of movement is critical to this effect or how the interval between action and outcome influences this phenomenon will be examined in future experiments.

Acknowledgements

This study was supported by a grant-in-aid for scientific research from the Japanese Ministry of Education, Culture, Sports, Science, and Technology (No. 14710044).

References

[1] M. Jahanshahi, M. Hallett, The Bereitschaftspotential: movement-related cortical potentials, Kluwer Academic Publishing/Plenum, New York, 2003.

[2] E.W.P. Schafer, M.M. Marcus, Self-stimulation alters human sensory brain responses, Science 181 (1973) 175–177.

[3] G. McCarthy, E. Donchin, The effects of temporal and event uncertainty in determining the waveforms of the auditory event related potential (ERP), Psychophysiology 13 (1976) 581–590.

[4] D. Papakostopoulos, A no-stimulus, no-response, event-related potential of the human cortex, Electroencephalogr. Clin. Neurophysiol. 48 (1980) 622–638.

[5] H. Nittono, P. Ullsperger, Event-related potentials in a self-paced novelty oddball task, NeuroReport 11 (2000) 1861–1864.

[6] G.A. Chiarenza, A critical review of physiological and clinical aspects of movement related brain macro-potentials in humans, Ital. J. Neurol. Sci. 12 (1991) 17–30.

[7] H. Nittono, A. Hamada, T. Hori, Brain potentials after clicking a mouse: a new psychophysiological approach to human–computer interaction, Hum. Factors 45 (2003) 591–599.

[8] E. Halgren, K. Marinkovic, P. Chauvel, Generators of the late cognitive potentials in auditory and visual oddball tasks, Electroencephalogr. Clin. Neurophysiol. 106 (1998) 156–164.

[9] R.T. Knight, D. Scabini, Anatomic bases of event-related potentials and their relationship to novelty detection in humans, J. Clin. Neurophysiol. 15 (1998) 3–13.

[10] H. Nittono, Event-related potentials elicited by self-initiated auditory and visual events, Int. J. Psychophysiol. 45 (2002) 132–133.

[11] B. Hommel, et al., The theory of event coding (TEC): a framework for perception and action planning, Behav. Brain Sci. 24 (2001) 849–937.

International Congress Series 1270 (2004) 32–37

ELSEVIER

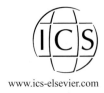

www.ics-elsevier.com

Clinical applications of the signal space separation method

Samu Taulu*, Juha Simola, Matti Kajola

Elekta Neuromag Oy, Software Development, Elimaenkatu 22 B, Helsinki 00510, Finland

Abstract. Conventional biomagnetic measurements suffer from the extreme sensitivity of the method to external and subject-related interference. Especially difficult to remove artifacts are caused by magnetic sources inside the shielded room and especially by magnetization associated with the subject. Such artifacts are encountered, e.g. with subjects having braces, magnetic stimulators and pacers or magnetic impurities in the lungs or in the head, etc. These problems, typical to patients, may severely reduce the clinical applicability of magnetoencephalography (MEG). The Signal Space Separation (SSS) method introduces a revolutionary improvement in feasibility and robustness of MEG measurements in the presence of such sources of artifacts. SSS allows recordings in environments with external interference of arbitrary geometry. With SSS, the compensation of subject-related artifacts typically arising from unintentional movements of the body and head is possible. With this method, every measurement can be uniquely decomposed into device-independent components with separate components for the interesting biomagnetic signals and external interference signals irrespective of the temporal or statistical nature of the sources. The device independence of this decomposition enables compensation of movement artifacts and analysis of DC phenomena. © 2004 Elsevier B.V. All rights reserved.

Keywords: Magnetoencephalography; Interference suppression; Movement compensation; DC phenomena

1. Introduction

Traditional biomagnetic measurements require extreme magnetic hygiene in the vicinity of the measurement device and cooperative subjects capable of avoiding movements during the measurement. This limits the feasibility of magnetoencephalography (MEG) for clinical measurements as nonmagnetic stimulus equipment and demagnetized personnel are required. Furthermore, patients seldom can stay still throughout the measurement.

There are several methods to suppress external interference signals, such as SSP [1] and reference channels [2], but their performance is limited by unpredictably changing interference, especially from sources inside the shielded rooms. SSP provides a good

* Corresponding author. Tel.: +358-9-756-24083; fax: +358-9-756-24011.
E-mail address: Samu.Taulu@neuromag.fi (S. Taulu).

0531-5131/ © 2004 Elsevier B.V. All rights reserved.
doi:10.1016/j.ics.2004.05.004

shielding factor, but with changing interference sources (e.g. magnetic impurities on the subject's head) it typically requires defining a new interference subspace. The reference channel method is based on assumptions about the smoothness of the interference fields, which are never met in the case of nearby sources.

Even more difficult artifacts are field distortions caused by movement of the subject or artifacts from possible magnetized particles attached to the moving head of the subject. Minimum norm estimate taking the head movement into account has been used to compensate for field distortions [3], but there have been no efficient solutions to cope with moving magnetic impurities.

In this paper, we introduce utilization of Signal Space Separation (SSS) to improve the clinical applicability of MEG. With this method, we can suppress any external interference with practically no a priori information about its source distribution. We also show that SSS can be used for movement correction, DC measurements, and calibration of the MEG device. The orientation of this paper is practical, with emphasis on demonstrations using real data collected with Elekta Neuromag™.

2. Materials and methods

2.1. Background of SSS

The SSS method [4] is based on a general model for biomagnetic multichannel measurement spanning all measurable signals of magnetic origin. SSS is a purely spatial method in which the measured signal is uniquely decomposed into elementary field components. This decomposition has two benefits. First, the biomagnetic signals arising from inside of the sensor array and signals arising from external interference sources consist of different elementary field components allowing one to resolve between them. Second, the SSS basis can be related to the head coordinates so that the decomposition encodes the signals in a device-independent manner. This allows compensation for movement of the subject, movement artifact suppression, and DC measurements.

The only assumption in SSS is that there are no sources in the volume where the sensors are located, so that the field can be expressed as a gradient of a harmonic scalar potential. Consequently, the elementary fields, from which the SSS basis vectors are composed, are derived from such potentials. The basic solutions associated with the biomagnetic sources and external interference sources correspond to harmonic potentials diverging inside or outside of the MEG helmet volume, respectively. This allows the decomposition of the signal space to different subspaces for these two kinds of sources. Thus, in SSS the biomagnetic signals and the external interference are modelled at the same time allowing a unique separation of biomagnetic signals from interference.

2.2. External interference suppression

Disturbances caused by any external interference sources (e.g. stimulators, assisting personnel, pacers, electrical equipments, etc.) can be removed by SSS by keeping the components corresponding to the biomagnetic signals only in the signal reconstruction. In this way, the only thing one needs to know about the biomagnetic and the interference sources is that they are inside and outside of the MEG helmet, respectively. The method simply recognizes these two different source types from the measurement. Thus, SSS performs well even with arbitrarily changing interference patterns.

2.3. Compensation for distortions caused by movement of the subject

Movement compensation requires a method for tracking the head position and a source model attached to the coordinate system of the head. One possible source model is the minimum norm estimate [3]. SSS provides a better source model for movement compensation as it also automatically suppresses the external interferences.

By modelling the movement of the subject as movement of the sensor array, the subject can be considered static in terms of the decomposed elementary field components. Thus, virtual signals corresponding to any reference head position can be calculated based on estimated SSS components, and these movement-compensated signals can be used for further data analysis as if the subject had not moved during the measurement.

Furthermore, any movement artifacts caused by magnetic impurities on the subject's head will be suppressed in this compensation method as their signals are deconvoluted with the movement information. In this way, the movement artifacts transform to DC-signals and can be removed from the data by a simple baseline correction. The next section describes generation of the signals caused by static, biomagnetic sources.

2.4. DC measurements

Stationary SQUID sensors record relative values of the magnetic field only. Consequently, DC sources, such as magnetic impurities on the scalp or physiological DC currents, are invisible in conventional MEG. However, movement of the subject relative to the measurement device transforms the DC fields into time-varying MEG signals. These signals can be transformed to DC by tracking the head movement and using the recorded movement information to decompose the signals into device-independent SSS components. After this demodulating with the movement information, the measured physiological DC signals can be studied and movement artifacts eliminated.

2.5. Calibration accuracy

The SSS method is based on the physics of magnetic fields and geometry. Therefore, its performance in the data analysis—ability to resolve between sources inside and outside of the helmet—depends crucially on the calibration accuracy of the sensor array used in the data acquisition. By calibration, we mean knowledge of the sensitivity, location, orientation, and imbalance of the individual sensors, as well as cross talk between the sensors in the entire array. Any inaccuracy in this information leads to mixing of the signals from internal and external field sources when data recorded with the array are analyzed. By simulated data, it can be shown that an overall relative inaccuracy of calibration leads to mixing of the signals from external and internal sources in the SSS processed data by the same relative amount. This is a rough rule of thumb.

3. Results

3.1. Effect of calibration accuracy on the SSS reconstruction

When using SSS for rejection of external interference, the achievable software magnetic shielding factor is roughly the inverse of the relative calibration accuracy. A 1% overall calibration accuracy results in a shielding factor of about 100. This property of the SSS method can be utilized effectively in the calibration of a sensor array. All the calibration parameters are fine tuned until the mixing of external and internal sources vanishes. This is demonstrated by aid of an empty room recording in Fig. 1. The software-shielding factor, obtained after SSS-based fine-tuning in this case, is about 1000, corresponding to an overall calibration accuracy of 1‰

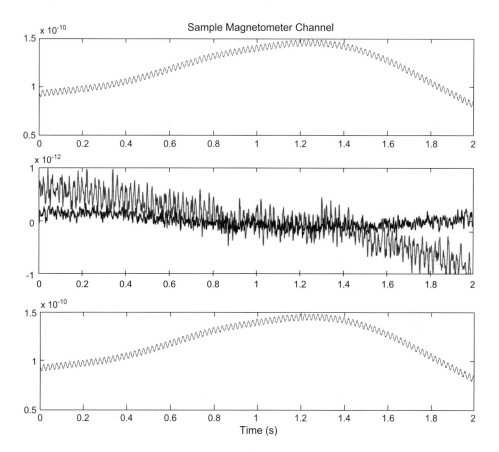

Fig. 1. Use of SSS for software magnetic shielding and calibration. The raw empty room recording in the uppermost frame shows a superposition of a slow magnetic interference with a 50 Hz contribution on top of it. The middle and lowermost frames show the signal from inside and outside of the helmet, respectively, as obtained by using SSS. In an empty room, recording the signal from inside the helmet should be zero. The red curve shows the internal signal corresponding to the as received calibration and the blue curve is obtained after SSS-based fine tuning of the calibration of the entire array. The fields are in Teslas.

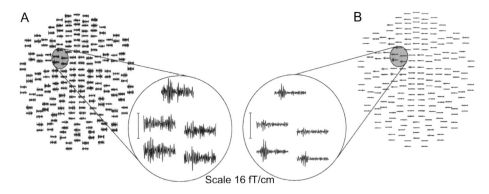

Fig. 2. Gradiometer waveforms from a high-frequency SEF measurement. (A) Shows the original waveforms and (B) shows the SSS reconstructed waveforms. The pass-band is 300–900 Hz. The time scale is 10–60 ms and amplitude scale −8.0–8.0 fT/cm. The number of averages is 800.

The calibration can be fine-tuned with SSS only if the pickup antennas of the sensors can be reliably characterized with a reasonably small number of free parameters. This is the case for modern thin film pickup antennas fabricated with photolithography on silicon. When used for data obtained with less accurately known pickup geometry-like wire wound axial gradiometers—the applicability of SSS is rather limited.

3.2. SSS reconstruction of a high frequency SEF measurement

Fig. 2 shows the original and SSS reconstructed waveforms of a high frequency SEF measurement. The original data are dominated by interference making the analysis very challenging. Only an experienced physician could recognize the SEF burst from these data in Fig. 2A. However, a rapid visual inspection of the SSS reconstructed waveforms of Fig. 2B clearly reveals the SEF response. This is especially clear from the close-ups. Fig. 3 shows the corresponding field maps at 20 ms latency. Again, for the unprocessed data an experienced physician would be required, whereas the SSS reconstruction reveals a clear dipolar field.

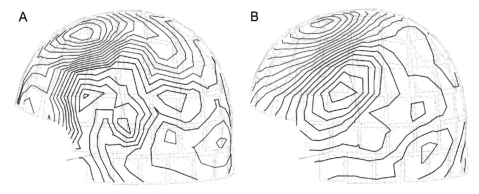

Fig. 3. Field distributions from the high-frequency SEF measurement of Fig. 2. (A) Shows the original field distribution based on gradiometer signals and (B) shows the SSS reconstructed distribution.

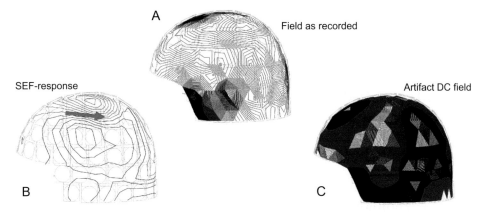

Fig. 4. Original and SSS reconstructed field distributions of an averaged SEF response from a moving, magnetic head of a subject are shown in (A) and (B), respectively. (B) Shows baseline-corrected data after demodulation of the motion, and the baseline (DC) field is shown in (C).

3.3. Compensation for movement artifacts

SSS-based compensation for movement artifacts was demonstrated by an SEF measurement of a voluntarily moving subject with magnetized particles attached to the head. The subject moved his head about 3 cm and raw data were recorded with continuously activated head position indicator coils. The head positions were calculated from the raw data as described in Ref. [3] and the SEF response was averaged by demodulating the head movement with SSS. Fig. 4A shows the averaged field without movement compensation. The field is dominated by the DC field of the magnetized particles modulated by the head motion. However, the demodulation of the movement transforms the fields of the particles to DC, and their contribution can be removed by baseline correction revealing the SEF response as shown in Fig. 4B. In addition, Fig. 4C shows the demodulated DC field related to the DC sources.

4. Discussion

Conventional MEG suffers from several practical restrictions in routine clinical examinations. The SSS method discussed here removes many of these restrictions and greatly facilitates clinical usage of MEG. Specifically, SSS relaxes the strict requirements on demagnetization of the personnel and usage of nonmagnetic equipment. Also, signal distortions caused by movement of the subject and artifacts caused by magnetized particles attached to the body can be removed by SSS. Physiological DC phenomena can be analyzed by using SSS and voluntary head movements.

References

[1] M.A. Uusitalo, R.J. Ilmoniemi, Signal-space projection method, Med. Biol. Eng. 32 (1997) 35–42.
[2] J. Vrba, S.E. Robinson, Signal processing in magnetoencephalography, Methods 25 (2001) 249–271.
[3] K. Uutela, S. Taulu, M. Hamalainen, Detecting and correcting for head movements, NeuroImage 25 (2001) 249–271.
[4] S. Taulu, M. Kajola, J. Simola, The signal space separation method, Biomed. Tech. (2004) 48 (in press).

International Congress Series 1270 (2004) 38–43

ELSEVIER

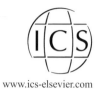

www.ics-elsevier.com

Solving the "neuroimaging puzzle" with the multimodal integration of EEG and functional magnetic resonance recordings

Fabio Babiloni[a,*], Claudio Babiloni[a,b], Filippo Carducci[a,c], Paolo Maria Rossini[b,c,d], Alessandra Basilisco[a], Laura Astolfi[a], Febo Cincotti[e]

[a] Department of Human Physiology and Pharmacology, University of Rome "La Sapienza", P.le A. Moro 5, 00185 Rome, Italy
[b] AFaR and CRCCS Ospedale Fatebenefratelli, Isola Tiberina, Rome, Italy
[c] IRCCS "San Giovanni di Dio" Istituto Sacro Cuore di Gesù, Brescia, Italy
[d] Cattedra di Neurologia, Università Campus Bio-Medico, Rome, Italy
[e] IRCCS Fondazione "Santa Lucia", Rome, Italy

Abstract. In this paper, advanced methods for the modeling of human cortical activity from combined high-resolution electroencephalography (EEG) and functional magnetic resonance imaging (fMRI) data are reviewed. These methods include a subject's multicompartment head model (scalp, skull, dura mater, cortex) constructed from magnetic resonance images, multidipole source model, and regularized linear inverse source estimates. Determination of the priors in the resolution of the linear inverse problem was performed with the use of information from the hemodynamic responses of the cortical areas as revealed by block-designed fMRI. © 2004 Elsevier B.V. All rights reserved.

Keywords: Linear inverse source estimate; EEG and fMRI integration; Movement-related potentials

1. Introduction

It is well known that high-resolution electroencephalography (HREEG) and magneto-encephalography (MEG) are two brain imaging techniques that present a high temporal resolution adequate to follow the cortical activity. Both techniques have a relatively modest spatial resolution on the centimeter scale. In spite of a lack of spatial resolution, neural sources can be localized from EEG or MEG data by making a priori hypotheses on their number and extension. It is worth noting that the spatial resolution of the HREEG/MEG techniques is fundamentally limited by the intersensor distances and by the fundamental laws of electromagnetism [1]. On the other hand, the use of a priori

* Corresponding author. Tel.: +39-64-9910317; fax: +39-64-9910917.
E-mail address. Fabio.Babiloni@uniroma1.it (F. Babiloni).

information from other neuroimaging techniques, such as functional magnetic resonance imaging (fMRI), which have high spatial resolution, has suggested a way of improving the localization of sources from HREEG/MEG data [2,3]. In fact, human neocortical processes involve temporal and spatial scales spanning several orders of magnitude, from the rapidly shifting somatosensory processes characterized by a temporal scale of milliseconds and a spatial scale of a few square millimeters to the memory processes, involving time periods of seconds and a spatial scale of square centimeters. Information about the brain activity can be obtained by measuring different physical variables linked to the brain processes, such as the increase in consumption of oxygen by the neural tissues or the variation of the electric potential over the scalp surface. It is worth noting that all these variables have their own spatial and temporal resolution. The different neuroimaging techniques are then confined to the spatiotemporal resolution offered by the measured variables. Today, no neuroimaging method allows a spatial resolution on a millimeter scale and a temporal resolution on a millisecond scale. As a consequence of the previous statement, the functional brain images obtained with the several techniques at our disposal (fMRI, HREEG, MEG) are like the pieces of a puzzle, the "neuroimaging puzzle", that we have to put together to retrieve a unique picture of the underlying brain activity. Hence, it is of interest to study the possibility to integrate the information offered by the different physiological variables related to the brain functions in a unique mathematical context. This operation is called the "multimodal integration" of variable X and Y, when the X variable has typically particular appealing spatial resolution property (on a mm scale) and the Y variable has particular attractive temporal properties (on a ms scale).

This paper deals with the multimodal integration of electromagnetic and hemodynamic data to locate neural sources responsible for the recorded EEG/MEG activity. The rationale of the multimodal approach based on fMRI, MEG and EEG data to locate brain activity is that neural activity generating EEG potentials or MEG fields increase glucose and oxygen demands [4]. This results in an increase in the local hemodynamic response that can be measured by fMRI [5,6]. On the whole, such a correlation between electrical and hemodynamic concomitants provides the basis for a spatial correspondence between fMRI responses and HREEG/MEG source activity. In the following, we present the mathematical principle underlying such multimodal integration.

2. Methods for the multimodal integration of EEG, MEG and fMRI data

Taking into account the measurement noise $\mathbf{n}$, supposed normally distributed, an estimate of the dipole source configuration $\mathbf{x}$ that generated the measured EEG potential distribution b can be obtained by solving the linear system:

$$\mathbf{Ax} = \mathbf{b} + \mathbf{n} \tag{1}$$

where $\mathbf{A}$ is the lead field matrix, in which each jth column describes the potential distribution generated on the scalp electrodes by the jth unitary dipole. Among the several equivalent solutions for the underdetermined system (1), the current density solution vector ξ was chosen by solving the following problem for the sources $\mathbf{x}$ [7]:

$$\xi = \arg \min_x \left(\| \mathbf{Ax} - b \|_{\mathbf{M}}^2 + \lambda^2 \| x \|_{\mathbf{N}}^2 \right) \tag{2}$$

where **M**, **N** are the matrices associated to the metrics of the data and of the source space, respectively, λ is the regularization parameter and $\|x\|_\mathbf{M}$ represents the **M** norm of the vector **x**. The solution of the variational problem, under the hypothesis of **M** and **N** positive definite, is given by computing the inverse operator **G** according to the following expressions:

$$\xi = \mathbf{G}b, \quad \mathbf{G} = \mathbf{N}^{-1}\mathbf{A}' (\mathbf{A}\mathbf{N}^{-1}\mathbf{A}' + \lambda\mathbf{M}^{-1})^{-1} \tag{3}$$

The metric **M**, characterizing the idea of closeness in the data space, can be particularized by taking into account the sensor's noise level, by using either the Mahalanobis distance [7] or the identity matrix [8]. The source metric **N** can be also particularized by a priori taking into account the information from the hemodynamic responses of the single voxels as derived from fMRIs, as shown in the following section. The introduction of fMRI priors into the linear inverse estimation produces a bias in the estimation of the current density strength of the modeled cortical dipoles. Statistically significant activated fMRI voxels, which are returned by the percentage change approach [9], are weighted to account for the EEG measured potentials. The inverse of the resulting metric is then proposed as follows [10]:

$$(\mathbf{N}^{-1})_{ii} = g(\alpha_i)^2 \|\mathbf{A}_{\cdot i}\|^{-2} \tag{4}$$

in which $(\mathbf{N}^{-1})_{ii}$ is the ith term on the diagonal of the square matrix N^{-1} and $\mathbf{A}_{\cdot i}$ is the ith column vector of the lead field matrix **A**. Furthermore, $g(\alpha_i)$ is a function of the statistically significant percentage increase of the fMRI signal assigned to the ith dipole of the modeled source space [9]. This function is expressed as

$$g(\alpha_i)^2 = 1 + (K-1)\frac{\alpha_i}{\max\alpha_i}, \quad K \geq 1, \quad \alpha_i \geq 0 \tag{5}$$

where α_i is the percentage increase of the fMRI signal during the task state for the ith voxel and the factor K tunes fMRI constraints in the source space. Fixing $K = 1$, let us disregard fMRI priors, thus returning to a purely electrical solution; a value of $K \gg 1$ allows only the sources associated with fMRI active voxels to participate in the solution. It was shown that a value of K in the order of 10 (90% of constraints for the fMRI information) is useful to avoid mislocalization due to overconstrained solutions [2,3].

3. Results

Fig. 1 illustrates the cortical distributions of the current density estimated with the described linear inverse approaches from the potential distribution relative to the movement preparation, about 200 ms before a right middle finger extension. Such an approach used no-fMRI constraint as well the fMRI constraints based on Eq. (5). The cortical distributions are represented on the realistic subject's head volume conductor model. Linear inverse solution obtained with the fMRI priors presents more localized spots of activations with respect to those obtained with the no fMRI priors. Remarkably, the spots of activation were localized in the hand region of the primary somatosensory (post-central) and motor (pre-central) areas contralateral to the movement. In addition, spots of minor activation were observed in the frontocentral medial areas (including supplementary

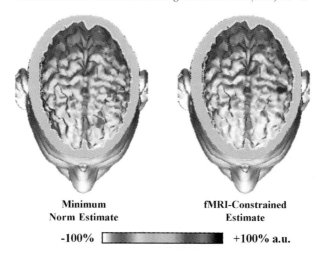

Minimum Norm Estimate   **fMRI-Constrained Estimate**

-100% [gradient bar] +100% a.u.

Fig. 1. Cortical distributions of the current density estimated with the linear inverse approaches from the potential distribution relative to the movement preparation, about 200 ms before a right middle finger extension. The cortical distributions are represented on the realistic subject's head volume conductor model. Left: cortical estimate obtained without the use of fMRI constraints, based on the minimum norm solutions. Right: cortical estimate obtained with the use of fMRI constraints based on Eq. (5) (see text for details).

motor area) and in the primary somatosensory and motor areas of the ipsilateral hemisphere.

4. Discussion

Any neuroimaging technique has its own visible and invisible sources. The visible sources for a particular neuroimaging technique are those neuronal pools whose spatio-temporal activity can be at least in part detected. In contrast, invisible sources are those neural assemblies that produce a pattern of the spatiotemporal activity not detectable by the analyzed neuroimaging technique. In the case of HREEG (or MEG) technique, it is clear that the visible sources are generally located at the cortical level, because the cortical assemblies are close to the recording sensors, and the morphology of the cortical layers allows the generation of open (rather than closed) electromagnetic fields. On the other hand, it is often poorly understood that the invisible sources for the EEG (or MEG) are all those cortical assemblies that do not fire synchronously together. In fact, in a dipole layer composed by M coherent sources and N incoherent ones, the potentials due to individual coherent sources are combined by linear superposition, while the combination of the incoherent sources is only due to statistical fluctuations. The ratio between the contributions of coherent to incoherent source can be expressed by $M N^{-0.5}$ [11]. Hence, if N is very large, say about 10 million of incoherent neurons that fire continuously, and M is a small percentage of such neurons (say 1%; about 100,000 neurons) that instead fire synchronously, we obtain that the potential measured at the scalp level will be determined by $10^5 \, 10^{-7/2}$, with a net result of about 30. Hence, only 1% of the active sources produce a potential larger than the other 99% by a factor of 30 just because of the synchronicity property. This means that the metabolic requirements occurring in cortical regions in which substantial EEG activity has been detected can be really modest, interestingly just 1% of the local neural population. As a consequence of that, neuroimaging techniques based on imaging of the metabolic/hemodynamic request of the neural assemblies may detect no relevant activity with respect to the baseline condition. However, there are other situations in which the visible sources for metabolic techniques such as fMRI and PET can be invisible for EEG or MEG techniques. Stellate cells are neurons present in the human cerebral cortex, and represent 15% of the neural population of the neocortex [12]. These cells occupy a spherical volume within the cortex, thus generating essentially a closed-field electromagnetic pattern. Such a field cannot be recorded at the scalp level by electrical or magnetic sensors, although the actual firing rate of such stellate neurons is rather high with respect to the other cortical neurons. This means that these neuronal populations present high metabolism requirements that can be detected by the fMRI technique, while at the same time they are "invisible sources" for the EEG and MEG techniques. Another example of invisible sources for the EEG and MEG techniques is represented by the neural assemblies located at the thalamic level, as they are also arranged in such a way to produce closed electromagnetic field, while having high metabolic requirements. The results for the multimodal integration of EEG/MEG and fMRI presented in this paper are in line with those regarding the coupling between cortical electrical activity and hemodynamic measure as indicated by a direct comparison of maps obtained using voltage-sensitive dyes (which reflect depolarization of neuronal membranes in superficial cortical layers) and maps derived from intrinsic optical signals (which reflect changes in light absorption due to changes in blood volume and oxygen consumption [13]. Furthermore, previous studies on animals have also shown a strong correlation between local field potentials, spiking activity, and voltage-sensitive dye signals [14]. Finally, studies in humans comparing the localization of functional activity by invasive electrical recordings and fMRI have provided evidence of a correlation between the local electrophysiological and hemodynamic responses [6]. It is worthy of note that, recently, a study aimed at investigating this link has been presented [15]. In this study, intracortical recordings of neural signals and simultaneous fMRI signals were acquired in monkeys. The comparisons were made between the local field potentials, the multiunit spiking activity and BOLD signals in the visual cortex. The study supports the link between the local field potentials and BOLD mechanism, which is at the base of the procedure of the multimodal integration of EEG/MEG with fMRI described above. This may suggest that the local fMRI responses can be reliably used to bias the estimation of the electrical activity in the regions showing a prominent hemodynamic response. Based on the evidences provided in literature and those presented here, it seems that the actual technologies for the multimodal integration of HREEG/MEG recordings and fMRI data are sufficiently accurate to solve, within the next years, the "neuroimaging puzzle" for the characterization of brain activity.

References

[1] P. Nunez, Electric Fields of the Brain, Oxford Univ. Press, New York, 1981.
[2] A.K. Liu, et al., Spatiotemporal imaging of human brain activity using functional MRI constrained magnetoencephalography data: Monte Carlo simulations, Proc. Natl. Acad. Sci. 95 (15) (1998) 8945–8950.

[3] A. Dale, et al., Dynamic statistical parametric mapping: combining fMRI and MEG for high-resolution imaging of cortical activity, Neuron 26 (2000) 55–67.

[4] P.J. Magistretti, et al., Energy on demand, Science 283 (5401) (1999) 496–497.

[5] A. Grinvald, et al., Functional architecture of cortex revealed by optical imaging of intrinsic signals, Nature 324 (6095) (1986) 361–364.

[6] A. Puce, et al., Comparison of cortical activation evoked by faces measured by intracranial field potentials and functional MRI: two case studies, Hum. Brain Mapp. 5 (4) (1997) 298–305.

[7] R. Grave de Peralta Menendez, S.L. Gonzalez Andino, Distributed source models: standard solutions and new developments, in: C. Uhl (Ed.), Analysis of Neurophysiological Brain Functioning, Springer Verlag, 1998, pp. 176–201.

[8] M. Hämäläinen, R. Ilmoniemi, Interpreting measured magnetic field of the brain: estimates of the current distributions. Technical report TKK-F-A559, Helsinki University of Technology, 1984.

[9] S. Kim, et al., Functional magnetic resonance imaging of motor cortex: hemispheric asymmetry and handedness, Science 261 (1993) 615–617.

[10] F. Babiloni, et al., Integration of high resolution EEG and functional magnetic resonance in the study of human movement-related potentials, Methods Inf. Med. 39 (2) (2000) 179–182.

[11] P.L. Nunez, Neocortical Dynamics and Human EEG Rhythms, Oxford Univ. Press, New York, 1995.

[12] V. Braitemberg, A. Schuz, Anatomy of the Cortex. Statistics and Geometry, Springer-Verlag, New York, 1991.

[13] D. Shoham, et al., Imaging cortical dynamics at high spatial and temporal resolution with novel blue voltage-sensitive dyes, Neuron 24 (1999) 791–802.

[14] A. Arieli, et al., Dynamics of ongoing activity: explanation of the large variability in evoked cortical responses, Science 273 (1996) 1868–1871.

[15] N.K. Logothetis, et al., Neurophysiological investigation of the basis of the fMRI signal, Nature 412 (6843) (2001) 150–157.

Cortical alpha rhythms in mild Alzheimer's disease. A multicentric EEG study

C. Babiloni[a,b,*], G. Binetti[c], E. Cassetta[b], D. Cerboneschi[b],
G. Dal Forno[d,e], C. Del Percio[a,c], F. Ferreri[b,d], R. Ferri[f], B. Lanuzza[f],
C. Miniussi[c], D.V. Moretti[a], F. Nobili[g], R.D. Pascual-Marqui[h],
G. Rodriguez[g], G.L. Romani[i], S. Salinari[j], F. Tecchio[k], P. Vitali[f],
O. Zanetti[c], F. Zappasodi[k], P.M. Rossini[b,c,d]

[a] Dipartimento di Fisiologia Umana e Farmacologia, Università "La Sapienza", Rome, Italy
[b] A.Fa.R. Osp. FBF Isola Tiberina, Rome, Italy
[c] IRCCS "S. Giovanni di Dio FBF, Brescia, Italy
[d] Università "Campus Biomedico", Rome, Italy
[e] Department of Neurology, Johns Hopkins University School of Medicine, Baltimore, USA
[f] Department of Neurology, Oasi Institute for Research on Mental Retardation and Brain Aging, Troina, Italy
[g] Division of Clinical Neurophysiology (DIMI), University of Genova, Genova, Italy
[h] The KEY Institute for Brain-Mind Research, University Hospital of Psychiatry, Zurich, Switzerland
[i] ITAB University Chieti and INFN, UdR L'Aquila, Italy
[j] Dipartimento Informatica e Sistemistica Università "La Sapienza", Rome, Italy
[k] IFN-Consiglio Nazionale delle Ricerche (CNR) Unità MEG-Osp. FBF Isola Tiberina, Rome, Italy

Abstract. The study aimed at mapping (i) the distributed alpha (8–13 Hz) electroencephalography (EEG) sources specific for mild Alzheimer's disease (AD) compared with vascular dementia (VaD) in normal, elderly people (Nold) and (ii) the distributed alpha EEG sources sensitive to mild AD at different stages of severity. Resting EEG (10–20 electrode montage) was recorded from 48 mild AD, 20 VaD and 38 Nold subjects. Both AD and VaD patients had 24–17 on their mini mental state examinations (MMSE). Alpha bands were subdivided in alpha 1 (8–10.5 Hz) and alpha 2 (10.5–13 Hz) subbands. Cortical alpha EEG sources were modeled by "low resolution brain electromagnetic tomography" (LORETA). Regarding issue (i), there was a decline of central, parietal, temporal and limbic alpha 1 sources specific to the mild AD group with respect to Nold and VaD groups. On the other hand, occipital alpha 1 sources showed a strong decline in mild AD compared with the VaD group. However, this finding was "unspecific" because a certain decline of these sources was also recognized in VaD compared with Nold. Regarding issue (ii), there was a lower power of occipital alpha 1 sources in the mild AD more severely diseased subgroup. On the whole, these findings stress the reliability of

* Corresponding author. Dipartimento di Fisiologia Umana e Farmacologia, Università "La Sapienza", P.le Aldo Moro 5, Rome 00185, Italy. Tel.: +39-6-49910989; fax: +39-6-49910917.
  E-mail address: claudio.babiloni@uniroma1.it (C. Babiloni).

modern technologies for EEG analysis as the LORETA approach to the study of cortical rhythmicity in resting mild AD. © 2004 Elsevier B.V. All rights reserved.

Keywords: Mild Alzheimer's disease (mild AD); Vascular dementia (VaD); Electroencephalography (EEG); Alpha rhythm; Low resolution brain electromagnetic tomography (LORETA)

1. Introduction

Electroencephalographic (EEG) rhythms are affected by Alzheimer's disease (AD) [1–3]. Compared with normal elderly subjects, Alzheimer's disease (AD) patients present an increase of delta (about 0.5–4 Hz) and theta (about 4–8 Hz) mean power, along with a decrease of alpha (about 8–13 Hz) and beta (about 13–30 Hz) mean power. EEG rhythms are also sensitive to the severity of dementia. Delta and/or theta rhythms do increase even in the earlier stages of AD [3] and seem to predict disease progression [4,5]. In normal subjects, the magnitude of alpha rhythm is maximal in scalp occipital areas. While alpha rhythm still peaks in the posterior scalp areas in mild AD patients, it is either equally distributed over the scalp or localizes more anteriorly with disease progression [5–7].

From a physiological point of view, EEG rhythms reflect the opening/closure ("gating function") of bidirectional connections among several cortical and subcortical (i.e., brain stem, thalamus) structures [8–10]. Therefore, a single dipole source indicates the "center of gravity" of the distributed cortical sources generating the EEG rhythms. An alternative approach for the modeling of these sources is called "low resolution brain electromagnetic tomography" (LORETA) [11,12], which uses thousands of dipole sources within a 3D brain model coregistered into Talairach space [13].

The present multicentric study was aimed at defining (i) the distributed alpha (8–13 Hz) EEG sources specific for mild AD compared with Vascular dementia (VaD) or normal aging (Nold) and (ii) the distributed alpha EEG sources sensitive to mild AD progression. For these aims, resting EEG was recorded from a large group of mild AD, VaD and normal elderly (Nold) subjects. Alpha bands were subdivided into alpha 1 (8–10.5 Hz) and alpha 2 (10.5–13 Hz) subbands. Cortical sources of alpha EEG rhythms were modeled by LORETA solutions in macrocortical regions.

2. Materials and methods

We recruited 48 mild AD patients, 20 VaD patients and 38 Nold subjects. All patients had a Mini Mental State Evaluation (MMSE) [14] with results ranging from 24 to 17. The mild AD patients were further subdivided into mild AD " − " (MMSE 24–21, 23 subjects) and mild AD " + " (MMSE 20–17, 25 subjects) to address the issue of the increase of the severity of mild AD. Table 1 shows a report of the mean values of relevant personal and clinical parameters of mild AD, VaD and Nold subjects.

Specialized, clinical units recorded EEG in resting subjects (eyes closed) whose vigilance was continuously controlled to avoid drowsiness. EEG data were recorded (0.3–70 Hz band pass) from 19 electrodes positioned, according to the international 10–20 system (Fp1, Fp2, F7, F3, Fz, F4, F8, T3, C3, Cz, C4, T4, T5, P3, Pz, P4, T6, O1, O2).

Table 1
Personal and neuropsychological data of interest of the Nold, AD, VaD subjects

	Nold	Mild AD	VaD
N	38	48	20
AGE (years)	67.5 (± 1.3 S.E.)	73.7 (± 1.3 S.E.)	76.4 (± 1.2 S.E.)
GENDER (F/M)	19/19	39/9	10/10
MMSE	29.2 (± 0.2 S.E.)	20.2 (± 0.3 S.E.)	20.4 (± 1.1 S.E.)
EDUCATION (years)	8 (± 0.7 S.E.)	5.5 (± 0.5 S.E.)	9.7 (± 1 S.E.)

A digital FFT-based power spectrum analysis (Welch technique, Hanning windowing function, no phase shift) computed the power density of alpha EEG rhythms with 0.5 Hz frequency resolution. The following alpha subbands were considered: alpha 1 (8–10.5 Hz) and alpha 2 (10.5–13 Hz).

We employed LORETA for the EEG source analysis, which has been extensively tested with simulation paradigms [11,12]. LORETA computed 3D linear solutions (LORETA solutions) for the EEG inverse problem within a three-shell spherical head model including scalp, skull and brain compartments. The brain compartment was restricted to the cortical gray matter/hippocampus. This compartment included 2394 voxels (7 mm resolution), each voxel containing an equivalent current dipole. LORETA solutions consisted of current voxel density values able to predict EEG spectral power density at scalp electrodes. To enhance the "topographical" results, a "spatial" normalization was obtained by normalizing the LORETA current density at each voxel for the LORETA power density averaged across all frequencies (0.5–30 Hz)/voxels of the brain volume. These normalized, relative current values were then log transformed. We collapsed LORETA solutions at the frontal, central, temporal, parietal, occipital and limbic regions of the brain model coded into Talairach space.

Regional, normalized LORETA solutions were compared by two ANOVA analyses, using relative current density values as the dependent variable and subjects' age and education as covariates. The first ANOVA design focused on distributed alpha EEG sources specific to mild AD. Its factors (levels) were Group (mild AD, VaD, Nold), Band (alpha 1, alpha 2) and ROI (central, frontal, parietal, occipital, temporal, limbic). The second ANOVA design focused on distributed alpha EEG sources sensitive to the severity of mild AD. Its factors (levels) were Group (Nold, mild AD −, mild AD+), Band (alpha 1, alpha 2) and ROI (central, frontal, parietal, occipital, temporal, limbic).

3. Results

Fig. 1 maps the grand average of LORETA solutions modeling distributed alpha EEG sources in Nold, mild AD (MMSE 24–17) and VaD groups. In the Nold group, alpha sources had strong magnitude and were distributed mainly in the parieto–occipital regions. Relative current density prevailed in alpha 1 compared with alpha 2 sources. Compared to the Nold group, the mild AD group showed a dramatic reduction of parieto–occipital alpha 1 sources. Compared to the AD group, the VaD group was characterized by a less dramatic decrease of parieto–occipital alpha 1 sources with respect to the Nold group.

Fig. 2 maps the grand average of LORETA solutions, modeling distributed alpha EEG sources in mild AD − (MMSE 24–21) and mild AD+ (MMSE 20–17) groups. Compared

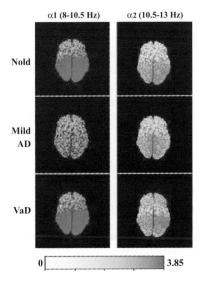

Fig. 1. Grand average of LORETA solutions (grey scale) modeling distributed alpha EEG sources in Nold, mild AD (MMSE 24–17) and VaD groups. The left side of the maps (top view) corresponds to the left hemisphere.

to the Nold group (see Fig. 1), occipital alpha 1 sources decreased in magnitude with the maximal severity of the disease (mild AD − to mild AD+).

The ANOVA analysis, focusing on distributed alpha EEG sources specific to mild AD, showed a statistical ANOVA interaction ($p = 0.03$) among Group (mild AD, VaD, Nold), Band (alpha 1, alpha 2) and ROI (central, frontal, parietal, occipital, temporal, limbic) factors. Duncan post hoc showed a strong decline of central, parietal, temporal and limbic alpha 1 sources specific to mild AD with respect to Nold and VaD. Furthermore, occipital alpha 1 sources showed a strong decline in mild AD compared with VaD. However, this

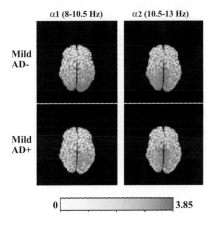

Fig. 2. Grand average of LORETA solutions (grey scale) modeling distributed alpha EEG in sources AD − (MMSE 24–21) and mild AD+ (MMSE 20–17). The left side of the maps (top view) corresponds to the left hemisphere.

finding was "unspecific" because a certain decline of these sources was also recognized in VaD compared with Nold.

The ANOVA analysis, focusing on distributed alpha EEG sources sensitive to the severity of mild AD, showed a statistical ANOVA interaction ($p = 0.01$) among Group (Nold, mild AD −, mild AD+), Band (alpha 1, alpha 2) and ROI (central, frontal, parietal, occipital, temporal, limbic) factors. Duncan post hoc indicated that the occipital alpha 1 sources had lower magnitude in mild AD − than Nold groups and lower magnitude in mild AD+ than mild AD − groups.

4. Discussion

Cortical alpha 1 sources characterized mild AD from VaD and normal aging. Compared to VaD and normal aging, mild AD showed a significant decrease of alpha 1 sources in all cortical regions. In particular, the most specific marker for mild AD was the reduction in magnitude of central, parietal, temporal and limbic alpha 1 sources compared with normal aging and VaD. Thus, it could be considered a marker specific for mild AD. On the other hand, the reduction of the alpha 1 sources in the mild AD group respect to the control groups was clearly less evident in the central cortical region when compared with the parietal, occipital and temporal cortical regions. Furthermore, it was practically absent in the frontal region. The present results enlighten the so-called "anteriorization" of scalp alpha rhythms in AD, repeatedly reported in previous studies using EEG mapping and single dipole localization [5,6,14,15]. Such an "anteriorization" may result from the fact that, in mild AD, alpha 1 sources decline in magnitude much more in parieto–occipital than frontal cortical regions, thus producing a "virtual displacement" of the "center of gravity" of the alpha rhythm.

Compared to normal aging, magnitude reduction of widespread alpha 1 sources in mild AD can be explained in terms of an abnormal increase of cortical excitation or disinhibition during the resting state. This explanation is in line with previous evidence showing abnormal central EEG rhythms or evoked potentials in AD subjects who performed voluntary movements or received somatosensory stimuli [16,17].

In the present study, another important focus was on specific features characterizing distributed cortical sources of EEG rhythms during the different stages of severity of mild AD. Occipital alpha 1 sources had a stronger magnitude in Nold than mild AD − and in mild AD − than mild AD+. These results, localized to the occipital cortical region, confirm previous scalp EEG evidence showing decreased alpha during AD progression [1,2,7,15,18–20]. The present abnormal sources of occipital EEG rhythms between mild AD at different stages of severity may be due to early pathological changes in extrastriate occipital areas [21] and their connections [22–24].

References

[1] C. Besthorn, et al., Discrimination of Alzheimer's disease and normal aging by EEG data, Electroencephalogr. Clin. Neurophysiol. 103 (2) (1997) 241–248.
[2] R. Chiaramonti, et al., Correlations of topographical EEG features with clinical severity in mild and moderate dementia of Alzheimer type, Neuropsychobiology 36 (3) (1997) 153–158.
[3] U. Schreiter-Gasser, T. Gasser, P. Ziegler, Quantitative EEG analysis in early onset Alzheimer's disease:

correlations with severity, clinical characteristics, visual EEG and CCT, Electroencephalogr. Clin. Neurophysiol. 90 (4) (1994) 267–272.

[4] F. Nobili, et al., Timing of disease progression by quantitative EEG in Alzheimer' s patients, J. Clin. Neurophysiol. 16 (6) (1999) 566–573.

[5] R. Ihl, et al., Topography of the maximun of the amplitude of EEG frequency in dementia of the Alzheimer type, Biol. Psychiatry 39 (1996) 319–325.

[6] R. Ihl, et al., Segmentation of the spontaneous EEG in dementia of the Alzheimer type, Neuropsychobiology 27 (4) (1993) 231–236.

[7] J.J. Claus, et al., The diagnostic value of electroencephalography in mild senile Alzheimer's disease, Clin. Neurophysiol. 110 (1999) 825–832.

[8] G. Pfurtscheller, C. Neuper, Event-related synchronization of mu rhythm in the EEG over the cortical hand area in man, Neurosci. Lett. 174 (1) (1994) 93–96.

[9] P. Nunez, Neocortical Dynamics and Human EEG Rhythms, Oxford Univ. Press, New York, 1995.

[10] G. Pfurtscheller, F.H. lopes da Silva, Event-related EEG/MEG synchronization and desynchronization: basic principles, Clin. Neurophysiol. 110 (11) (1999 Nov.) 1842–1857 (Review).

[11] R.D. Pascual-Marqui, C.M. Michel, LORETA (low resolution brain electromagnetic tomography): new authentic 3D functional images of the brain, ISBET Newsl. ISSN 5 (1994) 4–8.

[12] R.D. Pascual-Marqui, et al., Low resolution brain electromagnetic tomography (LORETA) functional imaging in acute, neuroleptic-naive, first-episode, productive schizophrenia, Psychiatry Res. 90 (3) (1999) 169–179.

[13] J. Talairach, P. Tournoux, Co-planar Stereotaxic Atlas of the Human Brain, Thieme, Stuttgart, 1988.

[14] J.J. Claus, et al., Slowing on quantitative spectral EEG is a marker for rate of subsequent cognitive and functional decline in early Alzheimer disease, Alzheimer Dis. Assoc. Disord. 12 (3) (1998) 167–174.

[15] T. Dierks, et al., Spatial pattern of cerebral glucose metabolism (PET) correlates with localization of intracerebral EEG-generators in Alzheimer's disease, Clin. Neurophysiol. 111 (2000) 1817–1824.

[16] C. Babiloni, et al., Movement-related electroencephalographic reactivity in Alzheimer disease, NeuroImage 12 (2) (2000) 139–146.

[17] R. Ferri, et al., Scalp topographic mapping of middle-latency somatosensory evoked potentials in normal aging and dementia, Neurophysiol. Clin. 26 (5) (1996) 311–319.

[18] F. Nobili, et al., Timing of disease progression by quantitative EEG in Alzheimer's patients, J. Clin. Neurophysiol. 16 (6) (1999) 566–573.

[19] G. Rodriguez, et al., EEG spectral profile to stage Alzheimer's disease, Clin. Neurophysiol. 110 (1999) 1831–1837.

[20] C. Huang, et al., Discrimination of Alzheimer's disease and mild cognitive impairment by equivalent EEG sources: a cross-sectional and longitudinal study, Clin. Neurophysiol. 11 (2000) 1961–1967.

[21] R.A. Armstrong, et al., Neuropathological changes in the visual cortex in the Alzheimer's disease, Neurosci. Res. Commun. 6 (1990) 163–171.

[22] A. Cronin-Golomb, et al., Visual dysfunction in Alzheimer's disease: relation to normal aging, Ann. Neurol. 29 (1) (1991) 41–52.

[23] A. Cronin-Golomb, et al., Incomplete achromatopsia in Alzheimer's disease, Neurobiol. Aging 14 (5) (1993) 471–477.

[24] J.H. Morrison, P.R. Hof, C. Bouras, An anatomic substrate for visual disconnection in Alzheimer's disease, Ann. N. Y. Acad. Sci. 640 (1991) 36–43.

International Congress Series 1270 (2004) 50–55

ELSEVIER

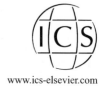

www.ics-elsevier.com

Structural and functional abnormalities of the auditory cortex in schizophrenia

Kiyoto Kasai*

Department of Neuropsychiatry, Graduate School of Medicine, University of Tokyo, 7-3-1 Hongo, Bunkyo, Tokyo 113-8655, Japan

Abstract. We used the combination of magnetic resonance imaging (MRI), event-related potentials (ERPs), and magnetoencephalography (MEG) to track structural and functional abnormalities of the superior temporal gyrus (STG) and its subdivisions of Heschl's gyrus (HG; primary auditory cortex) and planum temporale (PT; language-related association cortex) in schizophrenia. We found a significantly progressive decrease of left posterior STG gray matter volume at 1.5-year follow-up in first-episode patients with schizophrenia. When STG was divided into HG and PT, both showed a similar degree of volume reduction over time in patients with schizophrenia. Structural abnormalities of HG at the first-hospitalization and their progression were tightly coupled with the amplitude of mismatch negativity (MMN) elicited by tones, an ERP index of auditory sensory memory with the major generator in HG, in patients with schizophrenia. Moreover, in independent samples of schizophrenia, we showed that patients were associated with pronounced reduction of MMN amplitude elicited by speech sounds and its MEG counterpart (magnetic mismatch field, MMF). Finally, we found a significant correlation between MMF powers elicited by speech sounds and gray matter volumes of PT in patients with schizophrenia but not in control subjects. These converging results suggest a presence of progressive process in the structure and function of the auditory cortex in schizophrenia. © 2004 Elsevier B.V. All rights reserved.

Keywords: Schizophrenia; Auditory cortex; Superior temporal gyrus; Magnetic resonance imaging (MRI); Event-related potentials (ERPs); Magnetoencephalography (MEG); Mismatch negativity (MMN); Progression

1. Introduction

Schizophrenia is a syndrome in which auditory hallucinations, paranoid symptoms, and thought disorder are core features of clinical manifestations. Structural and functional neuroimaging studies have localized the basis for auditory hallucinations and thought disorder to abnormalities, at least in part, in the superior temporal gyrus (STG) (reviewed in Ref. [1]), largely corresponding to the auditory cortex and Wernicke's area. Moreover, converging evidence suggests that schizophrenia is asso-

* Tel.: +81-3-5800-9263; fax: +81-3-5800-6894.
  E-mail address: kasaik-tky@umin.ac.jp (K. Kasai).

0531-5131/ © 2004 Elsevier B.V. All rights reserved.
doi:10.1016/j.ics.2004.04.052

ciated with post-onset progressive deterioration in the structure and function of the brain (reviewed in Ref. [2]). In this paper, we will first describe structural abnormalities of the auditory cortex in schizophrenia and evidence for their progression. Next, we will focus on an abnormal link between structure and function of the auditory cortex, further suggesting the presence of a post-onset progressive process in this key region in schizophrenia.

2. Structural abnormalities of the auditory cortex and their progression

Smaller temporal lobe cortical gray matter volumes, including the left STG, have been reported in magnetic resonance imaging (MRI) studies of patients with chronic schizophrenia and, more recently, in patients with first-episode schizophrenia (reviewed in Ref. [3]). However, it remains unknown whether there are progressive decreases in temporal lobe cortical gray matter volumes in patients with first-episode schizophrenia and whether similarly progressive volume decreases are present in patients with affective psychosis. High-spatial-resolution MRI scans at initial hospitalization and 1.5 years later were obtained from 13 patients with first-episode schizophrenia, 15 patients with first-episode affective psychosis (mainly manic), and 14 healthy comparison subjects [4]. MRI volumes were calculated for gray matter of STG and for the amygdala-hippocampal complex. Patients with first-episode schizophrenia showed significant decreases in gray matter volume over time in the left STG compared with patients with first-episode affective psychosis or healthy comparison subjects. This progressive decrease was more pronounced in the posterior portion of the left STG (mean = 9.6%) than in the anterior portions (mean = 8.4%). No group differences in the rate of change over time were present in other regions. These findings demonstrate a progressive volume reduction of the left posterior STG gray matter in patients with first-episode schizophrenia but not in patients with first-episode affective psychosis.

Heschl's gyrus (HG) and the posteriorly adjacent planum temporale (PT) are located on the middle-posterior portion of the STG. HG is primary auditory cortex (Brodmann's area [BA]41/42), playing a crucial role in auditory perception [5]. The anterior portion of PT is part of unimodal auditory association cortex (part of BA22) surrounding HG, while the posterior portion adjacent to the temporoparietal junction (other portions of BA22 and part of BA39-40) is partially coextensive with Wernicke's area, consisting of heteromodal association cortex [6,7]. PT evinces the most prominent left–right asymmetry in the human brain [8], which is thought to reflect PT's critical role in language processing [9].

A previous investigation using volumetric MRI indicated smaller gray matter volumes bilaterally in HG and in left PT in first-episode patients with schizophrenia but not in first-episode patients with affective psychosis [10]. We sought to determine whether or not there are progressive decreases in gray matter volumes of HG and PT in first-episode schizophrenia, and whether or not such decreases are also present in first-episode affective psychosis. Twenty-eight patients at their first-hospitalization (13 with schizophrenia and 15 with affective psychosis, 13 of whom had a manic psychosis), and 22 healthy control subjects were tested at baseline and approximately 1.5 years later [11]. The degree of change over time in MRI volumes was compared between groups for gray matter of left and right HG and PT. First-episode patients with schizophrenia showed significant decreases in gray matter volume over time in left HG (6.9%) and left PT (7.2%) compared with first-episode affective psychosis or control samples. These findings demonstrated a left-biased progressive volume reduction in HG and PT gray matter in first-episode schizophrenia in contrast to first-episode affective psychosis and control subjects. Schizophrenia but not affective psychosis appears to be characterized by a post-onset progression of neocortical gray matter volume loss in subdivisions of left STG, and thus may not be developmentally fixed.

3. Abnormal structure–function relationship in HG

Salisbury et al. [12] suggested that the functional event-related brain potential mismatch negativity (MMN) elicited by tones, with a major generator in HG, showed normal mean group amplitude in first-episode schizophrenia, but was reduced in chronic patients. If schizophrenia involves peri-onset progressive process in HG, then the MMN amplitudes at first hospitalization and the degree of amplitude reduction over time could be tightly coupled to the structural index, i.e., HG volume.

Salisbury et al. [13] examined at first hospitalization for schizophrenia whether MMN amplitude indexed cortical gray matter volume in left hemisphere HG. Twenty first-episode schizophrenia patients, 21 first-episode psychotic mania patients, and 32 normal controls from the general community underwent MMN testing (1600 tones, 1 kHz standard tones 95%, 1.2 kHz deviant tones, 5%, visual distractor task), and high-resolution structural MRI. First-episode schizophrenia patients showed a correlation between left hemisphere HG volume and MMN amplitude $[R = -0.51]$, and between left hemisphere HG volume and the age first hospitalized $[R = -0.47]$. These correlations were not present in either controls or first hospitalized psychotic mania patients. These abnormal relationships are consistent with the presence of a pre-hospitalization progressive process that has differentially affected primary auditory cortex in schizophrenia.

They further investigated whether progressive reduction in HG volume was correlated with progressive amplitude reduction of MMN [13]. In fact, MMN amplitude became reduced in schizophrenia patients within approximately 1.5 years of first hospitalization ($p < 0.05$). Furthermore, the MMN reductions in 10 patients that also received structural MRI were significantly correlated with reduction in left HG gray matter volume ($N = 10$, $R = 0.73$, $p < 0.02$).

4. Abnormal structure–function relationship in PT

Cognitive dysfunction in schizophrenia is characterized by that in language processing. We predicted that reduction of MMN amplitude in response to across-phoneme change (i.e., vowel /a/ vs. /o/) was more pronounced than that in response to change in physical features (i.e., duration) of phoneme or tone in patients with schizophrenia. MMN topography using a high-density recording system was evaluated in 23 right-handed schizophrenic patients and in 28 comparison subjects [14]. Three types of MMN (duration change of pure-tone stimuli; duration change of Japanese vowel /a/; change between vowel /a/ versus /o/]) were recorded. As predicted, the schizophrenic patients had more reduced amplitude of the MMN under the across-phoneme change condition than under the conditions of duration change of vowel or tone. During the across-phoneme change condition, the schizophrenia group showed a significant bilateral reduction in MMN amplitude, in accordance with scalp current density mappings, which revealed that the schizophrenic patients showed significantly weaker left temporal sink/source combination and right frontal/temporal sink than the comparison subjects. These results demonstrate impaired frontotemporal cortical networks for preattentive change detection of speech sounds in schizophrenia. The language-related dysfunction in schizophrenia may be present at the early stage of auditory processing of relatively simple stimuli such as phonemes, and not just at stages involving higher-order semantic processes.

Next, we conducted a replication study of these findings in an independent sample of schizophrenia using a whole-head magnetoencephalographic (MEG) recording. The magnetic counterpart of MMN (magnetic mismatch field; MMF) elicited by a phonetic change was evaluated in 16 right-handed patients with chronic schizophrenia and in 19 age-, sex-, and parental socioeconomic status-matched normal control subjects [15]. As in the ERP study, three types of MMF (MMF in response to a duration decrement of pure-tone stimuli; a vowel within-category change [duration decrement of Japanese vowel /a/]; vowel across-category change [Japanese vowel /a/ versus /o/]) were recorded. While the schizophrenia group showed an overall reduction in magnetic field power of MMF, a trend was found toward more distinct abnormalities under the condition of vowel across-category change than under that of duration decrement of a vowel or tone. The patient group did not show abnormal asymmetries of MMF power under any of the conditions. These results represent a complete replication of our ERP study and provide further evidence for impaired categorical perception of speech sounds in the bilateral auditory cortex in schizophrenia.

In contrast to evidence of HG as a major generator for tonal MMN, previous studies have indicated that MMN in response to speech sounds is localized to PT [16,17], compatible with PT's role in language processing. Therefore, we investigated whether phonetic MMN can serve as a physiological metric of PT volume reduction in schizophrenia. Thirteen patients with chronic schizophrenia and 19 matched control subjects were examined using MEG and high-resolution MRI, in order to evaluate both MMF, in response to change between vowel /a/ and /o/, and gray matter volumes of HG and PT [18]. The magnetic global field power of mismatch response to change in phonemes showed a bilateral reduction in patients with schizophrenia. The gray matter volume of left PT, but not right PT or bilateral HG, was significantly smaller in patients with schizophrenia compared with that in control subjects. Furthermore, the phonetic mismatch strength in the left hemisphere was significantly correlated with left PT gray matter volume in patients with schizophrenia only. These results suggest that phonetic MMN may index underlying structural abnormalities of PT in schizophrenia.

Although this cross-sectional study using a chronic sample does not answer the timing of the presence of the abnormal structure–function relationships, this may be already present pre- or peri-onset. Another possible explanation may be that progression of phonetic mismatch and PT volume reduction may occur concurrently, resulting in a strong association specific to patients with schizophrenia. Supporting this interpretation, Kasai et al. [11] reported progressive decrease of gray matter volume of left PT in patients with first-episode schizophrenia. These findings may support a concurrent deterioration of structure and function of PT in patients with schizophrenia. However, only longitudinal testing will definitively demonstrate a coupling of progressive structural and functional deterioration of PT in schizophrenia.

5. Possible neurobiological mechanisms

Previous findings from basic neuroscience suggest that MMN represents a selective current flow through open, unblocked *N*-methyl-D-aspartate (NMDA) channels on NMDA-type glutamate receptors [19]. Javitt et al. [19] used a combination of intracortical recording and pharmacological micromanipulations in awake monkeys to demonstrate that both competitive and noncompetitive NMDA antagonists block the generation of MMN without affecting prior obligatory activity in the primary auditory cortex. Furthermore, they suggested that the MMN generation depends on the functional interaction between excitatory and inhibitory processes within cortex mediated by NMDA and GABA$_A$ receptors, respectively. In addition, the underlying mechanism involved in the progressive superior temporal volume reduction seen in schizophrenia [4,11] may involve the failure of NMDA-dependent recurrent inhibition that inactivates GABA neurons, thereby disinhibiting cholinergic and glutamatergic pathways through which excitotoxic activity is expressed, with consequent damage to dendritic spines and cell bodies of cerebrocortical neurons [20,21]. These lines of evidence may suggest an ongoing NMDA-mediated pathological process surrounding the superior temporal neocortex in patients with schizophrenia.

6. Conclusions

We demonstrated a presence of structural (regional MRI volume) and functional (MMN) abnormalities in the auditory cortex in schizophrenia and their progression over the early course of the illness. Abnormal relationships specific to schizophrenia, between HG morphology and tonal MMN, and between PT and phonetic MMN, indicate that structural and functional deterioration of the auditory cortex are occurring in ensemble. These results suggest a presence of post-onset, ongoing neurotoxic effect on glutamatergic neurotransmission in the auditory cortex in schizophrenia.

References

[1] K. Kasai, et al., Neuroanatomy and neurophysiology in schizophrenia, Neurosci. Res. 43 (2002) 93–110.
[2] J.E. Anderson, et al., Progressive changes in schizophrenia: do they exist and what do they mean? Restor. Neurol. Neurosci. 12 (1998) 175–184.
[3] M.E. Shenton, et al., A review of MRI findings in schizophrenia, Schizophr. Res. 49 (2001) 149–200.
[4] K. Kasai, et al., Progressive decrease of left superior temporal gyrus gray matter volume in first-episode schizophrenia, Am. J. Psychiatry 160 (2003) 156–164.
[5] R.J. Zattore, J.R. Binder, Functional and structural imaging of the human auditory system, in: A.W. Toga, J.C. Mazziotta (Eds.), Brain Mapping. The Systems, Academic Press, San Diego, CA, 2000, pp. 365–402.
[6] G.D. Pearlson, Superior temporal gyrus and planum temporale in schizophrenia: a selective review, Prog. Neuro-Psychopharmacol. Biol. Psychiatry 21 (1997) 1203–1229.
[7] M.M. Mesulam, Behavioral Neuroanatomy, in: M.M. Mesulam (Ed.), Principles of Behavioral and Cognitive Neurology, Oxford Univ. Press, New York, NY, 2000, pp. 1–120.
[8] N. Geschwind, W. Levitsky, Human brain: left–right asymmetries in temporal speech region, Science 161 (1968) 186–187.

[9] A.M. Galaburda, F. Sanides, N. Geschwind, Human brain: cytoarchitectonic left–right asymmetries in the temporal speech region, Arch. Neurol. 35 (1978) 812–817.

[10] Y. Hirayasu, et al., Lower left temporal lobe MR volumes in patients with first-episode schizophrenia compared with psychotic patients with first-episode affective disorder and normal subjects, Am. J. Psychiatry 155 (1998) 1384–1391.

[11] K. Kasai, et al., Progressive decrease of left Heschl's gyrus and planum temporale gray matter volume in schizophrenia. A longitudinal MRI study of first-episode patients, Arch. Gen. Psychiatry 60 (2003) 766–775.

[12] D.F. Salisbury, et al., Mismatch negativity in chronic schizophrenia and first-episode schizophrenia, Arch. Gen. Psychiatry 59 (2002) 686–694.

[13] D.F. Salisbury, et al., Mismatch negativity as an index of peri-onset cortical reduction in schizophrenia, Biol. Psychiatry 55 (2004) 221S.

[14] K. Kasai, et al., Impaired cortical network for preattentive detection of change in speech sounds in schizophrenia: a high-resolution event-related potential study, Am. J. Psychiatry 159 (2002) 546–553.

[15] K. Kasai, et al., Neuromagnetic correlates of impaired automatic categorical perception of speech sounds in schizophrenia, Schizophr. Res. 59 (2003) 159–172.

[16] T. Rinne, et al., Analysis of speech sounds is left-hemisphere predominance at 100–150 ms after sound onset, NeuroReport 10 (1999) 1113–1117.

[17] M. Tervaniemi, et al., Lateralized automatic auditory processing of phonetic versus musical information: a PET study, Hum. Brain Mapp. 10 (2000) 74–79.

[18] H. Yamasue, H. Yamada, S. Kamio, et al., Abnormal association between phonetic mismatch and planum temporale volume in schizophrenia. Neuroimage (in press).

[19] D.C. Javitt, et al., Role of cortical N-methyl-D-aspartate receptors in auditory sensory memory and mismatch negativity generation: implications for schizophrenia, Proc. Natl. Acad. Sci. U. S. A. 93 (1996) 11962–11967.

[20] R.W. McCarley, et al., Neuroimaging and the cognitive neuroscience of schizophrenia, Schizophr. Bull. 22 (1996) 703–725.

[21] C. Konradi, S. Heckers, Molecular aspects of glutamate dysregulation: implications for schizophrenia and its treatment, Pharmacol. Ther. 97 (2003) 153–179.

International Congress Series 1270 (2004) 56–60

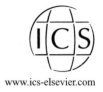

www.ics-elsevier.com

Dipole source localization of epileptic discharges in EEG and MEG

Hiroshi Otsubo*, Ayako Ochi, Ryota Sakamoto, Koji Iida

Division of Neurology, The Hospital for Sick Children, 555 University Avenue, Toronto, ON, Canada M5G 1X8

Abstract. The paper compares EEG with MEG dipoles to assess the importance of both the MEG and EEG for patients with intractable epilepsy. The combination of EEG and MEG dipole analysis provides more accurate and comprehensive information about epileptic activities than either method used alone and produces a full picture of not only epileptic discharges but epileptic neural behaviors in the brain. © 2004 Elsevier B.V. All rights reserved.

Keywords: EEG; MEG; Epileptic discharge; Dipole source localization; Simultaneous recording

1. Introduction

The usefulness of MEG dipole analysis [1] and EEG dipole analysis [2] in epilepsy surgery have recently been proven separately by comparing the data derived with those provided by intraoperative electrocorticography (ECoG) and intracranial video-EEG monitoring (IVEEG). We previously reported a systematic approach to EEG dipole analysis of interictal spikes that improves its reliability and accuracy, using 19-channel scalp prolonged video-EEG monitoring data [2].

The present study compares EEG with MEG dipoles derived from simultaneous short-term recording to assess the importance of these two analyses for patients with extratemporal lobe epilepsy. We clarified the relationship between both interictal MEG and EEG spike features as well as their dipole positions and moments. We hypothesized that the combination of MEG and EEG dipole localization of interictal spikes could delineate neurophysiological features of epileptic neuronal populations in extratemporal lobe epilepsy in children.

2. Patients and methods

We studied two patients with intractable extratemporal lobe epilepsies. Patient 1 was an 8-year-old right-handed girl with seizure since 6 months of age. Seizures

* Corresponding author. Tel.: +1-416-813-7855; fax: +1-416-813-6334.
E-mail address: hiotsubo@rogers.com (H. Otsubo).

consisted of left hand and facial twitching and staring. She had been treated with phenobarbital and is currently on carbamazepine. MRI was reported normal. Prolonged video EEG showed right central temporal spike discharges. Patient 2 was an 8-year-old right-handed girl with seizures since 5 years of age. Seizures consisted of right hand, arm and facial twitching, eye blinking, head bobbing and generalized tonic clonic seizures. She has been treated with multiple antiepileptic drugs. MRI was reported normal. Prolonged video EEG monitoring showed left central-temporal spike discharges.

2.1. MEG dipole analysis

We used a whole-head gradiometer-based Omega system (151 channels, CTF, Port Coquitalam, BC, Canada) at the Hospital for Sick Children in Toronto. We deprived patients of sleep the prior night and tested them in the supine position. At least fifteen 2-min periods of spontaneous data were recorded from each patient. The sampling rate for data acquisition was 625 Hz, with a band-pass filter of 3–70 Hz and a notch filter of 60 Hz. Head localization was performed at the beginning and end of each set. Three fiducial markers (preauricular points and nasion) and EEG electrodes were applied.

MEG epileptic events, spikes and waves, were visually identified by examining the MEG recordings and were cross-referenced with the simultaneous EEG recording. We applied a single moving dipole analysis with a single-shell, whole-head, individually created spherical model for a period of 50 ms before and after the peak of each spike. We defined the MEG dipoles for each spike as a single dipole fit from the earliest phase of each spike with the criteria of a residual error of less than 20%.

2.2. EEG dipole analysis

We collected EEG data simultaneously with the MEG recording using 19 electrodes (International 10-20 system). The scalp electrode positions and the three fiduciary points (nasion, right and left preauricular points) were registered using 3SPACE ISOTRAK II (Polhemus, Colchester, VT) combined with equivalent current dipole localization software for Windows, SynaPointPro (GE Marquette Medical System Japan, Tokyo). Measured electrode locations were then overlaid onto the realistic head model [3].

We analyzed the dipole localization of EEG spikes using a single moving dipole inverse-solution algorithm, a three-shell realistic head model and electrode-positioning data from 50 ms before to 50 ms after the maximum MEG peak in each spike. The dipole fits occurred every 1.6 ms. We defined the EEG dipoles for each spike as a single dipole fit from a peak of each spike with the criteria of a residual error of less than 5%.

2.3. MRI study

The dipole localizations were superimposed onto the MR images of each patient's brain. MRI (GE Signa 1.5 Tesla, General Electric Medical System, Milwaukee, WI) yielded continuous 124 T1-weighted coronal slices with a thickness of 2 mm, a pixel size

Table 1
Positions and moment strength of MEG and EEG dipoles in patients 1 and 2

	Dipoles	Position, mean ± S.D. and range (mm)			Moment strength, mean ± S.D. and range (nA m)
		x	*y*	*z*	
Patient 1	MEG	37.0 ± 5.4	− 13.5 ± 6.4	77.8 ± 5.9	164.6 ± 49.5
	(*n* = 10)	(29.6–47.0)	(− 24.6 to − 4.4)	(64.2–86.9)	(83.7–267.0)
	EEG	48.4 ± 12.4	− 19.9 ± 13.9	86.0 ± 15.7	302.9 ± 103.9
	(*n* = 6)	(26.6–67.5)	(− 42.1 to − 1.8)	(64.9–107.4)	(177.8–522.0)
Patient 2	MEG	− 49.2 ± 6.9	− 4.8 ± 4.4	66.6 ± 4.9	225.4 ± 68.3
	(*n* = 14)	(− 56.3 to − 34.1)	(− 14.6 to − 0.1)	(56.8–73.3)	(131.6–348.1)
	EEG	− 49.2 ± 0.9	7.8 ± 4.3	76.5 ± 2.7	630.0 ± 162.6
	(*n* = 14)	(− 50.4 to − 48.4)	(0.4–11.9)	(72.8–81.1)	(409.1–788.4)

X-axis, auricular line, with positive value right of center and negative value left of center; *Y*-axis, nasion-inion line; *Z*-axis, from the center toward the vertex of the head at a right angle.

of 0.781 mm and a 256 × 256 image matrix. The analyze marker (CTF) and SynaPointPro program were used for superimposition of the dipoles on the MR images (coronal, axial and sagittal views).

2.4. Comparison of EEG and MEG dipoles

After analyzing EEG and MEG dipoles, we compared them on each patient's MR image by visual inspection. We compared the actual values of time (milliseconds), positions (*x*-, *y*- and *z*-axis in millimeters), orientation angle (degrees) and moment strength (nA m) between EEG and MEG dipoles.

3. Results

We collected and analyzed both MEG dipoles and EEG dipoles in 22 spikes in patient 1 and 16 in patient 2. Table 1 describes positions and moment strength of MEG and EEG dipoles with certain criteria of error. MEG dipoles preceded to EEG dipoles with a mean of 8 ms in patient 1 (Fig. 1) and 23 ms in patient 2 (Fig. 2). In patient 1, we collected independently either MEG or EEG dipoles without simultaneous spike peaks. Patient 2 had double spike peaks of MEG and EEG, so we collected dipoles of first MEG spikes and second EEG spikes because of appropriate errors and moment strength. Dipole local-

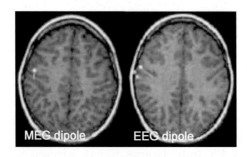

Fig. 1. MEG dipole and EEG dipole from a single interictal spike from patient 1.

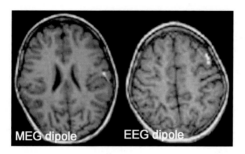

Fig. 2. MEG dipole and EEG dipole from a polyspikes and wave from patient 2.

izations of epileptic discharges between MEG and EEG dipoles differed with a mean of 29 mm in patient 1 and 19 mm in patient 2.

4. Discussion

The coexistence of different orientations and positions of EEG and MEG dipoles can identify the extent of the epileptic zone.

In patient 1, there was a short latency between maximum peaks of single MEG and EEG spikes. In addition, promptly following EEG, dipoles were localized with radial orientation in the same or neighboring gyrus. The results indicate that EEG and MEG depict activities of the neuronal discharges at close proximity without extensive propagation. MEG is sensitive to tangential dipoles, while EEG dipoles can supply the radial component of the epileptogenic zone. Merlet et al. [4], using simultaneously recorded MEG and EEG source localizations, demonstrated this phenomenon and showed further that an area including fissural and gyral cortices synchronizes immediately when MEG and EEG peaks are simultaneously seen. Baumgartner et al. [5] reported that tangential and radial dipoles represented propagation of epileptiform activity between two adjacent cortical areas.

In patient 2, longer latency between first MEG and second EEG spikes suggest propagation of the neuronal activity. Furthermore, the strength of EEG dipole moment of second spikes was larger than that of MEG dipole of the first spikes. A single source model from an MEG spike cannot determine the spatial extent of the epileptic zone because the model represents the center of activation by a point source rather than the area of activated cortex [6]. The enlarged moment strength of subsequent EEG dipoles indicates extended epileptic cortex within the single interictal discharge.

We combined the methods of EEG and MEG dipole analysis from simultaneous recordings to improve spatial and temporal resolution of interictal discharges to understand epileptic neuronal behaviors. On the basis of our study, albeit limited, it seems clear that combining EEG and MEG dipole analysis promises to be a reliable noninvasive method of detecting the epileptic zone in this group of patients.

References

[1] H. Otsubo, et al., MEG predicts epileptic zone in lesional extrahippocampal epilepsy: 12 pediatric epilepsy surgery cases, Epilepsia 42 (2001) 1523–1530.

[2] A. Ochi, et al., Systematic approach to dipole localization of interictal EEG spikes in children with extra-temporal lobe epilepsies, Clin. Neurophysiol. 111 (2000) 161–168.
[3] T. Yamazaki, et al., Multiple equivalent current dipole source localization of visual event-related potentials during oddball paradigm with motor response, Brain Topogr. 12 (3) (2000) 159–175.
[4] I. Merlet, et al., Apparent asynchrony between interictal electric and magnetic spikes, NeuroReport 8 (1997) 1071–1076.
[5] C. Baumgartner, et al., The functional organization of the interictal spike complex in benign rolandic epilepsy, Epilepsia 37 (12) (1996) 1164–1174.
[6] E. Pataraia, et al., Magnetoencephalography in presurgical epilepsy evaluation, Neurosurg. Rev. 25 (2002) 141–159.

International Congress Series 1270 (2004) 61–66

ELSEVIER

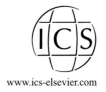

www.ics-elsevier.com

Brain mapping of evoked potential correlates of semantic meaning—cross-cultural studies

Wolfgang Skrandies *

Institute of Physiology, Justus Liebig University, D-35392 Giessen, Germany

Abstract. According to the "semantic differential technique" the affective meaning of words can be quantified in statistically defined, independent dimensions where every word is located on the three dimensions *evaluation* ("good–bad"), *potency* ("strong–weak"), and *activity* ("active–passive"). We studied how affective meaning of words is reflected in brain electric activity in German and Chinese subjects (a total of 52 German and 55 Chinese adults were investigated). Two experiments were performed on both subjects groups: (1) a list of words was rated on 12 adjective scales. All words had a comparable number of letters and frequency of occurrence in the Chinese or German language. Factor analysis followed by varimax rotation yielded three semantic dimensions. The correlation between languages ranged from 0.83 to 0.92. For each dimension, words were selected which scored highly positive or highly negative on one of the three dimensions, and had small scores on the others. This resulted in six semantically "clear" word classes. (2) Electrophysiological experiments were performed with 22 German and 23 Chinese healthy, right-handed adults. Stimuli were presented sequentially on a computer monitor in random order, and EEG was recorded from 29 channels. Evoked potentials were computed off-line for each semantic class. Significant differences in scalp topography between semantic word classes were not restricted to late "cognitive" components, but brain activity at latencies as early as 80 ms after stimulus onset was affected by semantic meaning of the stimuli in both groups. Comparison of the potential fields and spatial principal components analysis revealed very similar topographical components in German and Chinese subjects. These results show that early language-related neural activation occurs in subjects of different language and culture. © 2004 Elsevier B.V. All rights reserved.

Keywords: Language; Brain electrical topography; Event-related potential; Semantic differential

1. Introduction

The study of language processing has a long tradition in neuroscience research, and in addition to clinical studies performed during neurosurgery [1], there are many experiments on event-related brain activity and processing of language. The recording of electrical brain activity with high time resolution elicited by linguistic material yields sensitive neuronal indicators of semantic [2] or syntactic language processing [3]. Many recent studies on

* Tel.: +49-64147470; fax: +49-64147479.
E-mail address: Wolfgang.Skrandies@physiologie.med.uni-giessen.de (W. Skrandies).

0531-5131/ © 2004 Elsevier B.V. All rights reserved.
doi:10.1016/j.ics.2004.04.021

language-related electrical brain activity were concerned with the so-called N400 component that is elicited at a latency of approximately 400 ms after the presentation of a word stimulus which unexpectedly closes a sentence [4]. In a similar line, there are differences in electrical brain activity elicited by verb and noun interpretations of homophone words: Brown and Lehmann [5] statistically determined principal components that discriminated verb and noun stimuli. Early studies on semantic meaning of single word effects on event-related brain activity have been described [6] where electrophysiological data were obtained from very few recording channels. In the present paper, we will illustrate the influence of semantic meaning on topographic features of evoked electrical brain fields.

In evoked potential studies, the definition and control of stimuli are most crucial. For the present experiments, we used language stimuli which were statistically defined in terms of independent meaning dimensions. It is known that verbal material can be classified according to its connotative (affective) meaning, and the use of the semantic differential technique has proven to be of universal value [7]. In addition to the rating of single words, it has been demonstrated that the classification of emotions can be reduced to three independent dimensions [8]. The connotative meaning of words rated by subjects on adjective scales can be reduced in dimensionality by factor analysis, and commonly three factors explain more than 50% of the variance. The dimensions of *evaluation* (E), *potency* (P), and *activity* (A) have been repeatedly identified. We employed the semantic differential technique in order to define the stimulus material and test its reliability over different groups of subjects (a total of 52 German and 55 Chinese adults was studied). We will illustrate that brain electric fields recorded during word processing are affected by meaning already at latencies of about 100 ms.

2. Methods

We studied various groups of young and healthy adults. All subjects were right-handed. In order to produce reliable and valid stimulus material for evoked potential recordings, subjects were first investigated with the semantic differential technique. About 200 nouns

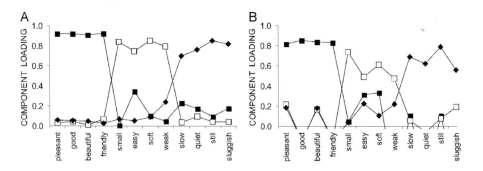

Fig. 1. Results of principal components analyses (PCA) computed on questionnaire data: Varimax-rotated component loadings. Note that component 1 (filled squares) is identified as *evaluation*, component 2 (open squares) corresponds to *potency*, and component 3 (diamonds) is related to *activity*. In all data sets, three components explain more than 60% of the variance. A is the result of 30 German subjects, B is the result of 32 Chinese adults. There is a high correlation between the German and Chinese data ($0.83 < r < 0.92$).

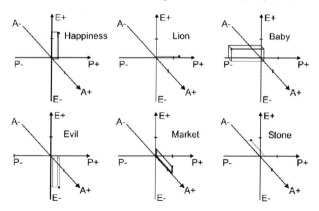

Fig. 2. Examples of semantically "clean" words. Mean component scores on the components *evaluation, potency,* and *activity* of 30 German subjects. Note that each word shows extreme values only on one dimension and has low values on the other two dimensions.

were rated on 12 adjective scales of opposite descriptors (see Fig. 1). Each scale extended over seven points. Principal component analysis on the questionnaires extracted three varimax-rotated orthogonal components which corresponded to the E, P, and A dimensions of Osgood et al. [7]. Next, component scores of each word were computed for all subjects, and words that scored highly positive (or negative) on one component but had only low scores on the other two dimensions were selected (i.e., stimuli were clearly associated with only one of the semantic dimensions). This allowed words to be defined as semantically "pure" which then were used in the electrophysiological experiments (see Fig. 2).

For the ERP recordings these words were presented in random order on a computer monitor, and averaged according to word class. The EEG was measured from 29 channels simultaneously from electrodes distributed between the inion and Fz (see Fig. 3). Stimuli were presented sequentially on a computer monitor for 1 s each. All words had comparable physical characteristics (length, luminance, contrast, occurrence frequency). The subjects' task was to visualize the words, and recall was tested at the end of the experiment in order to assure that subjects had actively processed the stimuli.

3. Results

3.1. Questionnaire data and the semantic differential

In all subjects groups we found very comparable factors which were identified according to Osgood et al. [7] as reflecting *evaluation* (E), *potency* (P), and *activity* (A). The results from a group of 30 German and 32 Chinese subjects is illustrated in Fig. 1. Here we show the loadings (the correlation between the components and each adjective scale) of three different components. The first component is clearly associated with "pleasant–unpleasant", "good–bad", "beautiful–ugly", and "friendly–unfriendly" (i.e., *evaluation*) while the other components display high loadings on the other adjective scales. These components can be clearly identified as *potency* and *activity.* Although the data illustrated in Fig. 1 stem from different subjects and languages, and different single

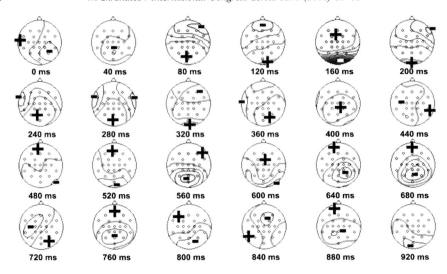

Fig. 3. Potential fields elicited by German words between 0 and 920 ms after stimulus presentation. Stimuli had extreme scores on the dimension A − (i.e., words were associated with passivity). Maps are shown every 40 ms. Recordings from 29 electrodes as indicated by head scheme. Lines are in steps of 0.5 μV, relative polarity with respect to the average reference as indicated. Mean data of a typical subject.

words were employed, the factor structure is remarkably similar. We observed correlation coefficients ranging between $r = 0.83$ and $r = 0.92$ indicating that the semantic dimensions in groups of German and Chinese subjects are nearly identical.

The three semantic dimensions accounted for more than 60% of the variance in each of the four subjects groups. In addition, we could also confirm that the dimension evaluation (E) explains most of the variance (>30% in each group).

Fig. 2 illustrates examples of semantically "clean" words, i.e., words that had high component scores on one dimension, and very small scores on the other two dimensions. For example, the word "Lion" scores very low on *evaluation* (0.068) and *activity* (0.057) while there is a high value on the dimension *potency* (1.364). Thus, this word is best characterized as very powerful. In a similar line, "Happiness" appears to be associated mainly with a high score on *evaluation* (1.32) indicating its overall positive affective meaning. Fig. 2 also displays examples of the other semantic categories, and it is obvious that six different classes can be identified on the basis of the semantic differential.

3.2. Evoked potential fields and the semantic differential

A sequence of potential fields evoked by semantic stimuli between 0 and 920 ms after the presentation of words is illustrated in Fig. 3. Maps are shown every 40 ms. Stimuli scored high on the dimension A − (i.e., words were associated with "passivity"). Primary visual processing is reflected by the occurrence of an occipitally positive component at 80 ms latency in Fig. 3.

It is evident that several different topographical distribution patterns occur sequentially, and there are components around 80, 160, or between 240 and 280 ms. In addition, late

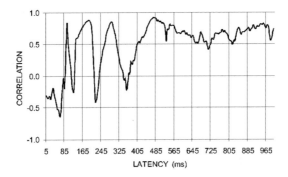

Fig. 4. Correlation between potential fields elicited by German or Chinese words between 5 and 1000 ms after stimulus presentation. Note that there are long intervals where topography is globally very similar ($r>0.36$ corresponds to $p<0.05$). Computation was performed on the grand mean data.

components can be identified 400 or 560 ms latency. Note how field strength (reflected by the number of field lines and the steepness of potential gradients) is changing over time, and epochs of stable field configuration can be seen at component latency. Steps in processing are reflected by the occurrence of so-called components that are associated with high field strength (defined by global field power, [9]) and stable topography. The occurrence of a given component was identified at the peak latency of maximal field strength. Quantitative analysis of global field power of all subjects for all conditions yielded 10 components occurring between 80 and 975 ms for the semantic stimuli. We analyzed how latencies, field strength and scalp field topography (positive or negative centroid locations in the anterior–posterior or in the left–right direction) of the components were influenced by the semantic dimensions (see Ref. [10]).

In both German and Chinese data we observed similar effects. Affective meaning had some influence on component latency, amplitude (field strength), and topography starting very early [10,11], and Fig. 4 illustrates the similarity of evoked potential fields in German and Chinese subjects. Here we show the correlation between maps at corresponding time points (200 maps between 5 and 1000 ms after the stimulus were correlated). From Fig. 4, it is obvious that there is a high overall similarity of data recorded in the groups of subjects (note that a correlation of $r>0.36$ is significant with $p<0.05$).

4. Discussion

In experiments performed with subjects of different languages there were significant effects of semantic meaning on brain electric activity occurring as early as at 80 ms latency, and we could also verify that this component is topographically different from the classical P100 [10,11]. The surprisingly early influence of semantic meaning on evoked potential fields may be explained in the general context of visual processing which is very fast [12].

Such results point to rapid processing in higher-level neural networks which may receive incoming information in parallel and, in turn, condition part of the visual cortex. Thus, semantic meaning classified in higher-level structures might represent top-down processing mechanisms. Components at mean latencies of 95 and 170 ms were topographically similar in German and Chinese subjects (with a significant correlation of 0.80 at 95 ms and 0.81 at 170 ms; $p < 0.001$). The overall similarity of the evoked potential fields could further be demonstrated by the results of a spatial PCA [13] where we found a very similar topographical pattern of brain activity elicited by semantically "clean" word stimuli. Of course, the effects were not identical, but the congruence is quite remarkable indicating that the processing of affective meaning of verbal material is universal: Chinese and German languages are vastly different, not only according to linguistic categories but there are also large cultural differences. Thus, the dimensions of the semantic differential may be regarded as robust and culture-free. The same holds true at a physiological level reflected by the analysis of language-evoked electric brain topography.

Acknowledgements

The experiments on the Chinese subjects were performed in collaboration with Dr. M.J. Chiu and Ms Y. Lin from the Department of Neurology, NTUH, Taipei. Supported by DAAD D/9922885 and NSC.

References

[1] G.A. Ojemann, The neurobiology of language and verbal memory: observations from awake neurosurgery, Int. J. Psychophysiol. 48 (2003) 141–146.

[2] F. Pulvermüller, B. Mohr, H. Schleichert, Semantic or lexico-syntactic factors: what determines word-class specific activity in the human brain? Neurosci. Lett. 275 (1999) 81–84.

[3] A.D. Friederici, S.A. Kotz, The brain basis of syntactic processes: functional imaging and lesion studies, NeuroImage 20 (2003) S8–S17.

[4] M. Kutas, K.D. Federmeier, Electrophysiology reveals semantic memory use in language comprehension, Trends Cogn. Sci. 4 (2000) 463–470.

[5] W.S. Brown, D. Lehmann, Verb and noun meaning of homophone words activate different cortical generators: a topographic study of evoked potential fields, Exp. Brain Res. (Suppl. 2) (1979) 159–168.

[6] R.M. Chapman, et al., Behavioral and neural analyses of connotative meaning: word classes and rating scales, Brain Lang. 11 (1980) 319–339.

[7] C.E. Osgood, W.H. May, M.S. Miron, Cross-Cultural Universals of Affective Meaning, University of Illinois Press, Urbana, IL, 1975.

[8] M.M. Bradley, P.J. Lang, Measuring emotion: the self-assessment manikin and the semantic differential, J. Behav. Ther. Exp. Psychiatry 25 (1994) 49–59.

[9] D. Lehmann, W. Skrandies, Reference-free identification of components of checkerboard-evoked multichannel potential fields, Electroencephalogr. Clin. Neurophysiol. 48 (1980) 609–621.

[10] W. Skrandies, Evoked potential correlates of semantic meaning: a brain mapping study, Cogn. Brain Res. 6 (1998) 173–183.

[11] W. Skrandies, M.J. Chiu, Dimensions of affective semantic meaning of Chinese language—behavioral and evoked potential correlates in Chinese subjects, Neurosci. Lett. 341 (2003) 45–48.

[12] W. Skrandies, Early effects of semantic meaning on electrical brain activity, Behav. Brain Sci. 22 (1999) 301–302.

[13] W. Skrandies, D. Lehmann, Spatial principal components of multichannel maps evoked by lateral visual half-field stimuli, Electroencephalogr. Clin. Neurophysiol. 54 (1982) 662–667.

International Congress Series 1270 (2004) 67–73

ELSEVIER

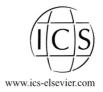

www.ics-elsevier.com

Tonotopic maps and short-term plasticity in the human auditory cortex

Isamu Ozaki*

Department of Physical Therapy, Faculty of Health Sciences, Aomori University of Health and Welfare, 58-1 Hamadate, Mase, Aomori 030-8505, Japan

Abstract. We showed tonotopic maps in the human auditory cortex based on the analysis of auditory evoked magnetic fields (AEFs) and rapid changes in tonotopic maps during auditory attention tasks. The location and strength of the N100m dipole for 400- and 4000-Hz tones were successively calculated before and at around the peak latency. In the right hemisphere, the current dipoles for 400 and 4000 Hz moved toward anterolateral direction before the N100m peak, showing parallel arrangement of the isofrequency bands. In the left hemisphere, the movement direction of 400-Hz dipoles was anterolateral, while that of 4000-Hz dipoles was lateral. This difference in the layout of isofrequency bands between right and left auditory cortices reflects distinct functional roles in auditory information processing such as pitch vs. phonetic analysis. In addition, when subjects tried to discriminate the differences in pitch or laterality, N100m amplitude increased. The N100m dipole distance between 400- and 4000-Hz tones was enlarged during pitch discrimination tasks especially in the right auditory cortex but was unchanged during laterality discrimination tasks. These dynamic changes in the N100m dipole presumably reflect a short-term plasticity in the primary auditory cortex. © 2004 Elsevier B.V. All rights reserved.

Keywords: Auditory evoked magnetic field; AEF; Isofrequency band; Auditory attention; Tonotopic map; Pitch discrimination; Laterality discrimination

1. Introduction

In an earlier study of steady-state auditory evoked magnetic fields (AEFs), Romani et al. [1] proposed that high-frequency tone is represented in the medial portion of Heschl gyrus. However, there remain debates as to tonotopic representation in the human auditory cortex. The N100m dipole for high-frequency tones reportedly is located more medially [2–6] or more posteriorly [4,7,8] than that for low-frequency tone. Other studies on AEFs claim that there is no tonotopic representation [9–11]. We suppose that these divergent results on human tonotopy have two sources [12]; one is that the location of the N100m dipole is determined at the peak latency; and the other is that there is a significant inter-individual or inter-hemispheric variety in 3D morphology of the human AI cortex [13]. We have reported

* Tel./fax: +81-17-765-2070.
E-mail address: isamu@auhw.ac.jp (I. Ozaki).

0531-5131/ © 2004 Elsevier B.V. All rights reserved.
doi:10.1016/j.ics.2004.05.083

that N100m dipole dynamically moves as a result of sequential activation of the neural columns that form the isofrequency bands [14,15] and that the isofrequency bands extend along the long axis of Heschl gyrus. In the present article, we will show two representative cases in which N100m dipole dynamically moves in a mostly lateral direction or a mostly anterior direction, reflecting the difference in 3D morphology of Heschl gyrus. Also, we will show rapid changes in N100m response during auditory attention.

2. Tonotopic maps as dynamic movement of N100m dipole

Here, we will demonstrate two cases from our previous studies [15]. AEFs (band-pass 0.1–330 Hz) were taken with a Neuromag system (4-D Neuroimaging, Helsinki, Finland), which has 204 planar first-order gradiometers at 102 measurement sites on a helmet-shaped surface, covering the whole scalp. Monaural 400- or 4000-Hz tone pips of 80 dB SPL (sound pressure level) and 50-ms duration with 2 ms rise–fall times were delivered by a plastic tube terminating in a molded ear insert. The stimuli were presented, with an interstimulus interval of 1 s, to the subject's right or left ear. The N100m current sources at each sampling point during the period between 25 ms before the peak and 5 ms after the peak were calculated from the AEFs recorded from the hemisphere contralateral to the stimulation site using a single equivalent current dipole (ECD) model in a spherical volume conductor. The details about data analysis including 3D MRI study appeared elsewhere [12,14,15].

Fig. 1 shows the case in which N100m dipole moves in a mostly lateral direction. When the AEFs become augmented from 70 to 90 ms, the distribution of the magnetic fields on the lateral view changes dynamically. That is, the distance between the extremas of flux out and flux in is shortening, suggesting that the dipole is approaching the recording device; i.e., the N100m dipole dynamically moves in medio-lateral direction. In Fig. 2, the dipoles for 400- and 4000-Hz tones, calculated sequentially up to the peak latency with continuity of the goodness-of-fit (GOF) value >90%, are superimposed onto the brain MRI of this subject. They are located on the supra-temporal plane of the right hemisphere; the dipoles for high-frequency tone are mapped

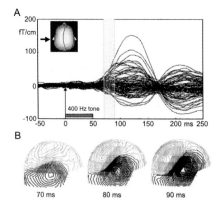

Fig. 1. (A) Superimposed AEF waveforms of the right hemisphere following left ear 400-Hz-tone stimulation in a 25-year-old man. (B) Magnetic fields at 70, 80 and 90 ms. Note that the distance between the extrema of flux out (thick traces) and flux in (thin traces) is shortening, suggesting that the dipole is approaching the recording device.

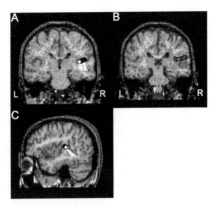

Fig. 2. Mediolateral movement of the N100m dipole for a 4000-Hz tone (A) and for a 400-Hz tone (B), obtained from the same subject in Fig. 1. Note that the dipoles for high-pitched tone are located more anteriorly.

anteriorly and travel with shorter distance. In the owl monkey AI cortex, the isofrequency bands are roughly parallel to the lateral fissure, the anterolateral border of the AI [16]. It is, therefore, supposed that in humans, the isofrequency bands are roughly parallel to the anterior border of the Heschl gyrus. So, we suggest that in this subject, Heschl gyrus mostly extends in the lateral direction and that the N100m dipoles for high-frequency tone at the peak latency is located more anteriorly.

The results of another subject in which N100m dipole moves in a mostly anterior direction are illustrated in Fig. 3. As shown in Fig. 3B, the border between flux out and flux in is displaced in the anterior direction in the rising phase of the N100m response (between 56 and 70 ms poststimulus). The estimated dipoles at 56 and 70 ms with the GOF value >90% are located on the supratemporal plane of the right hemisphere. We, therefore, suppose that in this subject, Heschl gyrus mostly extends in the anterior direction.

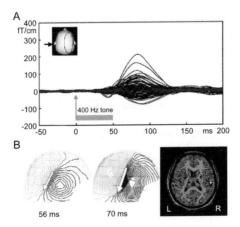

Fig. 3. (A) Superimposed AEF waveforms of the right hemisphere following left ear 400-Hz-tone stimulation in a 33-year-old woman. (B) Magnetic fields at 56 and 70 ms and the N100m dipoles from 56 to 70 ms superimposed on to the subject's MRI. Note that the estimated dipoles (white arrows or circles) move in the anterior direction.

Based on analysis of the N100m dipole movement in the rising phase of N100m response recorded from 31 healthy subjects, we obtained the layout of the isofrequency bands for 400 and 4000 Hz as shown in Fig. 4. They are in good agreement with the probability map of the primary auditory cortex based on the morphological analysis of 27 postmortem brains [13]. Firstly, the bands for the left hemisphere are located more posteriorly than for the right hemisphere. Secondly, in the right hemisphere, the isofrequency bands for 400 and 4000 Hz extend in an anterolateral direction. The parallel arrangement of the isofrequency bands for high-pitched and low-pitched tones in the right AI cortex are in line with the distinct functional role of the right hemisphere where the differences in pitch of the tones and music are analyzed [15].

The transverse temporal gyri of Heschl in the postmortem brain have an area of ca. 10 mm width $\times$ 30 mm length. We suppose that the isofrequency bands extend along the long axis of Heschl gyrus. Since the axis of the frequency is orthogonal to each band for the different frequencies represented, the axis of the frequency for 20–20,000 Hz tones that are audible for humans presumably occupies up to ca. 10 mm. Since each isofrequency band for the frequency representation is displaced with a function of the logarithm of the frequency [16,17], the isofrequency bands representing the frequencies with a difference of a factor of 10 in human will be ca. 3 mm apart from each other, which is in line with the results of the analysis of AEFs in right auditory cortex (Fig. 4, right panel).

Fig. 5 illustrates schematic drawing of tonotopic map when Heschl gyrus extends mostly in anterior direction. In these subjects, the bands for high-pitched tones are located more medially and are shorter than those for low-pitched tones. Therefore, when one determines N100m dipole location at the peak latency, one can obtain the difference in the locations such as Δx and Δy, i.e., a high-pitched tone can be concluded to be located more posteriorly by the difference of Δy. However, this reflects isofrequency band-dependent tonotopy but not classical tonotopy (Δt). If one examines the subjects whose Heschl gyrus mostly extends in lateral direction, tonotopic representation as the locations of the N100m dipoles at the peak latency for different pitches of the tones examined may differ. On the other hand, when

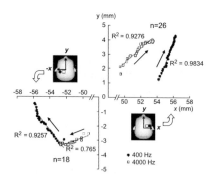

Fig. 4. Isofrequency bands for 400-Hz (closed circle) and 4000-Hz (open square) tones represented as normalized movement of the N100m dipoles on the x–y plane in left and right hemispheres. Arrows indicate the direction of N100m dipole movement from the starting time analyzed to the peak latency In the right hemisphere, the isofrequency bands for two frequencies are in parallel arrangement and the distance between the two bands is ca. 3 mm (modified from Ref. [15]).

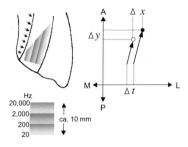

Fig. 5. Schematic drawings of the tonotopic maps when a subject's Heschl gyrus in the right hemisphere extends in a mostly anterior direction (modified from Ref. [12]). In the left panel, the layout of the isofrequency bands for different frequency tones is illustrated in the Heschl gyrus (small arrows, the first transverse temporal sulcus). In the right column, open and closed circles represent the locations of the N100m dipoles at the peak latency for high-pitched and low-pitched tones, respectively. The movements of the N100m dipole along the isofrequency bands are indicated by arrows. On the other hand, the differences in the locations (Δx or Δy) of the N100m dipoles at the peak latency (open and closed circles) for the different tone frequencies indicate "isofrequency band dependent tonopy". "Classical tonotopy" is expressed by Δt that is nearly 3 mm when a difference of the tone frequencies examined is a factor of 10. A, anterior; P, posterior; M, medial; L, lateral.

one determines dynamic movement of N100m dipole, one can obtain Δt, classical tonotopy, as the distance between the bands. To our knowledge, most previous papers on human tonotopy have argued tonotopic representations based on the locations of the N100m dipoles at the peak and neglected a significant inter-subject or inter-hemispheric variety in 3D morphology of Heschl gyrus, resulting in the divergent results on human tonotopy.

3. Rapid changes in tonotopic maps during auditory attention

We examined whether tonotopic maps are changed during auditory attention task. Our hypothesis was that since cortical representation of tone is fundamentally distributed but *not focal* along the primary auditory cortex [17], the activated areas of the AI cortex for the tones with different pitches will be segregated when subjects try to discriminate the difference in pitch of the tones as short-term plastic changes. We also hypothesized that segregation of tonotopic maps for the different pitches will not occur when subjects try to discriminate laterality of the tones but not the differences in pitch. To test the above hypotheses, we examined 23 right-handed, normal subjects [12]; we presented a 400- or a 4000-Hz tone to the subject's right or left ear with a random sequence. Subjects performed pitch discrimination tasks in which the target was high-pitched (right or left 4000-Hz tone, 10% each) or low-pitched (right or left 400-Hz tone, 10% each) and then laterality discrimination tasks in which the target was right (right 400- or 4000 Hz-tone, 10% each) or left (left 400- or 4000-Hz tone, 10% each). The details of the experimental design and results appear elsewhere [12].

We analyzed N100m responses as control or non-target responses; since in each task, subjects attend four categories of stimuli, non-target responses include effects of attention but not influence of finger extension to the target stimuli. As a result, attention produced an increase of dipole strength in pitch and laterality discriminating condition (Fig. 6) as well as shortening of the peak latency. On the other hand, the Euclidian dipole distance between 400- and 4000-Hz tones was enlarged in pitch discriminating condition especially

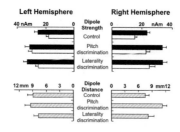

Fig. 6. Upper panel: the mean dipole strengths of the N100m responses for 400-Hz (closed bars) and 4000-Hz (open bars) tones in control and pitch or laterality discriminating conditions. The mean N100m dipole strength is augmented in pitch and laterality discriminating conditions. Lower panel: the N100m dipole distance between 400- and 4000-Hz tones in the three conditions. The mean dipole distance for pitch discriminating condition was larger. Note that enlargement of the dipole strength is marked in the right hemisphere. Results demonstrate mean ± S.E.M. $N = 18$ for the data for the left hemisphere, $N = 23$ for the right hemisphere (modified from Ref. [12]).

in the right hemisphere, but not in laterality discriminating condition (Fig. 6). These results suggest short-term plastic changes in the human auditory cortex during selective attention, which is in line with experimental data of the owl monkey showing that the accuracy of the performance is correlated with an enlargement of tonotopic map during training to discriminate the small difference of pitch of the tones [18]. Therefore, topographically organized neurons in the primary sensory cortex presumably play an important role in analyzing or storing the features of sensory stimuli.

Acknowledgements

We thank Drs. C.Y. Jin, Y. Suzuki, M. Baba, M. Matsunaga and I. Hashimoto for their valuable help. This study was supported by a Special Research Project Grant, Aomori University of Health and Welfare.

References

[1] G.L. Romani, S.J. Williamson, L. Kaufman, Tonotopic organization of the human auditory cortex, Science 216 (1982) 1339–1340.
[2] C. Pantev, et al., Tonotopic organization of the human auditory cortex revealed by transient auditory evoked magnetic fields, Electroenceph. Clin. Neurophysiol. 69 (1988) 160–170.
[3] C. Pantev, et al., Specific tonotopic organizations of different areas of the human auditory cortex revealed by simultaneous magnetic and electric recordings, Electroenceph. Clin. Neurophysiol. 94 (1995) 26–40.
[4] C. Pantev, et al., Study of the human auditory cortices using a whole-head magnetometer: left vs. right hemisphere and ipsilateral vs. contralateral stimulation, Audiol. Neuro-otol. 3 (1998) 183–190.
[5] M. Huotilainen, et al., Sustained fields of tones and glides reflect tonotopy of the auditory cortex, Neuro-Report 6 (1995) 841–844.
[6] D.C. Rojas, et al., Alterations in tonotopy and auditory cerebral asymmetry in schizophrenia, Biol. Psychiatry 52 (2002) 32–39.
[7] S. Arlinger, et al., Cortical magnetic fields evoked by frequency glides of a continuous tone, Electroenceph. Clin. Neurophysiol. 54 (1982) 642–653.
[8] T. Rosburg, et al., Tonotopy of the auditory-evoked field component N100m in patients with schizophrenia, J. Psychophysiol. 14 (2000) 131–141.
[9] T.P. Roberts, D. Poeppel, Latency of auditory evoked M100 as a function of tone frequency, NeuroReport 7 (1996) 1138–1140.

[10] B. Lütkenhöner, Single-dipole analyses of the N100m are not suitable for characterizing the cortical representation of pitch, Audiol. Neuro-otol. 8 (2003) 222–233.

[11] B. Lütkenhöner, K. Krumbholz, A. Seither-Preisler, Studies of tonotopy based on wave N100 of the auditory evoked field are problematic, NeuroImage 19 (2003) 935–949.

[12] I. Ozaki, et al., Rapid change of tonotopic maps in the human auditory cortex during pitch discrimination. Clin. Neurophysiol. 115 (2004) 1592–1604.

[13] J. Rademacher, et al., Probabilistic mapping and volume measurement of human primary auditory cortex, NeuroImage 13 (2001) 669–683.

[14] I. Ozaki, et al., Dynamic anterolateral movement of N100m dipoles in evoked magnetic field reflects activation of isofrequency bands through horizontal fibers in human auditory cortex, Neurosci. Lett. 329 (2002) 222–226.

[15] I. Ozaki, et al., Dynamic movement of N100m dipoles in evoked magnetic field reflects sequential activation of isofrequency bands in human auditory cortex, Clin. Neurophysiol. 114 (2003) 1681–1688.

[16] G.H. Recanzone, et al., Functional organization of spectral receptive fields in the primary auditory cortex of the owl monkey, J. Comp. Neurol. 415 (1999) 460–481.

[17] C.E. Schreiner, Spatial distribution of responses to simple and complex sounds in the primary auditory cortex, Audiol. Neuro-otol. 3 (1998) 104–122.

[18] G.H. Recanzone, C.E. Schreiner, M.M. Merzenich, Plasticity in the frequency representation of primary auditory cortex following discrimination training in adult owl monkey, J. Neurosci. 13 (1993) 87–103.

International Congress Series 1270 (2004) 74–78

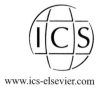

www.ics-elsevier.com

Sound-induced activation of auditory cortices in patients with inner-ear hearing loss

Yasushi Naito*

Department of Otolaryngology, Kobe City General Hospital, 4-6 Minatojima Nakamachi, Chuo, Kobe 650-0046, Japan

Abstract. Studies on sound-induced activation of auditory cortices in patients with inner-ear hearing loss were reviewed. First, we recorded auditory evoked magnetic fields (AEFs) by presenting 1-kHz pure tone at four different intensities in normal subjects and in patients with inner-ear hearing loss. Increment of dipole moment of N100m was more rapid according to the stimulus intensity in patients compared with that in healthy subjects. Next, we measured AEFs by presenting white noise and speech-related sounds. AEF responses in patients were less dependent on the acoustic structure of the stimuli than in normal subjects. Although the N100m moments were larger in the right hemisphere in normal subjects, such interhemispheric differences were not identified in the patient group. In the third study, we made two word lists, well-perceived and poorly perceived words, and measured rCBF during their monaural presentation. Well-perceived words activated bilateral temporal lobes and left angular gyrus (AG), while poorly perceived words activated only the temporal lobe contralateral to the stimulated ear and little or no activation was observed in AG. © 2004 Elsevier B.V. All rights reserved.

Keywords: Magnetoencephalogram (MEG); Positron emission tomography (PET); Auditory cortex; Hearing loss; Inner-ear

1. Introduction

Sound-induced activation of auditory cortices in subjects with mild to moderate inner ear hearing loss, which is common and experienced by most people with age, has rarely been reported. In this article, our three previous studies are reviewed to investigate how the disorder in the peripheral auditory organ influences the brain activation pattern, which may provide further information about the strategy used by the brain to process and recognize incomplete sensory signals delivered to it.

2. AEF in patients with loudness recruitment phenomenon

We measured auditory evoked magnetic fields (AEFs) in patients who had mild to moderate inner-ear hearing loss with loudness recruitment, a rapid rise in loudness

---

* Tel.: +81-78-302-4321; fax: +81-78-302-7537.
E-mail address: naito@kcgh.gr.jp (Y. Naito).

0531-5131/ © 2004 Elsevier B.V. All rights reserved.
doi:10.1016/j.ics.2004.06.024

sensation with increase in stimulus intensity, and compared them with those of normal-hearing subjects to elucidate the cortical correlates of abnormal loudness sensation [1].

2.1. Subjects

Eight patients with inner-ear hearing loss were studied. They had bilateral sensori-neural hearing impairment, and their hearing thresholds at 1 kHz ranged from 30 to 50 dB hearing level (HL). All patients exhibited loudness recruitment in both ears. AEFs were measured in each ear. The control group consisted of 14 healthy adults with normal audiograms.

2.2. Stimulus and measurement

A 1-kHz pure tone was presented monaurally and the intensity was set at 40, 50, 60 or 70 dB HL.

2.3. Moment of ECD for N100m

The moment of ECD for N100m increased as a function of sound intensity in both groups. Overall, the moment was larger to contralateral than to ipsilateral stimuli and larger in patients than in healthy subjects. The ratio of the ECD moment for N100m at 60 and 70 dB to that at 50 dB was 1.91 and 2.51 in patients, and 1.22 and 1.33 in healthy subjects.

2.4. Source location for N100m

All the source areas were located over the superior temporal auditory cortices in each hemisphere. No systematic change was observed as a function of stimulus intensity in either the healthy or the patient group.

2.5. Comments

In a previous study, which used electroencephalography, patients with sensorineural hearing loss exhibited larger amplitude of responses at the threshold level, with greater increase as a function of stimulus intensity than in healthy hearing subjects [2], a finding consistent with our results.

Loudness recruitment is a symptom commonly associated with inner-ear hearing impairment, but the neural mechanisms responsible for it are poorly understood. In our study, increase in cortical activation as a function of stimulus intensity was more prominent in patients. This larger increase in activation of auditory cortex in patients with inner-ear hearing loss is analogous to psychological characteristics of loudness recruitment, which can be considered one of the cortical correlates of subjective symptoms accompanying inner-ear hearing loss.

3. Effects of acoustic structures of sound stimuli on AEF

We measured AEFs by presenting white noise and speech-related sounds in normal subjects and in patients with mild inner-ear hearing loss [3]. The purpose of this study was to investigate the effects of acoustic structures of sound stimuli on AEFs and their alteration induced by inner-ear hearing loss.

3.1. Subjects

Eight normal subjects and seven patients with mild sensorineural hearing loss were examined. The mean hearing levels of the right and left ear among the patients were 29.4 and 33.7 dB.

3.2. Sound stimulation

Sound stimuli applied were: (1) white noise, (2) 170 Hz pure tone (the fundamental frequency (F0) of the vowel /a/), (3) synthetic complex sound (F0123) composed of F0 and three formants of the vowel /a/, and (4) the vowel /a/. The intensity of the sound stimuli was adjusted to 80 dB SPL.

3.3. MEG recording

AEFs were recorded with a whole-head magnetometer which has 122 first-order planar gradiometers.

3.4. N100m dipole moment

In normal subjects, the dipole moments of N100m for F0123 and /a/ stimuli were significantly larger than that for noise stimulus in the left hemisphere, and the N100m moment for F0123 was significantly larger than that for noise in the right hemisphere. The dipole moments in the right hemisphere with the left ear stimulation were significantly larger than those in the left hemisphere with the right ear stimulation.

In patients with hearing loss, the dipole moment of N100m for F0123 stimulus was significantly larger than that for noise stimulus in both hemispheres. No significant interhemispheric difference of the N100m dipole moment was noted in the patient group. The dipole moments in the patient group were significantly smaller than those in normal subjects in the right hemisphere, while the difference was not significant in the left hemisphere.

3.5. Comments

In normal subjects, N100m dipole moments evoked by a noise were smaller than those evoked by F0123 in both hemispheres. Such differences in AEF between noise and other stimuli, however, were less prominent in the patient group. The right hemispheric dominance observed in the present normal subjects was lost in patients for N100m. The N100m moments in the right hemisphere in the patient group were significantly smaller than in normal subjects. In contrast, the differences in these parameters between normal subjects and patients were not significant in the left hemisphere. Reduced AEF responses in the right hemisphere and subsequent disappearance of the right hemispheric dominance in the patient group might be related to an impairment in the processing of tone quality and loudness in inner-ear hearing loss.

4. Cortical activation by speech in patients with moderate hearing loss

We examined cortical activation by speech in patients with moderate inner ear hearing loss using positron emission tomography (PET) to investigate the influence of inner ear hearing loss on auditory networks in the brain [4].

4.1. Subjects

Five right-handed Japanese subjects were involved in the present study. All subjects were diagnosed as having inner ear hearing loss, and average pure-tone threshold was 55.6–75.3 dB HL in the right ear, and 53.7–73.6 dB HL in the left ear.

4.2. Sound stimulation paradigm

A pre-scan examination was performed for each subject to distinguish words that were perceived well from those that were perceived poorly. According to the result of the pre-scan examination, well-perceived words and poorly perceived words were picked from the word list for each ear for each subject.

4.3. Regional cerebral blood flow measurement and data analysis

For each stimulation condition, 15-O labelled water was injected into the right cubital vein and the rCBF was measured for 60 s. Each subject's brain was scanned using a PET scanner, and the data acquired were analyzed with the Statistical Parametric Mapping software.

4.4. Brain activation

Well-perceived word stimulation induced rCBF increase in the bilateral superior and middle temporal gyri, left inferior frontal gyrus (Broca's area) and its right hemisphere homolog, and left angular gyrus. Poorly perceived word stimulation induced rCBF increase in the superior and middle temporal gyri contralateral to the stimulated ear, Broca's area and its right hemisphere homolog. There was no significant activation in left angular gyrus during poorly perceived word stimulation.

4.5. Comments

During listening to speech, speech sounds undergo acoustic–phonetic and lexico-semantic processing and are perceived as meaningful words. Patients with inner ear hearing loss have difficulty in identifying phonemes and in perceiving words correctly, suggesting that insufficient activation of ipsilateral temporal lobe in our study may be related to the failure of acoustic–phonetic or lexico-semantic processing. However, inactivation of the ipsilateral auditory cortex may not to be due to the failure of meaning comprehension, since hearing reverse-played speech, which has no meaning, is reported to activate the temporal lobes bilaterally. Thus, inactivation of the ipsilateral auditory cortex in our study may reflect an alteration of acoustic–phonetic processing caused by distorted information from the damaged cochlea. In the present results, activation of the temporal lobe by well-perceived words was symmetrical irrespective of the ear stimulated, while that of the angular gyrus was restricted to the left hemisphere. Left hemisphere dominance for language processing is widely accepted and many functional activation studies have shown left hemisphere lateralization in cortical activation during auditory word comprehension. However, some reports point to a bilateral temporal speech processing system, at least at the prelexical level. It is reported that temporal lobe activation was seen bilaterally in acoustic and phonetic processing, while left lateralized activation in the temporoparietal regions was recognized during processing lexical semantic and/or syntactic information [5]. These reports indicate that the bilateral temporal lobe is related to the prelexical processing of speech sound, which is consistent with our results.

5. Conclusions

We observed excessive activity in the auditory cortex at high stimulus intensities in patients with inner-ear hearing loss. AEF responses in patients were less dependent on the acoustic structures of the stimuli than in normal subjects. In patients with inner ear hearing loss, insufficient activation of the temporal lobe ipsilateral to the ear stimulated might correlate with less accurate word comprehension. Injury to the peripheral auditory organs modifies information processing in the auditory cortex, which may correlate with various subjective symptoms that accompany inner-ear hearing loss.

References

[1] T. Morita, et al., Enhanced activation of the auditory cortex in patients with inner-ear hearing impairment: an MEG study, Clin. Neurophysiol. 114 (2003) 851–859.
[2] D.T. Cody, T. Griffing, W.F. Taylor, Assessment of the newer tests of auditory function, Ann. Otol. Rhinol. Laryngol. 77 (1968) 686–705.
[3] Y. Naito, et al., Auditory evoked magnetic fields in patients with hearing disorders, in: T. Yoshimoto, M. Kotani, S. Kuriki, H. Karibe, N. Nakasato (Eds.), Recent Advances in Biomagnetism, Tohoku University Press, Sendai, 1999, pp. 521–524.
[4] I. Tateya, et al., Inner ear hearing loss modulates ipsi-lateral temporal lobe activation by monaural speech stimuli, NeuroReport 14 (2003) 763–767.
[5] R. Zahn, et al., Hemispheric lateralization at different levels of human auditory word processing: a functional magnetic resonance imaging study, Neurosci. Lett. 30 (287) (2000) 195–198.

"Seeing" through the tongue: cross-modal plasticity in the congenitally blind

Ron Kupers[a],*, Maurice Ptito[b]

[a] Center for Functionally Integrative Neuroscience (CFIN), Aarhus University, and Aarhus University Hospital,
Noerrebrogade 44, 8000 Aarhus Denmark
[b] School of Optometry, Université de Montréal, CP 6128 Montreal H3C 3J7, QC, Canada

Abstract. Sensory substitution refers to the capacity of the brain to replace the functions of a lost sense by another sensory modality. This cross-modal plasticity has been documented both in animals and humans deprived of a particular sensory modality, such as vision or audition. Discovering new ways to exploit this cross-modal plasticity may help to optimize the recovery of sensory loss. The most commonly used form of sensory substitution is Braille reading, which enables the blind to read by using the somatosensory system. Recently, a human–machine interface, the tongue display unit (TDU), which uses the tongue as a medium for visual substitution in blind subjects, has been developed. We trained six congenitally blind and five blindfolded, sighted controls to use the TDU to perform a visual orientation discrimination task. Subjects were positron emission tomography (PET) scanned before and after an intensive 1-week training program with the TDU. Before training, no increased activity was measured in the visual cortex of either group during the orientation detection task. However, after training, patterned stimulation of the tongue activated the visual cortex in congenitally blind subjects. Sighted controls did not show occipital activation post-training despite equivalent performance on the same task. These data reveal the development of cross-modal plasticity in the brains of congenitally blind subjects. They further show that the time course of neuroplasticity in humans can be remarkably rapid. © 2004 Elsevier B.V. All rights reserved.

Keywords: Cross-modal plasticity; Congenitally blind; Transcranial magnetic stimulation; Occipital cortex; Sensory substitution

1. Introduction

Sight is probably the most important of our senses. Since we live in a very visual world, the loss of vision is one of the most incapacitating events that may overcome a person. It is therefore not surprising that many attempts have been undertaken to develop artificial forms of vision. The best-known example of artificial vision is Braille reading. Although Braille is an important tool for the blind, a major limitation is that it does not allow one to convey information from objects placed outside the egocentric space.

---

* Corresponding author. Tel.: +45-8949-3081; fax: +45-8949-4400.
E-mail address: ron@pet.auh.dk (R. Kupers).

0531-5131/ © 2004 Elsevier B.V. All rights reserved.
doi:10.1016/j.ics.2004.04.053

Over the past few decades, many efforts have been undertaken to develop alternative forms of artificial vision. Some of these approaches are based on highly invasive procedures, such as electrical stimulation of the retina [1] or visual cortex [2] and stem cell transplants in the eyes [3]. However, new sensory substitution systems replacing vision with touch or audition have been developed recently, offering valuable non-invasive alternatives [4–7].

2. Tactile vision sensory substitution (TVSS) systems

The system that we have been using is based upon the principle of tactile image projection and was developed by Bach-Y-Rita [5]. The system uses the tongue as a substrate for electrotactile stimulation. There are several good reasons to use the tongue as a substrate for electrotactile stimulation. First, the tongue is permanently covered with saliva and the sensory receptors are located close to the surface. As a result, stimulation can be applied with much lower voltage and current than is required for the skin. Second, the tongue is more densely populated with touch-sensitive nerves than most other parts of the body. Therefore, the tongue can convey higher-resolution information than the skin can [8]. Finally, the tongue is in the protected environment of the mouth and is normally out of sight and out of the way, which makes it cosmetically acceptable.

3. Behavioral training and positron emission tomography (PET) study

3.1. Methods

Six congenitally blind and five blindfolded, sighted control subjects participated in a behavioral training program and a PET study that was conducted before and after the behavioral training program. During behavioral training, subjects learned to use a TVSS system to discriminate the orientation of a series of Snellen patterns. Our system consists of a laptop, a tongue display unit (TDU), an electrode array and special image processing software. The electrode array measures 3×3 cm and consists of 144 gold-plated electrodes arranged in a 12×12 square matrix. Subjects had to detect the orientation of Snellen T's, which were randomly presented in one of four possible orientations. The images were presented on a laptop and the subjects could use a computer mouse to explore the image (Fig. 1). Electrical pulses were generated when the cursor was superimposed on any of the pixels on the screen forming the letter T.

The first PET session (see further) took place before the onset of training. Thereafter, the behavioral training program started and subjects underwent a 1-h daily training session with the TDU on the orientation task. The criterion that was set for successful learning was an 85% correct response on two successive training sessions. Once subjects had reached the criterion, they were PET scanned for the second time.

Subjects were scanned under the following three conditions in a semi-random order: (1) Rest: the electrode array was placed on the tongue with no stimulation; (2) Noise: subjects were presented with a random noise pattern without meaningful shape and they were asked to detect potential changes in the stimulus; and (3) Orientation task: tumbling T's were randomly presented in four different orientations and subjects had to indicate the correct orientation using the left thumb. The presentation of the tumbling T's started simulta-

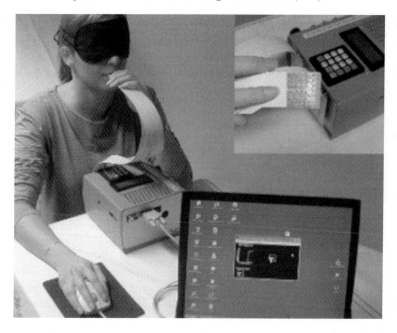

Fig. 1. Experimental setup. Subject uses a computer mouse to explore the image presented on the laptop. Insert shows the TDU control box and the electrode array with 144 contacts.

neously with tracer injection and was continued throughout the rest of the scanning time. Each scanning condition was repeated four times. The Aarhus Ethics Committee approved the study and subjects gave written, informed consent.

3.2. Results and discussion

During the first PET scanning session and at the beginning of training, subjects performed around chance level on the orientation detection task. The subjects' performance rapidly improved over time. At the end of the 1-week behavioral training period, there was no statistically significant difference in performance between both groups. Prior to training, significant increases in regional cerebral blood flow (rCBF) during the orientation detection task in both groups were restricted to parietal and prefrontal areas. In sharp contrast, the blind showed significant activations in large portions of occipital, occipito-parietal and occipito-temporal cortices post-training (Fig. 2). Blindfolded controls did not activate the visual cortex post-training despite equal performance on the orientation detection task. It is also noteworthy that the posterior parietal activation was significantly stronger in the congenitally blind following training.

These results indicate that the visual cortex is recruited in congenitally blind subjects who have learned to use the tongue in a visual orientation task. In contrast, trained, sighted, blindfolded controls showed a strong activation of the tongue area of the somatosensory cortex and of the prefrontal cortex. These results are reminiscent of those reported by others in a Braille reading task in blind subjects [9–11]. A difference with

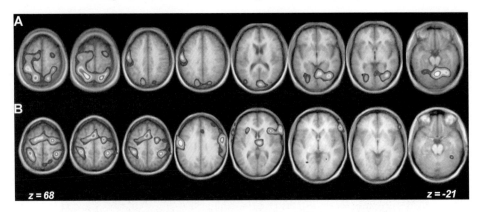

Fig. 2. PET results after training. Blind subjects activated large parts of the occipital cortex during the orientation detection task. RCBF increases in trained, blindfolded controls were restricted to parietal and prefrontal areas.

our study, however, is that blind subjects in these studies were already fluent in Braille reading at the time of scanning, thus making it impossible to delineate the time course of the plastic processes. Our results demonstrate that such plasticity can occur in a matter of hours.

It could be argued that mental imagery is at the basis of the visual cortex activation in blind subjects [12]. This is unlikely in the present experiment because our congenitally blind subjects never had any visual experience and never reported engaging in visual imagery. An alternative hypothesis is that the visual cortex activation in early blind subjects is mediated by the superior parietal lobe [10]. Tactile information is processed in the anterior part of the superior parietal cortex (area 7a), whereas visual information is processed more posteriorly, in area 7b. Therefore, tactile information may reach the visual system through increased connectivity between areas 7a and 7b after loss of vision, as suggested by the stronger activation of superior parietal areas in the blind. A pathway involving the lateral occipital tactile-visual region may also play a role in the activation of the visual cortex. This area is activated by visual and haptic exploration of objects [13]. Our results are, therefore, consistent with the hypothesis that somatosensory stimulation in the blind activates the occipito-temporal region and further expands into earlier retinotopic areas.

4. Trancranical magnetic stimulation (TMS) study

In order to study the functional relevance of the PET activations described above, we performed a TMS study in three early blind and five normal control subjects trained with the TDU device. Since preliminary TMS studies on some normal volunteers revealed possible contaminating attentional and motor effects during application of TMS pulses, we chose for a design using low frequency repetitive TMS (rTMS) with behavioral assessment after the TMS sequence. Previous studies showed long aftereffects of at least 20 min after a low-frequency rTMS train of 15 min over the occipital cortex [14].

We used a Magstim Rapid® magnetic stimulator connected to a double 9.0-cm figure-8-shaped coil with a maximal stimulator output of 1.2 T. We first identified the phosphene and motor thresholds using single TMS pulses. For occipital stimulation, the coil was positioned in a vertical position with its inferior limit 1 cm above the inion. For parietal stimulation, the coil was placed 2 cm anterior to the interaural line and 9 cm from the vertex on the left hemisphere, corresponding with the known representation of the tongue area [15]. Stimulus intensity was set to 110% of phosphene or motor threshold. One Hz rTMS was applied without interruption for 15 min (900 pulses). Before and after the TMS sequence, subjects performed the orientation detection task using the TDU. We measured reaction time and percentage of correct responses. Behavioral testing post-TMS started 2 min after the end of the TMS sequence.

No significant effects of rTMS on task performance were found in either group for both parietal and occipital rTMS. Reaction times and percentage of correct responses were not significantly different pre- and post-rTMS. In order to test whether a more dorsal stimulation site in the occipital cortex might produce different results, we retested the blind subjects with the coil positioned 2.5 cm above the inion. Also for this coil position, there was no interference with task performance. These data are different from those reported by Cohen et al. [16] showing interference with Braille reading when the occipital cortex was stimulated in early blind subjects. There are several important methodological differences between our study and the study by Cohen et al., which may explain the discrepancy in results.

Despite these negative data, we obtained some highly interesting results during the phosphene threshold assessment. In two of the congenitally blind subjects, single pulse TMS over the occipital cortex induced clear tactile sensations in the tongue. We mapped the area over which "tactile phosphenes" could be induced, and found a somatotopic representation of the tongue area with the left part of the tongue represented in the left occipital cortex, right part of the tongue in the right occipital cortex and middle part of the tongue on the medial occipital cortex. No such "tactile phosphenes" were elicited in any of the five trained, sighted subjects. These preliminary TMS data confirm our PET findings of the development of cross-modal plasticity and cortical reorganization in the early blind [17,18].

5. Conclusion

Our results reveal that the tongue can be used as a substitute for the eye and can act as a portal to the visual cortex of congenitally blind people. The TDU has the important advantage of being hands-free and providing sensory input corresponding to distal stimuli positioned beyond egocentric space. It would represent a major breakthrough in the quality of life of the blind.

Acknowledgements

This study was supported by a grant from the Danish Medical Research Council, the Danish Grundforskningsfonden and the FRSQ-Vision Network (Qc). We are indebted to Dr. E. Sampaio (Université de Strasbourg, France) for lending us the TDU device, S. Moesgaard (Aarhus University) for practical help during training of the subjects, Dr. P.-E. Buchholtz Hansen (Psychiatric Hospital Aarhus) for giving us access to his TMS laboratory and Dr. A. Fumal (University of Liège, Belgium) for helping us with the TMS experiments.

References

[1] M.S. Humayun, et al., Visual perception in a blind subject with a chronic microelectronic retinal prosthesis, Vis. Res. 43 (2003) 2573–2581.

[2] E.M. Schmidt, et al., Feasibility of a visual prosthesis for the blind based on intracortical microstimulation of the visual cortex, Brain 119 (1996) 507–522.

[3] I. Fine, et al., Long-term deprivation affects visual perception and cortex, Nat. Neurosci. 6 (2003) 1–2.

[4] P. Bach-y-Rita, et al., Vision substitution by tactile image projection, Nature 221 (1969) 963–964.

[5] P. Bach-Y-Rita, S.W. Kercel, Sensory substitution and the human–machine interface, Trends Cogn. Sci. 7 (2003) 541–546.

[6] C. Capelle, et al., A real time experimental prototype for enhancement of vision rehabilitation using auditory substitution, IEEE Trans. Biomed. Eng. 45 (1998) 1279–1293.

[7] P. Arno, et al., Occipital activation by pattern recognition in the early blind using auditory substitution for vision, NeuroImage 13 (2001) 632–645.

[8] R.L. Ringel, S.J. Ewanowski, Oral perception: 1. Two-point discrimination, J. Speech Hear. Res. 8 (1965) 389–398.

[9] N. Sadato, et al., Activation of the primary visual cortex by Braille reading in blind subjects, Nature 380 (1996) 526–528.

[10] C. Buchel, et al., Different activation patterns in the visual cortex of late and congenitally blind subjects, Brain 121 (1998) 409–419.

[11] H. Burton, et al., Adaptive changes in early and late blind: a fMRI study of Braille reading, J. Neurophysiol. 87 (2002) 589–607.

[12] A. Aleman, et al., Visual imagery without visual experience: evidence from congenitally totally blind people, NeuroReport 12 (2001) 2601–2604.

[13] A. Amedi, et al., Visuo-haptic object-related activation in the ventral visual pathway, Nat. Neurosci. 4 (2001) 324–330.

[14] A. Fumal, et al., Effects of repetitive transcranial magnetic stimulation on visual evoked potentials: new insights in healthy subjects, Exp. Brain Res. 15 (2003) 332–340.

[15] R.M. Rodel, R. Laskawi, H. Markus, Tongue representation in the lateral cortical motor region of the human brain as assessed by transcranial magnetic stimulation, Ann. Otol. Rhinol. Laryngol. 12 (2003) 71–76.

[16] L.G. Cohen, et al., Functional relevance of cross-modal plasticity in blind humans, Nature 389 (1997) 180–183.

[17] T. Kujala, K. Alho, R. Naatanen, Cross-modal reorganization of human cortical functions, Trends Neurosci. 23 (2000) 115–120.

[18] J.P. Rauschecker, Cortical map plasticity in animals and humans, Prog. Brain Res. 138 (2002) 73–88.

International Congress Series 1270 (2004) 85–90

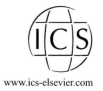

www.ics-elsevier.com

ELSEVIER

Principle and technique of NIRS-Imaging for human brain FORCE: fast-oxygen response in capillary event

Toshinori Kato[*]

*Ogawa Laboratories for Brain Function Research, Hamano Life Science Research Foundation,
12 Daikyo-cho, Shinjuku, Tokyo 160-0015, Japan*

Abstract. Two basic principles to measure positional information using photon have been discovered. The first one is the photon-CT (pCT) technique using straight-line light by Jobsis in 1977. The second is NIRS-Imaging of diffusion/scattering light that was discovered in 1991 by Kato. In the principle of NIRS-Imaging, a position of two probes and temporal responses of a measuring object determines each photon's functional pixels with border unclearness. As NIRS-Imaging uses uncertain light of positional information, it is thought of as a reversal to locate spatial information. At this point, for the pCT, which depends on precision of light for positional information, NIRS-Imaging is a completely opposite principle. It is difficult to penetrate the adult brain with light by pCT. With the discovery of the principle of NIRS-Imaging, which samples photon functional pixels, local blood physiology for oxygen exchange rapidly developed in brain and muscle studies. The sensibility of NIRS-Imaging is high for a signal of active oxygen exchange in capillaries. NIRS-Imaging is a non-invasive measurement for cerebral microcirculation in the capillary, not the vein. It is important to measure fast-oxygen response in capillary event (FORCE) related to neuronal responses, defined as the FORCE effect. Advanced NIRS-Imaging can distinguish the FORCE effect from a watering-the-garden effect. The slow blood change that defined a watering-the-garden effect can induce a strong signal in the vein by PET and fMRI. Therefore, oxygen consumption in tissues using fMRI and PET may be underestimated by the measurement of the passive washout flow in the vein. © 2004 Published by Elsevier B.V.

Keywords: Near-infrared spectroscopy (NIRS)-Imaging; Oxygen; Fast-oxygen response in capillary event (FORCE); Watering-the-garden effect; Photon functional pixel (PFP)

1. Introduction

Novelty in science is produced by access to the basic principle. Birth of a basic principle for functional imaging using light was similar too. Since 1977 the principle of NIRS-Imaging has acted as an antithesis to photon-CT (pCT). pCT uses straight-line light

* Tel.: +81-3-5919-3992; fax: +81-3-5919-3993.
E-mail address: kato@hlsrf.or.jp (T. Kato).

0531-5131/ © 2004 Published by Elsevier B.V.
doi:10.1016/j.ics.2004.05.052

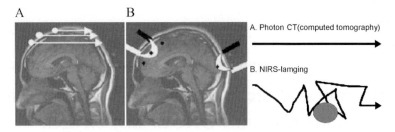

Fig. 1. Two basic principles to measure positional information, which used light. (A) Photon-CT of straight-line light by Jobsis in 1977. (B) NIRS-Imaging of diffusion/scattering light discovered in 1991 by Kato.

[1] (Fig. 1A). NIRS-Imaging by Kato and coworkers uses diffusion/scattering light [2,3] (Fig. 1B). Furthermore, Kato studied a principle of NIRS-Imaging more deeply. In the principle of NIRS-Imaging, a photon functional pixel (PFP) with border unclearness is decided by a position of two probes and local temporal responses of a measuring object. As NIRS-Imaging uses uncertain light of positional information, it is thought to be a reversal to locate spatial information. At this point, for the pCT, which depends on precision of light for positional information, NIRS-Imaging is a completely opposite principle. By discovery of a principle and the technique of NIRS-Imaging, which samples PFP, NIRS-Imaging was rapidly developed to measure local, temporal–spatial function from brain oxygenation monitoring. The physiological meaning of the changes in oxygenated hemoglobin (HbO$_2$) and deoxygenated hemoglobin (HbR) completely changed into local temporal–spatial information by this discovery.

2. Discovery of NIRS-Imaging

NIRS-Imaging, whereby near infrared rays (700–1300 nm, Fig. 2A) are irradiated from the skin of the head through the skull into the brain to measure changes of HbO$_2$ and HbR in the microvessel of the cortex, has progressed rapidly. NIRS-Imaging has the advantages that metabolism of separate tissue can be measured non-invasively and that this can furthermore be implemented with a simple apparatus (portability), unlike PET and fMRI. Using bedside NIRS-Imaging, it was possible to observe cerebral activity in a child and even a bedridden old person. It is the setting of a distance of 2.5 cm between

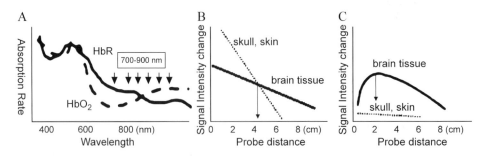

Fig. 2. The concept of NIRS-Imaging for shortening probe distance. (A) Absorption rates of HbO$_2$ and HbR. A qualitative simulation of light penetration into a brain during a resting state (B) and during an active state (C).

A B

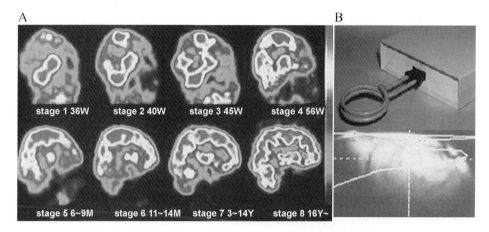

stage 1 36W stage 2 40W stage 3 45W stage 4 56W

stage 5 6~9M stage 6 11~14M stage 7 3~14Y stage 8 16Y~

Fig. 3. The concept of NIRS-Imaging of multiple surface probes for brain surface mapping. Differing cerebral blood flow distribution from neonates to adults [4]. (B) Surface coil for MR spectroscopy and brain surface imaging by surface coil [5].

probes that symbolized the birth of NIRS-Imaging. As the distance from the skull surface to the cortex is 1.5–2 cm, it was necessary to separate the distance of the probes more than 4.25 cm for sampling brain tissue during the resting state (Fig. 2B). Therefore, it is not exaggeration to say that the basic principle of NIRS-Imaging is a new technique, which can shorten the probe distance of 4.25 cm. Kato et al. found that they could shorten the distance of the probes to approximately 2.5 cm if they used a local cerebral response (Fig. 2C). In fact, Kato et al. conducted photo-stimulus experiments in humans in which near infrared light was irradiated to parts of the brain. As a result, they showed that it was able to monitor the distribution of localized brain function at the bedside and proved low resolution optical imaging using this bedside method of non-invasive detection of local brain function.

As for the pCT, measurement takes time. Even if we are going to use brain oxygen monitoring in neonates, it is weak for motion artifacts. In addition, Kato's 1988 thesis of brain development in neonates understood that a development pattern of cerebral blood flow distribution was associated with cerebral myelination, such as that shown in Fig. 3A [4]. Thus, we hypothesized that a cerebral oxygen state of neonates depended on the probe location for different cerebral blood flow distribution. MR spectroscopy using a surface coil is a non-invasive measurement of local cerebral metabolism for a functional pixel with border unclearness (Fig. 3B). Kato came up with the idea of NIRS-Imaging of multiple surface probes for brain surface mapping.

3. Fast-oxygen response in capillary event (FORCE)

As PFP with border unclearness is decided by the position of two probes and temporal responses of a measuring object using NIRS-Imaging, it is very important to understand the different physiological responses between resting and active states in the capillary and vein (Fig. 4). Signal increases in T2*-fMRI are believed to result from decreased paramagnetic HbR in the activation area. This mechanism has been described widely as

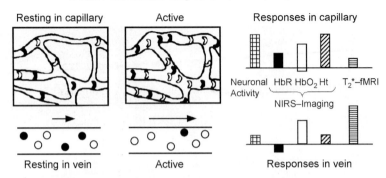

Fig. 4. Functional physiology in capillaries and veins using NIRS-Imaging and T2*-fMRI.

the blood oxygenation level dependent (BOLD) theory (Fig. 5A). The signal changes of T2*-fMRI may be paralleled with HbR by passive washout flow in the large vein. However, by oxygen exchange in the capillary, a simple washout flow hardly occurs in an active location. Therefore, the non-BOLD effect does not change in parallel with HbR in the capillary and micro-vein. A non-BOLD effect, which indicated discrepancies in this canonical BOLD theory, has been found in studies using optical techniques that directly measure hemoglobin changes (Fig. 5B) [6,8]. To understand different sensitivities between NIRS-Imaging and T2*-fMRI, the hematocrit (Ht) must be taken into account. In the blood in veins between resting and active states, there is less variation of hematocrit in comparison to the blood in capillaries [6]. The signal change in the vein is always larger than in the capillary when using T2*-fMRI [6–8]. In contrast, the signal change in the capillary is always larger than in the vein when using NIRS-Imaging. It is very difficult to detect a signal from the vein by using light for strong absorption.

The T2*-fMRI is sensitive to passive hemodynamic changes in a vein area where blood flow from both activated and non-activated areas is mixed, such as in the secondary watering-the-garden effect (a phenomenon of scattering water on a circumference in order to give water to one flower), but is less sensitive to active hemodynamic changes in a capillary area of an activation focus, such as the FORCE effect. Hemodynamics in capillaries differs greatly from that in veins. In veins, blood flow changes with a mild increase in blood volume and a constant hematocrit. In activation capillaries, the number of red

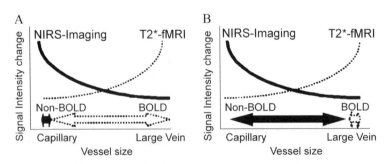

Fig. 5. Sensibility of NIRS-Imaging and T2*-fMRI for blood response in capillaries and veins. (A) Canonical BOLD hypothesis from blood physics; (B) hemodynamic bridging theory from blood physiology [6].

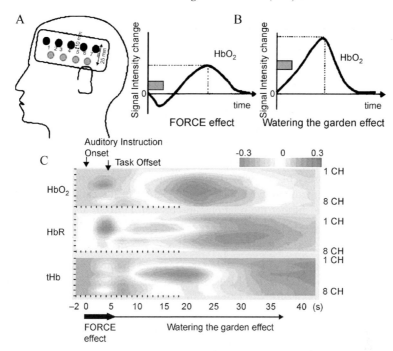

Fig. 6. Imaging for oxygen exchange in the capillary: distinguished FORCE effect from watering-the-garden effect. (A) The location of eight channels for NIRS-Imaging. The probes were placed on bilaterally front-temporal regions covered Broca's area. Sampling rate of data acquisition was 10 Hz. (B) The dynamic changes of HbO_2 in FORCE effect and watering-the-garden effect. The maximum peak of HbO_2 in FORCE effect was delayed and lower in comparison to watering-the-garden effect. (C) Temporal spatial mapping during a language task. An instructor speaks a word directly and exhibits it. Subject repeats immediately thereafter [9].

blood cells increases greatly with an increase in hematocrit. Therefore, the FORCE effect, measured by NIRS-imaging, is a good marker to observe the activation focus in comparison to secondary watering-the-garden effect (Fig. 6).

A

Intra-capillary
- Oxygen consumption
- Oxygen supply

Red blood cell

O_2 transport

Neuron
- Oxygen consumption
- Oxygen supply

Glia cell

B

Response order	Physiology	Location	Effective sampling
1st	Neuronal response	tissue	EEG, MEG
2nd	Oxygen exchange, consumption (FORCE effect)	in capillary	NIRS-Imaging
3rd	Active oxygen supply (1st watering-the-garden effect)	in capillary	NIRS-Imaging, PET
4th	Passive washout flow (2nd watering-the-garden effect)	in vein	fMRI, PET

Fig. 7. A schema of oxygen exchange and supply in capillaries and neurons (A) and sensitivity of modalities for functional response (B).

4. Tight linkage between FORCE and neuronal activity

Advanced NIRS-Imaging could distinguish the FORCE effect from a watering-the-garden effect during early language action. As blood responses were diffuse and broad, it is important to measure the FORCE effect related to neuronal response as a 2nd order response (Fig. 7A). The secondary watering-the-garden effect as a 4th-order response causes a big signal change in T2*-fMRI and PET studies (Fig. 7B). Our finding supported the technical insensibility in T2*-fMRI for the first 3–5 s [10] due to the non-BOLD effect in the capillary. Neuroimaging, using PET and MRI, should pay attention to the physiological misunderstanding and underestimation of oxygen consumption [11] due to the technical insensibility of the FORCE effect from NIRS-Imaging. NIRS-Imaging is a non-invasive measurement for cerebral microcirculation in the capillary, not in the vein. We need to understand further the relationship between FORCE and neuronal activity.

Acknowledgements

This study was partially supported by the research grant (14B-1) for nervous and mental disorders from the ministry of Health, Labor and Welfare, Japan. Thanks for useful discussion and analysis of NIRS-Imaging with Yoshimi Okawa, Toshihide Koike (Tokyo Gakugei University), Takanori Maesako (Osaka University), Miyoshi Kumoi (Kagoshima University) and of SPECT with Tsuyoshi Matsuo (Kameda Medical Center).

References

[1] F.F. Jobsis, Noninvasive infrared monitoring of cerebral and myocardial oxygen sufficiency and circulation parameters, Science 198 (1977) 1264–1267.

[2] S. Takashima, et al., Observation of changes in local brain blood flow by means of near-infrared spectros-copy, Comprehensive Research Report Concerning Medical Care for Children (People) with Disabilities from Japanese Ministry of Health and Welfare Grant, 1992, pp. 179–181(in Japanese).

[3] T. Kato, et al., Human visual cortical function during photic stimulation monitoring by means of near-infrared spectroscopy, J. Cereb. Blood Flow Metab. 13 (1993) 516–520.

[4] T. Kato, K. Okuyama, Assessment of maturation and impairment of brain by I-123 Iodoamphetamine SPECT and MR imaging in children, Showa Univ. J. Med. Sci. 5 (1993) 99–115.

[5] T. Kato, et al., Assessment of brain death in children by means of P-31 MR spectroscopy: preliminary note, Radiology 179 (1991) 95–99.

[6] T. Yamamoto, T. Kato, Paradoxical correlation between signal in functional magnetic resonance imaging and deoxygenated hemoglobin content in capillaries: a new theoretical explanation, Phys. Med. Biol. 47 (2002) 1121–1141.

[7] N. Pouratian, et al., Spatial/temporal correlation of BOLD and optical intrinsic signals in humans, Magn. Reson. Med. 47 (2002) 766–776.

[8] A. Hess, et al., New insights into the haemodynamic blood oxygenation level-dependent response through combination of functional magnetic resonance imaging and optical recording in gerbil barrel cortex, J. Neurosci. 20 (2000) 3328–3338.

[9] T. Kato, et al., Cerebral hemodynamics and local activity of Broca's area using high selectivity, near-infrared spectroscopic imaging—properties during the task of word repetitions aloud, Clin. Encephalogr. 46 (2004) 20–32(in Japanese).

[10] N.K. Logothetis, et al., Neurophysiological investigation of the basis of the fMRI signal, Nature 412 (2001) 150–157.

[11] P.T. Fox, et al., Nonoxidative glucose consumption during focal physiologic neural activity, Science 241 (1988) 462–464.

International Congress Series 1270 (2004) 91–96

ELSEVIER

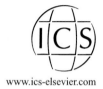

www.ics-elsevier.com

Tissue viability assessed by MRI

Leif Østergaard[a],*, Masaharu Sakoh[b]

[a] Department of Neuroradiology, Danish National Research Foundations Center for Functionally Integrative Neuroscience, Aarhus University Hospital, Nørrebrogade 44, DK-8000 Århus C, Denmark
[b] Department of Neurosurgery, Tokyo Women's Medical University, Tokyo, Japan

Abstract. In recent years, magnetic resonance imaging (MRI)-based methods have been developed that allow non-invasive measurements of cerebral haemodynamics (perfusion-weighted MRI) and cellular damage (diffusion-weighted MRI) in ischemia. These techniques provide powerful tools for assessing tissue viability in acute stroke. We review these techniques along with examples of their use in the study of stroke pathophysiology. © 2004 Elsevier B.V. All rights reserved.

Keywords: Magnetic resonance imaging (MRI); Perfusion-weighted imaging (PWI); Diffusion-weighted imaging (DWI); Cerebral ischemia; Tissue viability; Cerebral metabolism

1. Introduction

Perfusion measurements by dynamic susceptibility contrast magnetic resonance imaging (MRI) utilizes very rapid imaging (most commonly echo planar imaging [EPI]) to capture the first pass of intravenously injected paramagnetic contrast agent—hence, the term '*Bolus Tracking*'. By kinetic analysis of these data, haemodynamic indices, namely cerebral blood flow (CBF), cerebral blood volume (CBV) and mean transit time (MTT) can be derived.

2. Perfusion MRI

2.1. Theory

Bolus tracking is commonly carried out using dynamic susceptibility contrast imaging, tracking the passage of a rapidly injected paramagnetic Gd-based chelate by a T_2 (spin echo)- or T_2^* (gradient echo)-weighted sequence (often EPI). In the brain, the first pass extraction of contrast agent is zero when the blood–brain barrier is reasonably intact, and the intravascular compartmentalisation of contrast agent creates large, microscopic susceptibility gradients, and the dephasing of spins as they diffuse among these results in signal loss in T_2- and T_2^*-weighted images, described by Villringer in

---

* Corresponding author. Tel.: +45-89494091; fax: +45-89494400.
E-mail address: leif@pet.auh.dk (L. Østergaard).

0531-5131/ © 2004 Elsevier B.V. All rights reserved.
doi:10.1016/j.ics.2004.04.089

1998 [1]. Weisskoff et al. [2–4] performed a detailed analysis of these physical effects using Monte Carlo modelling as well as experimental data. They found that spin echo measurements are mainly sensitive to vessel sizes comparable with the water diffusion length during the time-of-echo (~ 10 μm), whereas gradient echo measurements are equally sensitive to all vessel sizes. Experimentally and clinically, this has the effect that to create similar signal losses during first pass, twice the amount of contrast agent (usually double dose of standard Gd chelate, 0.2 mmol/kg) must be injected if imaging is performed using SE EPI, relative to imaging with GE EPI (where 0.1 mmol/kg is generally injected). In return for this, the SE theoretically yields higher sensitivity in detecting changes in small vessel density. As important, they found that an approximate linear relationship exists between tissue contrast agent concentration and change in T_2 relaxation rate.

$$\Delta R_2(t) \propto C_t(t) \tag{1}$$

This is a central assumption in the subsequent kinetic analysis (below).

For gradient and spin echo sequences, signal intensity depends in an exponential fashion upon the transverse relaxation rate changes, ΔR_2 yielding the relation between concentration and signal intensity

$$C_t(t) = -k\log\left(\frac{S(t)}{S(t_o)}\right)/\text{TE} \tag{2}$$

The assumption of linearity in Eq. (1) has been confirmed by indirect measurements in vivo [5] and is now widely used in perfusion measurements, where $S(t_o)$ is determined from the baseline signal in the images prior to the contrast bolus arrival.

In a simulation study, Kiselev et al. [6–8] found that due to the complex physics of MR signal formation in perfused tissues, the linearity in Eq. (3) may not hold for all ranges of contrast agent concentrations or tissues. This non-linearity may cause overestimation of perfusion estimates [6,8].

2.2. Cerebral blood volume measurements

Rosen et al. [9–12] derived maps of relative CBV by kinetic analysis of the concentration–time curves (see above) while dynamically tracking the passage of a bolus high-susceptibility contrast agent. Note that the technique is applicable to any tracking of the passage of an intravascular tracer, irrespective of modality (dynamic CT is also suited for this purpose) with high temporal resolution. The key issue is temporal resolution of the dynamic imaging relative to the characteristic blood transit time of the tissue (typically 4–6 s). Upon a standard 5 ml/s injection into an antecubital vein, the tissue bolus passage duration is of the order of 12–20 s in adults. With echo planar imaging, a typical choice of temporal resolution is TR = 1.5 s or faster. With current high-performance gradient systems, this allows acquisition of 10–15 slices (typically with a spatial resolution of roughly 1.5 mm in-plane, 5–6 mm slice thickness) for every TR, providing good brain coverage. For purposes involving deconvolution (see below), temporal resolution slower than 1.5 s per image is not advised.

By detecting the arterial as well as the total tissue concentration as a function of time during a single transit, the CBV can be determined from the ratio of the areas under the tissue and arterial concentration–time curves, respectively [13–15].

$$CBV = \int_{-\infty}^{\infty} C_t(\tau)d\tau \bigg/ \int_{-\infty}^{\infty} C_a(\tau)d\tau \qquad (3)$$

With concentrations determined from Eq. (3), and as arterial measurements (due to limited spatial resolution) are not readily quantifiable, relative CBV values are usually reported. Assuming uniform arterial concentration profiles in all arterial inputs, relative CBV measurements are determined by simply integrating the area under the concentration–time curve [9–11], occasionally by the use of a gamma variate function to correct for tracer recirculation [16]. In a recent report, Perkiö et al. [17] concluded that numerically integrating the area of the tissue curve (over the full time range for which it was imaged) or integrating the area of the deconvolved tissue impulse response curve (see below) most accurately represents the most accurate methods of determining relative CBV.

2.3. The residue function—cerebral blood flow

The tissue concentration–time curves is the convolution of the impulse response (CBF times $R(t)$) and the shape of the arterial input function

$$C_t(t) = CBF\ C_a(t) \otimes R(t) \qquad (4)$$

In order to derive CBF from this equation, the impulse response has to be determined by deconvolution, essentially fitting CBF $R(t)$ from the experimental data. As $R(0)=1$, CBF is determined as the initial height of the impulse response function. The most commonly used technique for this deconvolution is *Singular Value Decomposition* [18,19]. See also Liu et al. [20] for details on noise suppression by SVD. The major disadvantage of the original SVD approach is a tendency to underestimate flow when tissue tracer arrival is delayed relative to the arterial input function [19,21]. This problem has been circumvented by the so-called circular SVD, recently published by Wu et al. [22].

2.4. The mean transit time

The calculation of MTT thereby requires knowledge of the transport function or CBF, as by the Central Volume Theorem [13]

$$MTT = \frac{CBV}{F_t} \qquad (5)$$

2.5. Delay and dispersion

Even though a straight delay of tracer arrival can be accounted for by, e.g., circular SVD, model-less approaches cannot distinguish tracer dispersion in feeding vessels from the tracer retention in the capillary bed: Large vessel dispersion will be interpreted as a low flow, although actual tissue flow is normal [19,21]. This is a more fundamental limitation that cannot be circumvented unless a specific model of major vessel dispersion is assumed (e.g., by a vascular operator as in Ref. [23]).

Utilizing the superior spatial resolution of the raw perfusion images, Alsop et al. [24] suggested detecting the arterial input function regionally, i.e., from arterial branches close to the tissue voxel being analysed. Although correctly assigning the arterial supply of a voxel to one of several nearby arterial branches may be difficult, e.g., in vascular watershed areas and in vascular occlusion (stroke), this may prove a promising approach in overcoming this inherent methodological problem.

3. Assessing tissue viability by perfusion- and diffusion-weighted MRI in acute stroke

3.1. Background

Acute stroke is the 3rd leading cause of death in the Western world and the major cause of adult disability. As the incidence of the disease increases exponentially with age, the increase in mean age will cause the incidence to roughly double within the next 50 years. In light of this, the study of stroke pathophysiology and the search for therapeutic strategies to limit tissue damage after acute stroke is intense. Treatment must be started promptly as neuronal damage progresses rapidly after onset of ischemia. Also, there is growing evidence that treatment must be tailored for the individual patient to optimise efficacy and avoid serious side-effects (e.g., haemorrhage after thrombolysis). This need for assessing tissue viability represents a challenge to current diagnostic imaging procedures in acute stroke patients. First, diagnostic imaging should provide not only rapid, precise diagnostic support, but also provide prognostic information to guide treatment. Secondly, diagnostic imaging should provide the means for supporting the development of novel pharmaceuticals, by identifying efficacious drugs in small patient populations.

3.2. Perfusion and diffusion MRI and tissue viability

The development of diffusion-weighted imaging (DWI) has provided a powerful tool for demonstrating cytotoxic oedema in severe ischemia in acute stroke [25]. There is evidence that the water diffusion reduction (quantified as the apparent diffusion coefficient, ADC) reflects the severity and duration of ischemia and may indeed be reversible if tissue is reperfused. DWI may thereby be of diagnostic as well as prognostic value. With the development of perfusion-weighted imaging (PWI) by dynamic susceptibility contrast-enhanced (DSCE) MRI, images obtainable on most clinical scanners may elucidate areas where CBF and thereby oxygen supply is compromised to such an extent that subsequent tissue damage is imminent [19]. Especially, PWI allows measurement of the blood MTT, a sensitive marker of decreased perfusion pressure. The tissue volume showing PWI abnormalities often exceed that of abnormal DWI, referred to as *perfusion–diffusion mismatch*. This is now known to be a strong prognostic tool (more than 90% of patients displaying such PWI–DWI mismatches typically experience lesion growth) [26]. The DWI–PWI mismatch, however, typically overestimates final infarct size. More recent PWI techniques, measuring quantities directly related to oxygen metabolism, have improved the accurate prediction of final infarct size and location [27].

3.3. Diffusion weighted MRI and residual metabolism

Sakoh et al. [28,29] measured cerebral oxygen and glucose metabolism ($CMRO_2$ and CMRglc) in a porcine middle cerebral artery occlusion (MCAO) model of acute stroke. It was found that the percent decrease in $CMRO_2$ is linearly correlated to the percent change in ADC, down to 70% of normal ADC. Below this limit, ADC decrease was accompanied by an abrupt decrease in glucose metabolism and further decrease in oxygen metabolism, signalling rapid neuronal death. Traditionally, ADC changes have been assumed to signal irreversible cell death [28]. The results indicate that—in the first hours following onset of ischemia—residual metabolism and possibly viable cells exist in areas of altered diffusion. More recent clinical studies suggest that DWI lesions may indeed be reversible, lending hope to these areas indeed being salvageable by early intervention.

3.4. Prognostic tools

The development multiple functional image modalities, all providing physiological or structural information relevant to subsequent infarct risk, represents a problem in terms of rapidly extracting relevant, regional prognostic information. This has led to an effort to develop the so-called *prognostic tools*. These are algorithms that provide the user with images of infarct risk, rather than the many underlying PWI and DWI images [30]. The algorithms are trained to predict risk of infarction on a large set of clinical cases in which acute as well as follow-up images are obtained. The tool then applies the resulting predictive model on subsequent data set, estimating infarct risk on a pixel-by-pixel basis. Thereby, highly specialised diagnosis and individualised treatment planning may poten-tially be carried out without the need for extensive training in interpreting acute functional MRI data. These tools may indeed in the future support the early identification of new therapeutic approaches: Risk estimates obtained from untreated and treated patients may be compared and drug action quantified directly in terms of infarct risk reduction. The use of this highly sensitive approach is believed to greatly reduce the size of patient population needed to establish drug efficacy.

References

[1] A. Villringer, et al., Dynamic imaging with lanthanide chelates in normal brain: contrast due to magnetic susceptibility effects, Magn. Reson. Med. 6 (2) (1988) 164–174.

[2] C.R. Fisel, et al., MR contrast due to microscopically heterogeneous magnetic susceptibility: numerical simulations and applications to cerebral physiology, Magn. Reson. Med. 17 (2) (1991) 336–347.

[3] J.L. Boxerman, et al., MR contrast due to intravascular magnetic susceptibility perturbations, Magn. Reson. Med. 34 (4) (1995) 555–566.

[4] R.M. Weisskoff, et al., Microscopic susceptibility variation and transverse relaxation: theory and experi-ment, Magn. Reson. Med. 31 (6) (1994) 601–610.

[5] C.Z. Simonsen, et al., CBF and CBV measurements by USPIO bolus tracking: reproducibility and com-parison with Gd-based values, J. Magn. Reson. Imaging 9 (1999) 342–347.

[6] V.G. Kiselev, On the theoretical basis of perfusion measurements by dynamic susceptibility contrast MRI, Magn. Reson. Med. 46 (2001) 1113–1122.

[7] V.G. Kiselev, S. Posse, Analytical theory of susceptibility induced NMR signal dephasing in a cerebrovas-cular network, Phys. Rev. Lett. 81 (1998) 5696–5699.

[8] V.G. Kiselev, S. Posse, Analytical model of susceptibility-induced MR signal dephasing: effect of diffusion in a microvascular network, Magn. Reson. Med. 41 (1999) 499–509.

[9] B.R. Rosen, et al., Perfusion imaging with NMR contrast agents, Magn. Reson. Med. 14 (2) (1990) 249–265.

[10] B.R. Rosen, et al., Susceptibility contrast imaging of cerebral blood volume: human experience, Magn. Reson. Med. 22 (2) (1991) 293–299.

[11] B.R. Rosen, et al., Contrast agents and cerebral hemodynamics, Magn. Reson. Med. 19 (2) (1991) 285–292.

[12] J.W. Belliveau, et al., Functional mapping of the human visual cortex by magnetic resonance imaging, Science 254 (5032) (1991) 716–719.

[13] G.N. Stewart, Researches on the circulation time in organs and on the influences which affect it: Parts I–III, J. Physiol. (Lond.) 15 (1894) 1–89.

[14] P. Meier, K.L. Zierler, On the theory of the indicator-dilution method for measurement of blood flow and volume, J. Appl. Phys. 6 (1954) 731–744.

[15] K.L. Zierler, Theoretical basis of indicator-dilution methods for measuring flow and volume, Circ. Res. 10 (1962) 393–407.

[16] H.K. Thompson, et al., Indicator transit time considered as a gamma variate, Circ. Res. 14 (1964) 502–515.

[17] J.P. Perkiö, et al., Evaluation of four postprocessing methods for determination of cerebral blood volume and mean transit time by dynamic susceptibility contrast imaging, Magn. Reson. Med. 47 (2002) 973–981.

[18] L. Østergaard, et al., High resolution measurement of cerebral blood flow using intravascular tracer bolus passages: Part II. Experimental comparison and preliminary results, Magn. Reson. Med. 36 (5) (1996) 726–736.

[19] L. Østergaard, et al., High resolution measurement of cerebral blood flow using intravascular tracer bolus passages: Part I. Mathematical approach and statistical analysis, Magn. Reson. Med. 36 (5) (1996) 715–725.

[20] H.L. Liu, et al., Cerebral blood flow measurement by dynamic contrast MRI using singular value decomposition with an adaptive threshold, Magn. Reson. Med. (1999) 167–172.

[21] F. Calamante, D.G. Gadian, A. Connely, Delay and dispersion effects in dynamic susceptibility contrast MRI: simulations using singular value decomposition, Magn. Reson. Med. (2000) 466–473.

[22] O. Wu, et al., Tracer arrival timing-insensitive technique or estimating flow in MR perfusion-weighted imaging using singular value decomposition with a block-circulant deconvolution matrix, Magn. Reson. Med. 50 (2003) 100–110.

[23] L. Østergaard, et al., Modeling cerebral blood flow and flow heterogeneity from magnetic resonance residue detection, J. Cereb. Blood Flow Metab. 19 (1999) 690–699.

[24] D. Alsop, Local input functions, Proc. International Society for Magnetic Resonance in Medicine (ISMRM), 2002, p. 497.

[25] M.E. Moseley, et al., Early detection of regional cerebral ischemia in cats: comparison of diffusion- and T2-weighted MRI and spectroscopy, Magn. Reson. Med. 14 (2) (1990) 330–346.

[26] J.H. Galicich, L.A. French, J.C. Melby, Use of dexamethasone in the treatment of cerebral edema associated with brain tumors, Lancet 81 (1961) 46–53.

[27] L. Østergaard, et al., Combined diffusion-weighted and perfusion-weighted flow heterogeneity magnetic resonance imaging in acute stroke, Stroke 31 (2000) 1097–1103.

[28] M. Sakoh, et al., Relationship between residual cerebral blood flow and oxygen metabolism as predictive of ischemic tissue viability: sequential multitracer positron emission tomography scanning of middle cerebral artery occlusion during the critical first 6 hours after stroke in pigs, J. Neurosurg. 93 (4) (2000) 647–657.

[29] M. Sakoh, et al., Prediction of tissue survival after middle cerebral artery occlusion based on changes in the apparent diffusion of water, J. Neurosurg. 95 (3) (2001) 450–458.

[30] O. Wu, et al., Predicting tissue outcome in acute human cerebral ischemia using combined diffusion- and perfusion-weighted MR imaging, Stroke 32 (4) (2001) 933–942.

Central regulation for oral function

International Congress Series 1270 (2004) 99–104

ELSEVIER

www.ics-elsevier.com

Cortical activation during tongue movement revealed by fMRI: fact and myth on chewing-side preference

Takashi Ono*

Maxillofacial Orthognathics, Graduate School, Tokyo Medical and Dental University, 1-5-45 Yushima, Bunkyo, Tokyo, 113-8549, Japan

Abstract. A chewing-side preference (CSP) is a preference for one side of the dentition during chewing. However, little is known about whether the CSP is associated with lateral tongue movement (TM). The aims of this study were: (1) to identify cortical areas responsible for producing TMs by using blood oxygenation level-dependent (BOLD) functional magnetic resonance imaging (fMRI) and their relations to the CSP and (2) to determine whether and how the TM-related cortical activation was affected by bilateral chewing. A marked increase in BOLD signals was detected in primary sensorimotor cortices (SM1) during TMs. In subjects with the CSP, the BOLD signal change in the SM1 was significantly greater on the side contralateral to the CSP. In subjects with the left CSP, the BOLD signal intensity was significantly increased in the left SM1 within 10 min after bilateral gum chewing. Moreover, this augmented activation significantly decreased within 20 min during tongue protrusion and leftward movement. In the right SM1, there were no marked changes during TMs. The results suggest that, in SM1 responsible for TMs, (1) there is a relationship between hemispheric dominance and CSP and (2) bilateral gum chewing enhances TM-related SM1 ipsilateral to the CSP. Thus, it appears that the CSP plays an important role in the organization of tongue and jaw movement at the cortical level. © 2004 Elsevier B.V. All rights reserved.

Keywords: Tongue movement; Cortical activation; Plasticity; Chewing-side preference; Functional magnetic resonance imaging (fMRI)

1. Introduction

Asymmetries in motor performance are most consistent for handedness (77%), and least consistent for footedness (49%) [1]. Later, another less known asymmetry in masticatory behavior was reported [2], namely chewing-side preference (CSP). Although handedness is the most easily observed expression of cerebral lateralization, little is known about the relationship between the CSP and cerebral influence. Rather, several studies have suggested that the CSP may be an expression of motivational and/or sensorimotor behavior influenced by peripheral factors [2–4].

* Tel./fax: +81-3-5803-5533.
E-mail address: t-ono.mort@tmd.ac.jp (T. Ono).

0531-5131/ © 2004 Elsevier B.V. All rights reserved.
doi:10.1016/j.ics.2004.05.006

The cerebral representation of the tongue encompasses bilaterally in the inferior region of the primary sensorimotor cortex (SM1) [5]. A functional magnetic resonance imaging (fMRI) study has shown that brain activation during tongue protrusion is found in several areas, including the SM1 [6]. However, it is unclear whether lateral movement of the tongue is associated with unilateral focal activation of the SM1. Therefore, the current body of knowledge regarding the cortical control of tongue movement (TM) does not permit a definite description of the hemispheric lateralization during voluntary TMs. Moreover, little is known about whether the CSP is associated with lateral TM, though it is known that the jaws and tongue show cyclic movement during chewing, suggesting a close functional connection [7–10].

On the other hand, it has been reported that there are no significant differences in regional cerebral blood flow in the SM1 before, during and after gum chewing [11], whereas it was demonstrated that the cortical temperature increased during and after gum chewing [12]. Since movements of the tongue and masticatory muscles are closely associated, it appears to be appropriate to perform TM without activation of masticatory muscles to avoid chewing-related motion artifacts to investigate chewing-related cortical activation. The aims of this study were: (1) to identify cortical areas responsible for producing TMs, including lateral excursion of the tongue by using blood oxygenation level-dependent (BOLD) fMRI and their relations to the CSP and (2) to determine whether and how cortical activation patterns during TM were affected by bilateral chewing.

2. Materials and methods

Fifteen healthy right-handed adults participated in Experiment 1. TMs were designed to produce minimal or no displacement of the tongue or jaw to minimize TM-related motion artifacts. A 1.5-T apparatus (Magnetom Vision, Siemens, Germany) was used to obtain MR images. Imaging with a T1-weighted sequence was performed to obtain structural brain images. Consequently, 40 transverse T2*-weighted slices were obtained. All of the subjects performed the following four tasks in the block design: tongue protrusion (T_P), TM to the right (T_R) and left (T_L) and "rest" as a control. One of the TM blocks occurred randomly between two "rest" blocks (Fig. 1A). The subject performed each TM block 6 times and the "rest" block 18 times. SPM99 software was used for fMRI data analysis. Subtraction was used in the following comparisons: (1) T_{P+R+L}-"rest", (2) T_P-"rest", (3) T_R-"rest" and (4) T_L-"rest". Second-level random effects analyses were used ($p < 0.001$, uncorrected). The statistically significant locations were superimposed on a standard brain atlas [13]. All of the subjects were also divided into two groups with ($n = 10$) and without ($n = 5$) an evident CSP. Subjects with CSP were further subgrouped to those with the right ($n = 5$) and left ($n = 5$) CSPs. The mean percentage change in BOLD signal (mBOLD) for a voxel containing the coordinate that showed maximum activation in the bilateral SM1 was calculated. A Mann–Whitney U test ($p < 0.05$) was used to compare the mBOLD in each SM1 for the group with an evident CSP. The TM paradigms, methods used for fMRI data acquisition and analysis, have been fully described elsewhere [14].

Seventeen healthy, right-handed adults were recruited for Experiment 2. Each subject was interviewed to determine the CSP, which was further confirmed by using a mandibular kinesiograph (K6-I, Myo-tronics, USA). Of the 17 subjects, six subjects who showed a

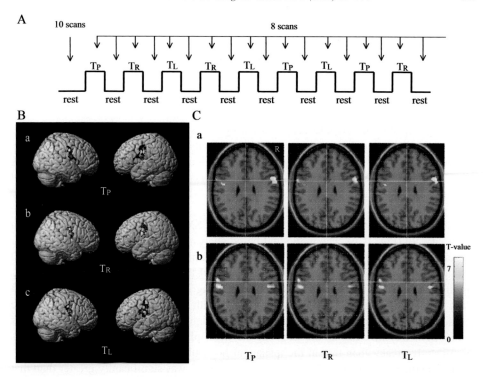

Fig. 1. Task design and brain activities. (A) The tongue movement (TM) paradigm. (B) The activation foci during TMs (T_P, T_R and T_L): (a) T_P-"rest"; (b) T_R-"rest"; and (c) T_L-"rest". Significant activations of the bilateral SM1 are shown. Note that there were no marked differences in activation foci for the three different TMs in terms of size or location. (C) Representative activation patterns in the SM1 of subjects with evident chewing-side preferences (CSPs) on the given sectional planes ($z = 30$): (a) subject with the left CSP and (b) subject with the right CSP. Significant activations of the bilateral SM1 are shown. Color code denotes T values. Abbreviations: T_P, tongue protrusion; T_R, TM to the right; T_L, TM to the left; R, right side; L, left side. Reproduced from Shinagawa et al. [14], with permission from IADR/AADR.

strong left CSP volunteered to participate in Experiment 2. General conditions and training session were identical to those in Experiment 1. After training the TMs, each subject performed two runs before and after gum chewing. First, the subject performed a run that consisted of 290 scans before gum chewing. The subject was then instructed to voluntarily chew a gum base (Recaldent, Warner-Lambert, Japan) on the bilateral dentition for 5 min. Immediately after chewing, the second run that consisted of the same number of scans was performed. The subject performed each of three randomized TM tasks six times, and each was followed by a "rest" period as a control. fMRI data obtained from each subject after gum chewing were divided into two phases, the first and second 10 min beginning immediately after gum chewing. Statistical comparisons were performed for the group and for each subject, and used to identify regions with significantly increased activation during TMs relative to "rest" in three conditions before and after gum chewing. The following subtractions were performed: (1) TM-"rest" before gum chewing, (2) TM-"rest" in the first 10 min after gum chewing and (3) TM-"rest" in the second 10 min after gum chewing. An unpaired t test was used to compare the mBOLD on the bilateral SM1 for TMs before and after gum chewing. The main and interaction effects of gum chewing and TMs on the mBOLD in each SM1 were tested by the F test, and repeated using two-way ANOVA followed by Fisher's test. Statistical significance was established at $p < 0.01$.

3. Results

In Experiment 1, the regions activated during T_{P+R+L} were detected bilaterally in the SM1, cerebellum, supplementary motor area, operculum, insula, putamen and thalamus. Further, to investigate the activation pattern in individual cortices, the tongue movements were segregated into T_P, T_R and T_L. Notable focal activations were seen in the bilateral SM1 during TMs (Fig. 1B). In the subject with left CSP, the right SM1 was more strongly activated than its left counterpart during T_P, T_R and T_L (Fig. 1Ca). On the other hand, the left SM1 was more strongly activated than the right SM1 during TMs in the subject with the right CSP (Fig. 1Cb). The individual-based analysis of BOLD signals in the SM1 for all subjects revealed that there were no significant hemispheric differences in the mBOLD during T_P, T_R, T_L and T_{P+R+L}. However, the mBOLD in the SM1 on the right side was significantly greater than that on the left side during T_{P+R+L} for subjects with the left CSP. On the other hand, in the SM1 for subjects with the right CSP, the mBOLD on the left side was significantly greater than that on the right side during T_{P+R+L}. In subjects with CSPs, the mBOLD in the SM1 in the hemisphere contralateral to the CSP was significantly greater than that in the ipsilateral hemisphere during T_{P+R+L}.

In Experiment 2, the BOLD signal in the right SM1 was significantly greater than that in the left before gum chewing. In the left SM1, the mBOLD significantly increased in the first 10 min after gum chewing compared with those before chewing during T_P, T_R and T_L. In the second 10 min after gum chewing, the mBOLD in the SM1 significantly decreased compared with those in the first 10 min during T_P and T_L, while there was no significant change during T_R. On the other hand, in the right SM1, there were no significant increases in the mBOLD during any TM in the first 10 min. In the second 10 min, there was no significant change during T_P or T_R, whereas there was a significant decrease during T_L. With regard to the main and interaction effects of gum chewing and TMs on the mBOLD in the SM1 of each hemisphere, only gum chewing ($p < 0.0001$) and not TMs, had an effect on the mBOLD in the bilateral SM1. On the other hand, there were no significant interaction effects of gum chewing and TMs on the mBOLD in the bilateral SM1.

4. Discussion

The two main findings in Experiment 1 are, first, areas of the bilateral SM1 were significantly activated regardless of the kind of TM, and, second, in subjects with an evident CSP, the signal intensity in the SM1 was significantly greater in the side contralateral to the CSP. No differences in the bilateral activation of the SM1 during the three kinds suggests that sensory inputs from intraoral structures of different locations during T_P, T_R and T_L may activate distinctive areas in the bilateral S1. Therefore, T_{P+R+L} as well as the individual tasks were analyzed to cancel the differential effects of trigeminal sensory inputs elicited by different tasks even though there appeared to be no significant differences in sensory inputs from the tongue to the bilateral S1 [15]. When the subjects were dichotomized and a group analysis was performed for the 10 subjects with an evident CSP regardless of the side, a significant contralateral dominance for T_{P+R+L} was found. This positive relationship between CSP and TM may indicate that the masticatory system concurrently maximizes jaw and tongue function.

Experiment 2 revealed that bilateral gum chewing enhanced activation of the SM1 ipsilateral to the CSP during TMs. It was found that there were no significant differences in the mBOLD in the SM1 during "rest" between the first and second 10 min after gum chewing. Therefore, a net increase in neuronal activities in the SM1 during TM might play a role. Although it is not clear why the area of activation in the SM1 increases after gum chewing, bilateral gum chewing may reinforce the sub-threshold chewing-related neuronal activity. It was shown that repetitive thumb movements induced rapid and short-term reorganization of the SM1 [16,17]. Bilateral jaw movement requires highly coordinated contraction and relaxation of many orofacial muscles. In addition, updated afferent information is always necessary to smoothly perform bilateral gum chewing. The increase in the TM-related activation of the SM1 after gum chewing may be comparable with that reported for thumb movement [16,17]. In Experiment 2, TM-related activation of the bilateral SM1 was equalized after gum chewing; a significant increase in the mBOLD was only seen on the left hemisphere. Although the neural mechanism for this is not clear, this finding is interesting in the context that chewing-related transient plasticity may be affected by long-term plastic change due to the left CSP. This assumption may be supported by the fact that there was no interaction effect between gum chewing and the TM pattern; there was only a main effect of gum chewing. Since there are several limitations in Experiment 2, including the small sample size and the unilateral CSP, further studies are necessary to understand the interaction among the CSP, hemispheres and chewing.

Acknowledgements

The author is grateful to Dr. Hideo Shinagawa, Dr. Yasuo Ishiwata, Prof. Ei-ichi Honda, Prof. Takehito Sasaki, Prof. Masato Taira, Prof. Atsushi Iriki, Prof. Takayuki Kuroda and Prof. Kimie Ohyama for their comments, guidance and collaboration to conduct the study. This research was supported by Grants-in-Aid 10307052 and 09470467 from the Japanese Ministry of Education, Culture, Sports, Science and Technology.

References

[1] C. Porac, S. Coren, Lateral Preferences and Human Behavior, Quintesscence, New York, 1981.
[2] L.V. Christensen, J.T. Radue, Lateral preference in mastication: a feasibility study, J. Oral Rehabil. 12 (1985) 421–427.
[3] E. Helkimo, G.E. Carlsson, M. Helkimo, Chewing efficiency and state of dentition: a methodologic study, Acta Odontol. Scand. 36 (1978) 33–41.
[4] L.H. Pond, N. Barghi, G.M. Barnwell, Occlusion and chewing side preference, J. Prosthet. Dent. 55 (1986) 498–500.
[5] W. Penfield, E. Boldrey, Somatic motor and sensory representation in the cerebral cortex as studied by electrical stimulation, Brain 60 (1937) 389–443.
[6] D.R. Corfield, et al., Cortical and subcortical control of tongue movement in humans: a functional neuro-imaging study using fMRI, J. Appl. Physiol. 86 (1999) 1468–1477.
[7] L. Mioche, K.M. Hiiemae, J.B. Palmer, A postero-anterior videofluorographic study of the intra-oral management of food in man, Arch. Oral Biol. 47 (2002) 267–280.

[8] J.B. Palmer, K.M. Hiiemae, J. Liu, Tongue–jaw linkages in human feeding: a preliminary videofluoro-graphic study, Arch. Oral Biol. 42 (1997) 429–441.

[9] K.M. Hiiemae, J.B. Palmer, Tongue movements in feeding and speech, Crit. Rev. Oral Biol. Med. 146 (2003) 413–429.

[10] K. Takada, et al., Tongue, jaw, and lip muscle activity and jaw movement during experimental chewing efforts in man, J. Dent. Res. 75 (1996) 1598–1606.

[11] T. Momose, et al., Effect of mastication on regional cerebral blood flow in humans examined by positron-emission tomography with ^{15}O-labelled water and magnetic resonance imaging, Arch. Oral Biol. 42 (1997) 57–61.

[12] M. Funakoshi, et al., Effects of mastication on post-natal development of brain, in: K. Kubota (Ed.), Mechanobiological Research on the Masticatory System, VEB Verlag fur Medizin und Biologie, Berlin, 1989, pp. 162–167.

[13] J. Talairach, P. Tournoux, Co-Planar Stereotaxic Atlas of the Human Brain, Thieme, New York, 1988.

[14] H. Shinagawa, et al., Hemispheric dominance of tongue control depends on the chewing-side preference, J. Dent. Res. 82 (2003) 278–283.

[15] J.V. Pardo, et al., PET study of the localization and laterality of lingual somatosensory processing in humans, Neurosci. Lett. 234 (1997) 23–26.

[16] J. Classen, et al., Rapid plasticity of human cortical movement representation induced by practice, J. Neuro-physiol. 79 (1998) 1117–1123.

[17] J. Liepert, C. Terborg, C. Weiller, Motor plasticity induced by synchronized thumb and foot movements, Exp. Brain Res. 125 (1999) 435–439.

International Congress Series 1270 (2004) 105–110

www.ics-elsevier.com

ELSEVIER

Cortical regulation during the early stage of initiation of voluntary swallowing ☆

Shinichi Abe[a,*], Yutaka Watanabe[b], Masuro Shintani[c],
Gen-yuki Yamane[b], Yoshinobu Ide[a],
Masaki Shimono[d], Tatsuya Ishikawa[e]

[a] Department of Anatomy, Tokyo Dental College, 1-2-2 Masago, Mihakma, Chiba 261-8502, Japan
[b] Department of Oral Medicine, Tokyo Dental College, Japan
[c] Brain Research Laboratory, Tokyo Dental College, Japan
[d] Department of Oral Physiology, Tokyo Dental College, Japan
[e] Department of Conservative Dentistry, Tokyo Dental College, Japan

Abstract. The aim of the present study was to reveal the spatiotemporal relations among cortical regions involved in the initiation of voluntary swallowing in humans, using magnetoencephalography (MEG). The swallowing-related activity was distributed widely for 2000 ms before the electromyogram (EMG) onset of the right suprahyoid muscle. The cingulate cortex, the insula and the inferior frontal gyrus were the main loci active prior to swallowing. These cortical loci coincide with those suggested by previous human brain mapping studies that investigated the brain mechanism, which controls swallowing. Activation in the cingulate cortex was registered in the early stage of swallowing and could be related to the cognitive process regarding the food being safe to swallow. The activation in the insula lasted for a long period of time before the initiation of swallowing. This suggests that the long-lasting activation in the insula prior to swallowing is essential for the initiation of swallowing. © 2004 Elsevier B.V. All rights reserved.

Keywords: Deglutition; Magnetoencephalography; Insula; Cingulate cortex; Inferior frontal gyrus

1. Introduction

The average age of the human population is increasing rapidly and as a result, certain health care issues have arisen. Because of increased care for the aged, dysphagia (difficulty in swallowing) has been recognized as a growing health problem to be treated and, accordingly, it calls attention to the mechanism of swallowing. Swallowing is regulated by "the swallowing center" in the brainstem [1], and the glossopharyngeal nerve [2] and the superior laryngeal nerve [3] have been identified as afferent fibers to

☆ A part of this study was published in two papers [8,9].
* Corresponding author. Tel.: +81-43-270-3571; fax: +81-43-277-4010.
E-mail address: shinabe@tdc.ac.jp (S. Abe).

0531-5131/ © 2004 Elsevier B.V. All rights reserved.
doi:10.1016/j.ics.2004.04.048

elicit swallows. However, the initiation of swallowing is partially a voluntary action that requires the integrity of sensorimotor areas of the cerebral cortex [4]. In this respect, non-invasive techniques, such as functional magnetic resonance imaging (fMRI) [5] and positron emission tomography (PET) [6], have been utilized to demonstrate the cortical neuroanatomy of swallowing. Previous studies in this area have suggested that various regions of the brain, including the cingulate cortex, the supplementary motor area, the premotor area, the motor area and the insula, are involved in the execution of voluntary swallowing.

The aim of the present study was to define spatiotemporal relations among regions of the brain involved in the central initiation of human voluntary swallowing, using the magnetoencephalography (MEG) technique.

2. Materials and methods

2.1. Subjects and tasks

The protocol was approved by the ethical committee of the Oral Health Science Center at the Tokyo Dental College. Nine healthy men (aged 25–30 years), who gave their informed consent, participated in the study. None of the subjects had a history of swallowing problems in terms of subjective or objective symptoms, and they were all right-handed as assessed with a modified version of the Edinburgh Inventory. The subjects were instructed to sit in a relaxed position in a magnetically shielded room with their heads supported against the helmet-shaped sensor array of the magnetometer.

2.2. Data recording

Magnetic brain signals were recorded non-invasively with pairs of gradiometers of 204 channels from 102 loci in the cerebral cortex using a MEG (4-D Neuroimaging, Vectorview, Helsinki, Finland). To monitor eye movements, an electrooculogram (EOG) was recorded with a pair of electrodes placed on the left upper and lower orbital regions. Electromyograms (EMGs) were recorded with a pair of surface electrodes attached to the right suprahyoid muscles and the right extensor digitorum muscle. During the recording session, subjects were asked to concentrate on performing the two tasks described above. Outside the shielded room and throughout the session, EOG, EMG and MEG signals were monitored with a computer display in an operating room. The behavior of the subject was also monitored from the operating room using a video camera. Raw data were stored on a CD-ROM disk for later, off-line analysis. All signals were digitized at 401 Hz and were bandpass filtered (0.03–15 Hz for MEG and EOG, and 100–200 Hz for EMG).

The MEG signal was 3000 ms in duration, starting 2500 ms prior to the EMG onset and ending 500 ms after the EMG onset, and was recorded during the two tasks. The onset was determined by the time when the suprahyoid or digitorum EMG activity exceeded a certain level. Before averaging, the spontaneous signals were reviewed off-line to exclude inadequate triggering signals, so that epochs containing eye motion artifacts, ambiguous EMG bursts or other artifacts were omitted from the analysis. Thirty epochs, considered to be acceptable under the abovementioned criteria, were averaged for one task. Dipole field patterns were automatically sought first at every 5 ms on the whole head, and separately in the left and right hemisphere. Isocontour maps were constructed at a time point within the analysis window from the field distribution of the cortex using the minimum-norm estimate. The equivalent current dipoles (ECDs) were determined from the MEG signals using single-dipole analysis. The ECDs were then superimposed on the subject's magnetic resonance images (MRIs) to show the source locations with respect to anatomical structure. Only ECDs over 75% of the field variance were accepted for the analyses.

3. Results

3.1. Signal configuration

Typical recordings of the magnetic component of brain electromagnetic activity during swallowing as shown in Fig. 1. Each contains 102 lines for 3000 ms of magnetic force recorded by 204 sets of SQUID aligned over the head. It is clear that the swallowing-related activities were distributed widely for 2000 ms before the EMG onset.

3.2. Activation foci with swallowing and finger movement

First, the cortical loci activated during voluntary swallowing were documented. Although there was little difference in the activity patterns among the subjects, activities were observed mainly at cortical loci of the anterior cingulate cortex (ACC: Brodmann's area (BA) 25, 24, 32, 33), the posterior cingulate cortex (PCC: BA31, 23), the middle frontal gyrus (MFG, i.e., premotor and motor area: BA8, 9), the inferior frontal gyrus (IFG: BA44) and the insula. Activation in the ACC, PCC and MFG was observed in four of the eight subjects, and activation in the IFG was observed in five of the eight subjects. Regarding the insula, seven of the eight subjects showed activation. Although the activity was found only in one or two of the eight subjects, the supplementary motor area (SMA:

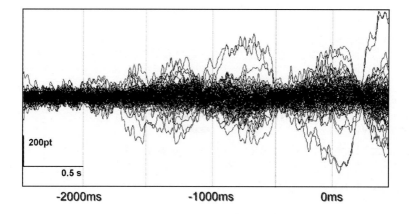

Fig.1. The time of the swallowing trigger was regarded as 0 ms, and all changes in the magnetic field in the cerebral cortex between 2500 ms before swallowing and 500 ms after swallowing overlapped [9].

BA8, 9), the superior frontal gyrus (SFG: BA8) and the primary motor cortex and premotor cortex (i.e., lateral precentral gyrus: BA4 or 6) were also activated during swallowing (Table 1).

3.3. Hemispheric asymmetry of cortical activation

From the previous imaging studies, we had expected the current source to be related to swallowing for multiple sites and for a long duration of the activity. Thus, ECDs were estimated automatically every 5 ms from 2500 ms before the EMG onset. Consequently, in the MFG, IFG and insula, long-lasting activations were found.

Our general observations can be described as follows. In the voluntary swallowing task, the activation sites deep in the frontal lobe, such as the ACC, the PCC and the SMA, were lateralized not only to be unilateral but also bilateral hemispheres as with the SFG (where only two subjects were involved). However, most of the activities in the MFG, the IFG and the insula were lateralized to the left hemisphere.

3.4. Temporal aspects of the cortical activities

In the voluntary swallowing, the cingulate cortex was activated in the early stage of the recording window (Fig. 2). The average latency from the onset of the suprahyoid muscle burst was obtained as -1682 ± 519 ms ($n=6$) for the ACC, -1969 ± 146 ms ($n=7$) for the PCC and -1259 ± 615 ms ($n=49$) for the insula. Obviously, activation in the PCC occurred prior to the insula ($p<0.003$, one way ANOVA and Bonferroni test). Activities in loci other than the cingulate cortex and the insula occurred shortly after the

Table 1
Activated regions of all subjects according to the process of time [9]

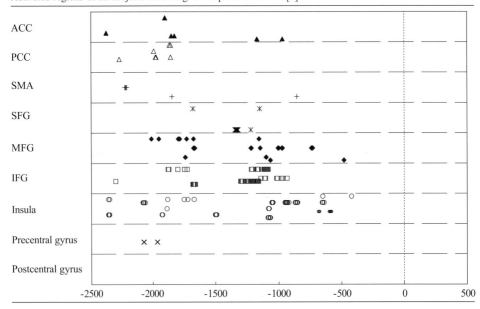

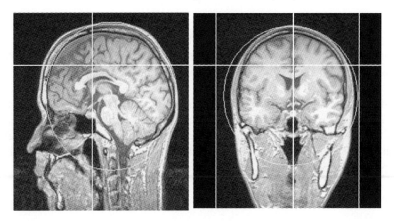

Fig. 2. Overlapping of the nerve activity sources on MRI images [8].(A): Frontal cross section. (B): Sagittal cross section. A nerve activity sources was estimated to be present at the position indicated with the arrow, which may be in the cingulate gyrus.

start of the recording. The mean latencies for the SMA, the SFG, the MFG and the IFG were measured as -1929 ± 545 ms $(n=6)$, -1338 ± 144 ms $(n=9)$, -1286 ± 439 ms $(n=25)$ and -1262 ± 249 ms $(n=52)$, respectively.

It should be noted that activities in the insula were generally consistent among the subjects. The activities also began during the early stage of the recording window and were distributed widely in the window as seen in the large standard deviation (i.e., activities in the insula were long-lasting prior to the initiation of swallowing). Activities observed in some of the ACC, the PCC and the SMA, i.e. the loci located on the inferior side of the frontal lobe, were distributed in the early stage of the recording window (2375–1825 ms before the EMG onset). Activities then began in the MFG or in the IFG at around 1055–2010 ms before the EMG onset. Activation at the precentral gyrus was rare and was observed in the early stage of the recording window (mean latency: -2018 ± 64 ms, $n=4$).

4. Discussion

Our study used MEG to demonstrate the temporal aspect of cortical activation which occurs during voluntary swallowing. As described in the introduction, MEG detects neural activity through magnetic field changes. Therefore, its temporal resolution may be better than that of other imaging devices, such as fMRI and PET, but while muscles are active, cortical activities may not be recorded due to the magnetic field arising from the muscles. Therefore, we focused this study on clarifying the cortical initiation of voluntary swallowing.

In this study, MEG revealed that the insula, the cingulate cortex and the inferior frontal gyrus were the main active loci prior to the voluntary swallowing movement. Those cortices are cytoarchitectonically and functionally distinct and coincide with the loci suggested by previous human brain mapping studies to be involved in the regulation of swallowing. In the present study, the left insula was the most pronounced locus among the loci activated prior to swallowing, and this was observed in nearly all the subjects that participated (seven out of eight subjects). This suggests that the insula may be essential for the initiation of swallowing. In this respect, Daniels and Foundas [7] studied unilateral stroke patients with discrete lesions of the insular cortex to determine the role of the insula in swallowing. They confirmed dysphagia using videofluoroscopy in three of the four patients. All patients had lesions that involved the anterior insula, whereas the only patient without dysphagia had a lesion restricted to the posterior insula. In the present study, the anterior insula was confirmed to be the locus activated in all subjects studied. This suggests that the long-lasting activation in the insula prior to swallowing is essential for the initiation of swallowing. We now think that the rise of motivation before swallowing is most important for patients receiving treatment for dysphagia.

References

[1] A. Jean, Brain stem control of swallowing: neuronal network and cellular mechanisms, Physiol. Rev. 81 (2001) 929–969.

[2] J. Kitagawa, et al., Pharyngeal branch of the glossopharyngeal nerve plays a major role in reflex swallowing from the pharynx, Am. J. Physiol., Regul. Integr. Comp. Physiol. 282 (2002) R1342–R1347.

[3] T. Sumi, Interrelation between rhythmic mastication and reflex deglutition as studied on the unitary activity of trigeminal motoneurons in rabbits, Jpn. J. Physiol. 27 (1977) 687–699.

[4] R.E. Martin, B.J. Sessle, The role of the cerebral cortex in swallowing, Dysphagia 8 (1993) 195–202.

[5] R.E. Martin, et al., Cerebral cortical representation of automatic and volitional swallowing in humans, J. Neurophysiol. 85 (2001) 938–950.

[6] S. Hamdy, et al., Identification of the cerebral loci processing human swallowing with $H2^{15}O$ PET activation, J. Neurophysiol. 81 (1999) 1917–1926.

[7] S.K. Daniels, A.L. Foundas, The role of the insular cortex in dysphagia, Dysphagia 12 (1997) 146–156.

[8] S. Abe, et al., Magnetoencephalographic study of the starting point of voluntary swallowing, Cranio 21 (1) (2003) 46–49.

[9] Y. Watanabe, et al., Cortical regulation during the early stage of initiation of voluntary swallowing in humans, Dysphagia (2004) (in press).

International Congress Series 1270 (2004) 111–116

ELSEVIER

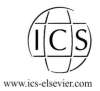

www.ics-elsevier.com

Involvement of chewing in memory processes in humans: an approach using fMRI

K. Sasaguri[a], S. Sato[a], Y. Hirano[a], S. Aoki[b], T. Ishikawa[b],
M. Fujita[c], K. Watanabe[c], M. Tomida[d], Y. Ido[e], M. Onozuka[a,*]

[a]Department of Physiology and Neuroscience, Kanagawa Dental College, 82 Inaoka-cho Yokosuka,
Kanagawa 238-8580, Japan
[b]Tokyo Dental College, Chiba, Japan
[c]Gifu University School of Medicine, Gifu, Japan
[d]Tokyo Women's Medical University School of Medicine, Tokyo, Japan
[e]Kizawa Memorial Hospital, Minokamo, Japan

Abstract. Using fMRI in young and aged human brains, we evaluated the link between masticatory function and senile processes. Chewing resulted in a bilateral increase in blood oxygenation level-dependent (BOLD) signals in the sensorimotor cortex, supplementary motor area, insula, thalamus, amygdala, and cerebellum in both age groups, but the increase was smaller in the first three regions and higher in the cerebellum in the aged subjects. Interestingly, only the aged subjects showed significant signal increases in the association areas, which received information from the primary sensorimotor cortex, supplementary area, or insula, and an increase in the hippocampal BOLD signal and memory acquisition. Similar effects in elderly subjects were seen as a result of more leisurely eating with increased chewing due to the wearing of dentures. The results indicate the involvement of chewing in the neuronal circuit to the hippocampus in the elderly, which plays an important role in preventing aged-related deterioration in the hippocampus. © 2004 Elsevier B.V. All rights reserved.

Keywords: Chewing; Memory; Aging; Brain; Hippocampus

1. Introduction

In recent years, much effort has been devoted to evaluating the interaction between masticatory function and senile dementia [8]. In previous experimental studies, masticatory dysfunction has been shown to be involved in the senile process of hippocampal mechanisms, e.g. reduced spatial cognition [14,15,19], decreased input activities [18], enhanced neuronal degeneration [3,12,14,15,19] and the decline in the cholinergic system [13]. In addition, a soft diet from the weanling stage causes later impairment of avoidance performance in mice [4], and differences in neuronal density between the right and left cerebral hemispheres are seen in rats with unilateral mastication [2]. These findings

* Corresponding author. Tel.: +81-46-822-9067; fax: +81-46-822-8869.
E-mail address: onozuka@kdcnet.ac.jp (M. Onozuka).

0531-5131/ © 2004 Elsevier B.V. All rights reserved.
doi:10.1016/j.ics.2004.04.046

strongly suggest that masticatory work may play an important role in neuronal function in the aged brain. However, in humans, the mechanism that links senile processes of memory to masticatory function has not been fully documented, although analysis using positron emission tomography (PET) has shown that chewing increases blood flow in various regions of the cerebral cortex [6].

Functional magnetic resonance imaging (fMRI) has provided a new tool for testing specific hypotheses about the anatomical and physiological regions involved in processing sensory and motor information in the human brain [16]. Blood oxygenation level-dependent (BOLD) contrast fMRI not only detects small signal changes that are related to changes in the magnetization of protons within the blood, but also provides enhanced spatial and temporal resolution [5]. We therefore used fMRI to assess the link between masticatory function and senile processes in the intact human brain.

2. Materials and methods

2.1. Subjects

Two groups of right-handed male subjects were studied, a young group (19–26 years) and an aged group (61–72 years). In the present study, the subjects with neurological or psychiatric disease were excluded from the study. Written informed consent was obtained from each subject after a full explanation of the study, and all subjects were studied with local ethical approval (Committees of Kizawa Memorial Hospital).

2.2. Task paradigm

The subject performed four cycles, each consisting of 32 s of rhythmic chewing of gums without odor or taste and 32 s without chewing.

In another experiment, to evaluate the involvement of chewing in hippocampal activity, BOLD signal changes in this region during picture encoding were examined before and after chewing of moderately hard gum for 2 min. Four cycles of 16 pictures of scenes (experimental) and 16 showing the " + " character on a blue background (control) were performed, with the subject trying to memorize a picture projected every 2 s.

2.3. Image acquisition

During this encoding, BOLD signals in the hippocampus were continuously recorded and compared before and after chewing of gum. For each subject, functional (T_2*-weighted) images, followed by an anatomical (T_1-weighted) image, were acquired using a 1.5-T Horizon MRI scanner (GE, USA). The functional images consisted of echo-planar image volumes, which were sensitive to BOLD contrast in the axial orientation (TE = 44 ms, TR = 4000 ms). The volume covered the entire brain with a 64×64 matrix and 42 slices (voxel size = $3.75 \times 3.75 \times 4$ mm, slice thickness = 3.8 mm, gap = 0.2 mm).

2.4. Data analysis

Data analysis was performed as described previously [10]. Briefly, motion artifacts, which may have been due to chewing, were removed by a low-pass filter of 1.5 s using

MEDx software. Furthermore, we confirmed that motion artifacts were less than 0.01 mm (0.267% of a voxel) in any direction. The successive functional images for each subject were normalized to the MNI template, and spatially smoothed with an 8-mm Gaussian kernel using SPM99. Statistical analysis, based on the general linear model approach [1], was employed. Global changes in the BOLD signal were removed using proportional scaling. The resulting areas of activation were characterized in terms of peak height and spatial extent. Group analysis [3] was used to characterize differences in brain neuronal activation during chewing between the two age groups, in addition to individual analysis.

3. Results

In all subjects, chewing was associated with increases in the BOLD signal in various regions of the brain, with significant increases being seen in the sensorimotor cortex, supplementary motor area, insula, amygdala, thalamus, and cerebellum (Fig. 1). The increase in the signal during chewing was dependent on biting force. In addition, in agreement with a previous finding [10], a study using hard and moderately hard types of gum showed that, in the sensorimotor cortex, supplementary motor area, insula, and amygdala, chewing of moderately hard gum resulted in a larger increase in the BOLD signal than the chewing of hard gum, whereas the converse was true for the signal in the cerebellum, while no difference in signal increase was seen in the thalamus.

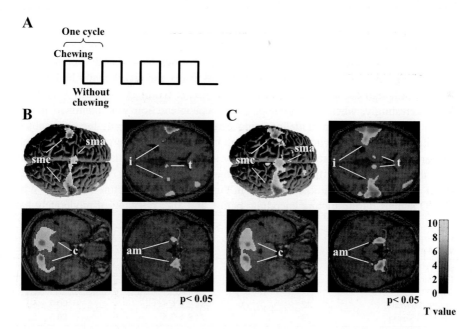

Fig. 1. Effect of aging on brain regional activity during gum chewing of moderately hard gum. (A) The task paradigm used. Significant signal increases associated with chewing were seen in a young adult subject (B) and an aged subject (C). Abbreviations: smc, primary sensorimotor cortex; sma, supplementary motor area; i, insula; t, thalamus; c, cerebellum; am, amygdala. Scale: *t* value.

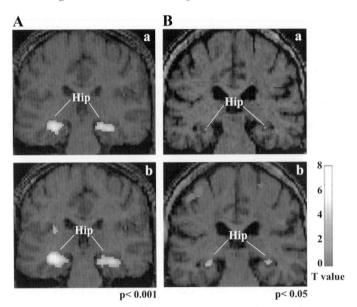

Fig. 2. Effect of aging on hippocampal activity before and after 2-min chewing of moderately hard types of gum. (A) Young subject; (B) aged subject. A significant signal increase associated with picture encoding between before (a) and after (b) chewing was seen in an aged subject. Hip, hippocampus. Scale: t value.

Using moderately hard gum, we also examined whether differences in chewing-induced brain activation were seen between the young and aged groups. When group analysis was employed, the increased signal intensity in the aged group was slightly smaller in the sensorimotor cortex, supplementary motor area, and insula and significantly higher in the cerebellum, although the activated volume was different (compare between A and B in Fig. 1). Interestingly, when the psychophysiological interaction was examined in each subject by structural equation modeling using AMOS software [3], only the aged subjects showed significant increases in various association areas, which receive information from the primary sensorimotor cortex, supplementary motor area, or insula (data not shown).

Since the hippocampus is indispensable for memory formation [17], we also evaluated the effect of chewing on neuronal activities in this region during picture encoding. When the BOLD signals during picture encoding, before and after chewing of moderately hard

Table 1
Effect of 2-min chewing on memory acquisition

Subjects	Number	Score (accuracy rate), %	
		Before chewing	After chewing
Young (19–26 years)	42	88.2 ± 6.6	90.7 ± 5.3
Aged (60–73 years)	33	73.8 ± 7.6	80.3 ± 8.8

The results are expressed as the mean value of accuracy rate (%) when the retrieval test was performed before or after chewing for 2 min. *$p < 0.01$ compared with corresponding score before chewing. Note that aged subjects showed a significant increase in memory acquisition after chewing for 2 min, whereas no effect was seen in young subjects.

gum were measured, we found that, in aged subjects, gum chewing not only enhanced hippocampal neuronal activities (Fig. 2), but also increased memory acquisition (Table 1). Young subjects, however, revealed no significant effect. Similar effects in elderly subjects were seen as a result of more leisurely eating, with increased chewing, or being fitted with dentures.

4. Discussion

This study demonstrates that chewing induces regional increases in BOLD signals in various regions of the brain, some of which are related to aging. In this study, in agreement with a previous PET finding [6], chewing significantly activated the oral region of the primary sensorimotor cortex, supplementary motor area, insula, thalamus, and cerebellum. These regions are believed to receive sensory information from the lips, tongue, oral mucosa, gingivae, teeth, mandibles, and temporomandibular joint, and to control masticatory movement and the lingual and facial muscles [7,8], and, thus, may be called the masticatory center [7]. Furthermore, from the results obtained using a gum, a moderate biting force may be most effective in maintaining neuronal activities within the brain.

Studies on aging and mastication have shown that the loss of teeth and deficits in masticatory muscle power with advanced age impair masticatory function, thereby causing a reduction in sensory input activity to the central nervous system [9]. Thus, the smaller BOLD signal increase seen in the sensorimotor cortex, supplementary motor area, and insula during chewing in aged subjects may be due to such age-related deterioration. In addition, based on our past finding [11] that the increase in the BOLD signal in some association areas was lost on continuous chewing, short periods of chewing separated by intervals of no chewing may be very important for increased neuronal activity in the association cortex, in which sensory information is projected via the perforant path onto the hippocampal formation, playing a crucial role in learning and memory [17]. Indeed, in the aged, gum chewing for 2 min enhanced hippocampal neuronal activity and increased memory acquisition. Taken together with the fact that these effects are also seen in the elderly as a result of more leisurely eating or the fitting of dentures, we propose the following mechanism. In the elderly, chewing indirectly activates the association areas through neuronal circuits within the mastication center. Sensory information in this center is projected through the perforant path onto the hippocampus, the first brain region to show neuropathological changes with advancing age, as well as playing a crucial role in learning and memory [17]. Input activities in the central nervous system are known to play an indispensable role in suppressing neuronal degeneration. In the present study, chewing was also found to activate the amygdala, which is closely related to the hippocampus [3].

In conclusion, we suggest involvement of chewing in the neuronal circuit to the hippocampus in the elderly, which plays an important role in preventing age-related deterioration in the hippocampus. Therefore, we strongly support that chewing is a useful therapy for preventing senile dementia.

Acknowledgements

This work was supported by Grants-in-Aid for Scientific Research from the Ministry of Education, Science and Culture of Japan (14370630; 15390590) and a grant from Lotte

(Tokyo, Japan). We also express our deep gratitude to K. Hasegawa, N. Muramatsu and Y. Nomura for their excellent assistance.

References

[1]   K.L. Friston, et al, Statistical parametric maps in functional imaging, Hum. Brain Mapp. 2 (1995) 189–210.

[2]   H. Fujisawa, The effect of mastication on post-natal development of the rat brain with a histological and behavioral study, J. Jpn. Oral Biol. 32 (1990) 495–508.

[3]   T. Iidaka, et al, Neural interaction of the amygdala with the prefrontal and temporal cortices in the processing of facial expressions as revealed by fMRI, Cogn. Brain Res. 9 (2000) 73–83.

[4]   S. Kawamura, The effect of food consistency on conditioned avoidance response in mice and rats, Jpn. J. Oral Biol. 31 (1989) 71–82.

[5]   E.M. Meisenzahl, R. Schlosser, Functional magnetic resonance imaging research in psychiatry, Neuroimag. Clin. N. Am. 11 (2001) 365–374.

[6]   I. Momose, et al, Effect of mastication on regional cerebral blood flow in humans examined by positron-emission tomography with 15O-labelled water and magnetic resonance imaging, Arch. Oral Biol. 42 (1997) 57–61.

[7]   Y. Nakamura, N. Katakura, Generation of masticatory rhythm in the brainstem, Neurosci. Res. 23 (1995) 1–19.

[8]   M. Nakata, Masticatory function and its effects on general health, Int. Dent. J. 48 (1998) 540–548.

[9]   K. Okimoto, et al, Ageing and mastication: the relationship between oral status and the progress of dementia at senile hospital, J. Jpn. Prosthodont. Soc. 35 (1991) 931–943.

[10] M. Onozuka, et al, Mapping brain region activity during chewing: a functional magnetic resonance imaging study, J. Dent. Res. 81 (2002) 743–746.

[11] M. Onozuka, et al, Age-related changes in brain regional activity during chewing: a functional magnetic resonance imaging study, J. Dent. Res. 82 (2003) 657–660.

[12] M. Onozuka, et al, Evidence for involvement of glucocorticoid response in the hippocampal changes in aged molarless SAMP8 mice, Behav. Brain Res. 131 (2002) 125–129.

[13] M. Onozuka, et al, Changes in the septohippocampal cholinergic system following removal of molar teeth in the aged SAMP8 mouse, Behav. Brain Res. 133 (2002) 197–204.

[14] M. Onozuka, et al, Reduced mastication stimulates impairment of spatial memory and degeneration of hippocampal neurons in aged SAMP8 mice, Brain Res. 826 (1999) 148–153.

[15] M. Onozuka, et al, Impairment of spatial memory and changes in astroglial responsiveness following loss of molar teeth in aged SAMP8 mice, Behav. Brain Res. 108 (2000) 145–155.

[16] F. Pulvermuller, Words in the brain's language, Behav. Brain Sci. 22 (1999) 253–336.

[17] B.H. Wainer, et al, Ascending cholinergic pathways: functional organization and implications for disease models, Prog. Brain Res. 98 (1993) 9–30.

[18] K. Watanabe, et al, The molarless condition in aged SAMP8 mice attenuates hippocampal Fos induction linked to water maze performance, Behav. Brain Res. 128 (2002) 19–25.

[19] K. Watanabe, et al, Evidence for involvement of dysfunctional teeth in the senile process in the hippocampus of SAMP8 mice, Exp. Gerontol. 36 (2001) 283–295.

International Congress Series 1270 (2004) 117–120

www.ics-elsevier.com

ELSEVIER

Relationship between cortical motor functions and orofacial disease: the mirror neuron system and temporomandibular disorders

Yoshiyuki Shibukawa [a,b,c,*], Tatsuya Ishikawa [a], Zhen-Kang Zhang [d],
Ting Jiang [e], Masuro Shintani [a], Masaki Shimono [a],
Toshifumi Kumai [a,f], Yutaka Kato [a], Takashi Suzuki [a,b],
Motoichiro Kato [a,g], Yoshio Nakamura [a]

[a] Laboratory of Brain Research, Oral Health Science Center, Tokyo Dental College, 1-2-2 Masago,
Mihama-ku, Chiba 261-8502, Japan
[b] Department of Physiology, Tokyo Dental College, Japan
[c] Department of Physiology and Biophysics, Faculty of Medicine, University of Calgary, 3330 Hospital Drive
N.W., Calgary, AB, Canada T2N 4N1
[d] Department of Maxillofacial Surgery, Stomatology School of Peking University, China
[e] Department of Prosthetic Dentistry, Stomatology School of Peking University, China
[f] Department of Oral Physiology, Matsumoto Dental University, Japan
[g] Department of Neuropsychiatry, Keio University School of Medicine, Japan

Abstract. A group of neurons in the monkey premotor cortex discharges both when the monkey is performing a given action as well as when it is observing the experimenter performing a similar action (mirror neuron system; action execution/observation matching system). Several brain imaging studies indicate that this system also exists in humans. The present study aimed to compare activation patterns of the cortical areas activated during observation of jaw movements between healthy normal subjects and patients with temporomandibular disorders (TMD). Whole-scalp neuromagnetic responses were recorded from five healthy volunteers and six patients with TMD. The subjects were instructed to carefully observe a pre-recorded video of bilaterally symmetrical jaw-opening movements performed by another individual. During the observation task in healthy subjects, we found magnetic signals generated by the region of the occipitotemporal region near the inferior temporal sulcus and maxillofacial area of the primary motor cortex. In patients, however, we found the attenuation of magnetic response from primary motor cortex. These findings suggest that the maxillofacial area of the primary motor cortex is included in the jaw movement-related action execution/observation matching system in humans, and provide new neuropathological evidence that

* Corresponding author. Department of Physiology and Biophysics, Faculty of Medicine, University of Calgary, 3330 Hospital Drive N.W., Calgary, AB, Canada T2N 4N1. Tel.: +1-403-220-4537; fax: +1-403-210-8743.

  E-mail address: yshibuka@tdc.ac.jp (Y. Shibukawa).

0531-5131/ © 2004 Elsevier B.V. All rights reserved.
doi:10.1016/j.ics.2004.04.096

TMD patients exhibit dysfunction of the jaw movement-related action execution/observation matching system. © 2004 Elsevier B.V. All rights reserved.

Keywords: Human; Magnetoencephalography; Mirror neuron system; Motor cortex; Temporomandibular disorder; Visual cortex

1. Introduction

Temporomandibular disorder (TMD) is a collective term embracing a number of chronic pain related problems that involve the masticatory musculature and/or the temporomandibular joint(s) [1]. Although the pathological mechanisms underlying TMD have remained poorly understood, convergent evidence has suggested that the development of TMD could result from pathological changes in neurophysiological functions in the central nervous system [2–4]. In this study, we hypothesized that patients with TMD may show dysfunction of the human motor related cortical regions that directly control orofacial motor behavior and the masticatory neuromuscular system.

It is well known that a group of neurons in the monkey premotor cortex (area F5) discharges while the monkey performs a given action as well as when the monkey observes the experimenter performing a similar action (mirror neurons) [5,6]. Mirror neurons play an important role in matching action observation and execution (an action observation/execution matching system), as well as in imitation and understanding for action. Neuroimaging studies have indicated that a similar system (MNS) also exists in the human brain. MEG recordings have shown that Brodmann's area 44 (Broca's area in the left hemisphere) and the primary motor cortex (M1) are included in the human MNS [7,8]. Shibukawa et al. [9] reported that the region in the human precentral gyrus activated during observation of simple jaw opening movements corresponded with the region activated in the execution of voluntary jaw opening movements. Therefore, they reported that the face region in the human primary motor cortex is involved in an action execution/observation matching system for voluntary jaw movement.

To have a better understanding of the possible modification of the cortical machinery for the orofacial motor functions in patients with TMD, we examined our hypothesis that patients with TMD may show dysfunction of the human motor cortical function related to the MNS associated with jaw movements.

2. Experimental procedures

Subjects consisted of five healthy adults who had no abnormal findings in oral function and six patients suffering from TMD. All of the subjects were right-handed. All of the subjects gave written informed consent to participate in the present study, which was approved by the Ethics Committee of Tokyo Dental College in accordance with the Declaration of Helsinki. The subjects were asked to carefully observe a series of video-clips (30 frames/s) of bilaterally symmetrical jaw opening movements performed by another person (Fig. 1A). A 306-channel neuromagnetometer (Vectorview, Neuromag, Helsinki, Finland) was used for recording magnetic fields. The magnetic signals recorded in 100 trials in a session were averaged. The analysis period was set to 1300 ms, from 500

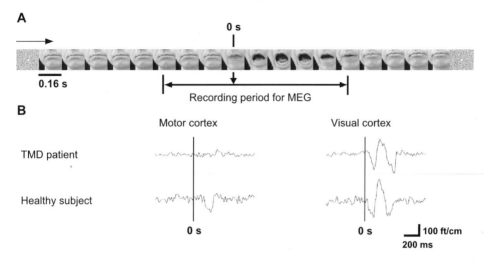

Fig. 1. (A) A sequential image shows a series of the video-clip representing one jaw opening movement sequence, moving from the left to right. Each image shows the first frame of every five consecutive frames with 1/6 s. The recording period was set to 1.3 s from 0.5 s preceding to 0.8 s following presentation of the frame showing the start of jaw opening movement. (B) Traces show the magnetic signals in the healthy subject (lower) and the TMD patient (upper) from the sensorimotor area (left traces) and occipital area (right traces). The straight lines indicate the start of jaw opening movement in video-stimuli which the subjects observed during the recordings.

ms preceding to 800 ms following the onset of the observing jaw movements. The sources of the dipolar magnetic field patterns were modelled as equivalent current dipoles (ECDs) whose three-dimensional location, orientation and strength were estimated in a spherical conductor model based on the individual MRIs obtained from each subject [10] (time-varying multi-dipole model [8,10]).

3. Results and discussion

Using a whole-head MEG, we obtained magnetic signals produced by neurons in the human cortex while the subjects observed videotaped jaw opening movements made by another individual (Fig. 1A). The signals were averaged with trigger pulses generated at the onset of the observed jaw opening movements. During the observation task of jaw opening movements, we found magnetic fields from the neuromagnetic sensor array located at the occipital region in the healthy subjects and TMD patients (Fig. 1B, right traces). In the TMD patients, however, we consistently found marked attenuation of magnetic signals from the sensors of sensorimotor regions compared with those from the same areas in the healthy subjects (Fig. 1B, left traces). In the multi-dipole analysis (not shown) on the healthy subjects, ECDs producing magnetic signals from the occipital and sensorimotor area were located in the occipitotemporal area near the inferior temporal sulcus (the human homologue of the monkey MT/V5) and the lateral part of the precentral gyrus (the maxillofacial region of the primary motor cortex; M1mx), respectively. In contrast, we could consistently detect the activities of magnetic fields from the MT/V5 in the TMD patients; however, the activation of those from M1mx were lacking (Fig. 1B).

M1mx activation in our healthy subjects is consistent with recent neurophysiological and neuroimaging evidence which has clearly shown that action observation is related to activation of cortical areas that are involved in motor control in humans [6,8,11]. Thus, our results indicate that the existence of jaw movement-related MNS (i.e. an action observation/execution matching system for jaw movements in humans) on M1mx and activities of the MNS (the M1mx) are attenuated in the TMD patients.

The attenuated cortical responses in the MNS in this study could explain the neuropathological mechanisms in TMD.

It has been reported that activation of the primary motor cortex by observation of jaw movements, as a MNS, plays a crucial role in orofacial motor functions including motor behavior and/or cognition [6,12,13]. In the present MEG recordings, therefore, it reasonably follows that the lack of primary motor cortex activation in association with jaw movement observation in the TMD patients reflects changes in cortical motor function. These cortical functional disturbances and/or disorders could result in uncontrolled orofacial motor behavior (e.g., teeth clenching and grinding, jaw thrusting) [1], and subsequent chronic pain in the TMD patients.

Acknowledgements

This work was supported by Grants (HRC 3A04, 3A12, 3A13) for High-Tech Research Center Projects from the Ministry of Education, Culture, Sports, Science and Technology of Japan to Y.N., M.K. and T.I.

References

[1] The American Academy of Orofacial Pain, in: J.P. Okeson (Ed.), Orofacial Pain: Guidelines for Assessment, Diagnosis, and Management, Quintessence Publishing, Carol Stream, Illinois, 1996, pp. 113–189.

[2] W. Maixner, et al., Sensitivity of patients with painful temporomandibular disorders to experimentally evoked pain, Pain 63 (1995) 341–351.

[3] C.R. Carlson, et al., Psychological and physiological parameters of masticatory muscle pain, Pain 76 (1998) 297–307.

[4] H.C. Tenenbaum, et al., Sensory and affective components of orofacial pain: is it all in your brain? Crit. Rev. Oral Biol. Med. 12 (2001) 455–468.

[5] V. Gallese, et al., Action recognition in the premotor cortex, Brain 119 (1996) 593–609.

[6] G. Rizzolatti, G. Luppino, The cortical motor system, Neuron 27 (2001) 889–901.

[7] G. Buccino, et al., Action observation activates premotor and parietal areas in a somatotopic manner: an fMRI study, Eur. J. Neurosci. 13 (2001) 400–404.

[8] N. Nishitani, R. Hari, Temporal dynamics of cortical representation for action, Proc. Natl. Acad. Sci. U. S. A. 18 (2000) 913–918.

[9] Y. Shibukawa, et al., Activation of human primary motor cortex during observation of jaw movements, in: H. Nowak, J. Haueisen, F. Giesler (Eds.), BIOMAG 2002, VDE-Verlag, Berlin, Germany, 2002, pp. 401–403.

[10] R. Hämäläinen, et al., Magnetoencephalography-theory, instrumentation, and applications to noninvasive studies of the working human brain, Rev. Mod. Phys. 65 (1993) 413–497.

[11] N. Nishitani, R. Hari, Viewing lip forms: cortical dynamics, Neuron 19 (2002) 1211–1220.

[12] G. Rizzolatti, M.A. Arbib, Language within our grasp, Trends Neurosci. 21 (1998) 188–194.

[13] R. Matsumoto, et al., Motor-related functional subdivisions of human lateral premotor cortex: epicortical recording in conditional visuomotor task, Clin. Neurophysiol. 114 (2003) 1102–1115.

International Congress Series 1270 (2004) 121–125

www.ics-elsevier.com

Ketamine inhibits pain-SEFs following CO_2 laser stimulation on trigeminally innervated skin region: a magnetoencephalographic study

Nobuyuki Matsuura[a,b,*], Yoshiyuki Shibukawa[a,c,d],
Tatsuya Ichinohe[a,b], Takashi Suzuki[a,c], Yuzuru Kaneko[a,b]

[a]Laboratory of Brain Research, Oral Health Science Center, Tokyo Dental College, Chiba, Japan
[b]Department of Dental Anesthesiology, Tokyo Dental College, Chiba, Japan
[c]Department of Physiology, Tokyo Dental College, Chiba, Japan
[d]Department of Physiology and Biophysics, Faculty of Medicine, University of Calgary, Canada

Abstract. Pain-related somatosensory-evoked magnetic fields (pain-SEFs) in the cerebral cortex are mainly detected in the secondary somatosensory cortex (SII) and the cingulate gyrus. However, there are no magnetoencephalography (MEG) studies that report the effects of analgesic agents on pain-SEFs. We therefore recorded the pain-SEFs, following CO_2 laser painful stimulation at 0.8 W on a trigeminally innervated skin region, and investigated the effects of ketamine hydrochloride (0.2 mg/kg IV), an N-methyl-D-aspartate (NMDA) receptor antagonist, on pain-SEFs in five healthy volunteers. Immediately after each recording, the magnitude of pain sensation was evaluated on a visual analogue scale (VAS). The equivalent current dipoles (ECDs) of pain-SEFs, following CO_2 laser painful stimulation, were estimated in the SII in the contralateral hemisphere with about 100-ms latency. Ketamine reversibly inhibited pain-SEFs and decreased VAS. The result suggests that ketamine blocked the NMDA receptors in the nociceptive relay station involved in the trigeminal caudal subnucleus, resulting in the reduction of cortical activation in the SII. © 2004 Elsevier B.V. All rights reserved.

Keywords: Ketamine; CO_2 laser; Magnetoencephalography; Pain-related somatosensory-evoked magnetic fields; Secondary somatosensory cortex

1. Introduction

In functional encephalic image research with nociceptive stimulation, cerebral activities are mainly recorded in the secondary somatosensory area (SII), insula and cingulate gyrus [1,2,3]. The initial response to noxious stimulation to the orofacial region is recorded at about 100-ms latency [1,4]. However, the participation of the cortical regions in pain

---

* Corresponding author. Department of Dental Anesthesiology, Tokyo Dentak College, 1-2-2, Masago, Mihama, Chiba 2618502, Japan. Tel.: +81-43-270-3970; fax: +81-43-270-3971.
E-mail address: matsuura@tdc.ac.jp (N. Matsuura).

0531-5131/ © 2004 Elsevier B.V. All rights reserved.
doi:10.1016/j.ics.2004.05.062

perception and information processing is still controversial. This may be partly attributable to difficulties in methods of appropriate recording of nociceptive stimulation. In recent years, many researchers are using laser beams for painful stimulation. Laser beam stimulation can selectively activate thermal-pain receptors [2,5]. In addition, laser beams do not produce error during stimulation and recording time because lasers consist of light.

In a treatment for pain in the orofacial region, various agents are used because of the complexity of the origin. In those cases, many researchers support that ketamine, an N-methyl-D-aspartate (NMDA) receptor antagonist, is effective for the treatment of orofacial pain [6,7].

We therefore used magnetoencephalography (MEG) to record the pain-related somato-sensory-evoked magnetic fields (pain-SEFs) evoked by nociceptive CO_2 laser stimulation to trigeminally innervated skin to investigate the effects of ketamine on pain-SEFs.

2. Materials and methods

The subjects were five healthy adult male volunteers, ages 25 to 35 years (mean age 29.4 years). All volunteers gave informed consent before the experiment. This study was approved by the Institutional Ethical Committee, and undertaken according to the Declaration of Helsinki.

Right mentally innervated skin (about 2 cm below the right angle of the mouth) was stimulated with a CO_2 laser stimulator, and pain-SEFs induced by the stimulation were recorded. For stimulation, a CO_2 laser emission device (modified from a laser unit used in dental treatment; OPELASER 03SIISP, Yoshida, Tokyo, Japan) was fitted with a hollow glass wave-guide. Its wavelength was 10.6 μm and the radiated area was 0.6 mm in diameter. Stimulus pulses were 50 ms in duration, 0.8 W in intensity and repeated at random intervals between 3 and 5 s.

For administration of pharmacological agents, a 24G Angiocath™ (Becton, Dickinson and Company, NJ, USA) was placed in the left cephalic vein, and acetated Ringer's solution containing glucose (Veen-3G®, Nikken-Kagaku, Tokyo, Japan) was continuously infused. Ketamine hydrochloride (Ketalar®, Sankyo, Tokyo, Japan) was administered at a dose of 0.2 mg/kg.

Pain-SEFs were recorded before, immediately and 20 min after the ketamine injection. The magnitude of pain sensation was evaluated on the visual analogue scale (VAS) [8] immediately after the recordings.

Recording of magnetic signals was undertaken in a magnetically shielded room with a 306-channel SQUID (Superconducting Quantum Interference Device) neuromagnetometer (Vectorview, Elekta-Neuromag, Helsinki, Finland) covering the entire head. The locations of coils with respect to the three anatomical landmarks on the head (left and right pre-auricular points and nasion) were determined with a three-dimensional digitizer for alignment of the MEG and MRI coordinate systems. The magnetic signals were band-pass filtered through 0.1–330 Hz, and signals in electro-oculograms (EOG) were band-pass filtered through 0.03–30 Hz. All signals were digitized at a sampling rate of 1 kHz. During each recording session, 100 sweeps were averaged. The analysis period was 900 ms, which included a pre-stimulus period of 50 ms and post-stimulus period of 850 ms. Only the equivalent current dipoles (ECDs) fulfilling goodness-of-fit values of more than

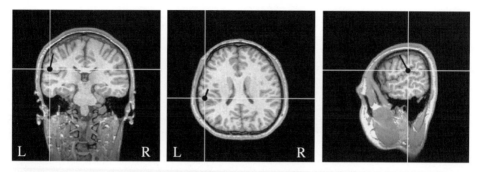

Fig. 1. Equivalent current dipoles (ECD) on a subject's MRI following CO_2 laser stimulation of the right mentally innervated skin at 0.8 W. ECD for 1M was estimated in the contralateral secondary somatosensory cortex (SII).

90% were used to search time-varying multi-dipoles in which the entire measurement time and all SQUID channels were taken into account as computing parameters [9,10].

All numerical values are expressed as mean ± S.E.M. The following tests were used for statistical analyses: Student's t-test and Mann–Whitney U-test, where appropriate. A P value less than 0.01 was considered significant.

3. Results

Pain-SEFs following nociceptive CO_2 laser stimulation at 0.8 W delivered to the mentally innervated skin were found to occur in the bilateral cerebral cortex. Latency at the initial peak was approximately 100 ms (1M), respectively, and was common to all subjects. A dipole estimated for 1M was located in the SII contralateral to the stimulated side in all subjects (Fig. 1).

In all subjects, intravenous administration of low doses of ketamine caused significant decreases in the amplitude of pain-SEFs and VAS corresponding to 1M following CO_2 laser stimulation (Fig. 2). The amplitude of pain-SEFs and VAS was almost recovered to control levels 20 min after ketamine administration (Figs. 2 and 3). Estimation of the ECD

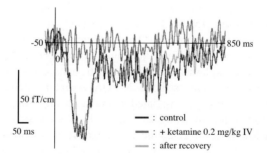

Fig. 2. Effect of an NMDA receptor antagonist (ketamine) on pain-SEFs. The amplitude of the first component of pain-SEFs (1M) following CO_2 laser stimulation decreased in all subjects immediately after intravenous administration of a low-dose of ketamine, but recovered to control levels 20 min after administration.

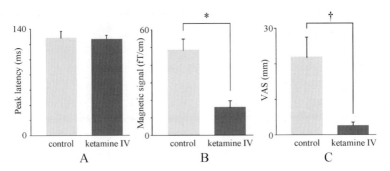

Fig. 3. Effect of an NMDA receptor antagonist (ketamine) on pain-SEFs. Column height represents mean peak latencies (ms) in (A), mean amplitudes of magnetic signals (fT/cm) in (B), and mean magnitude of pain sensation assessed with visual analogue scale (mm) in (C). The mean peak latency of 1M after ketamine hydrochloride administration was not significantly different from control (A). The mean amplitude of magnetic signals (fT/cm) after ketamine administration was significantly smaller than that before administration (*$P<0.01$; Student's t-test, B). The magnitude of pain sensation significantly decreased immediately after ketamine administration ($^{\dagger}P<0.01$; Mann–Whitney U-test, C).

location was impossible immediately after ketamine administration in all subjects, whereas an ECD could be located in SII after 20 min.

4. Discussion

The most appropriate method to study the mechanism of pain has been sought for many years. CO_2 laser stimulation allows us to selectively activate superficial nociceptive receptors in the skin. In the present study, pain-SEFs were recorded around 100-ms (1M) latency after painful CO_2 laser stimulation. In all subjects, an ECD for 1M could be estimated in the SII contralateral to stimulation. Some reports indicate an early or initial response to pain stimulation in the SII in the human cerebral cortex [1–3,11,12]. Our results are consistent with these earlier findings.

Ketamine is an antagonist for NMDA receptors and brings about an inhibition of the central nervous system, such as anesthesia and analgesia [13,14]. Ketamine is used clinically, not only as a general anesthetic, but also in the treatment of chronic intractable pain, phantom limb pain, neuropathic pain, and also in the management of postoperative pain in sub-anesthetic doses [15,16]. In the present study, low doses of ketamine were found to suppress pain-SEFs reversibly. An estimation of ECD location proved to be impossible under the reversible action of ketamine. The action of ketamine on pain-SEFs and pain sensation may be explained by its antagonistic action upon NMDA receptors. It is conceivable that ketamine suppressed the NMDA receptors mediating this excitatory transmission, thereby preventing pain-related neuronal activity from reaching the cerebral cortex, and finally exerting an analgesic effect. It is suggested that an intravenous administration of a low dose of ketamine was effective in suppressing pain sensations conveyed from the trigeminal, nerve-innervated, mandibular skin of the face.

In conclusion, the SII was activated by the application of noxious stimulation to the mentally innervated skin, and therefore suggested to participate in pain perception of noxious stimulation. Ketamine blocks the N-methyl-D-aspartate (NMDA) receptors in the nociceptive relay station, included in the trigeminal caudal subnucleus, resulting in the reduction of cortical activation in the SII.

Acknowledgements

The author would like to greatly thank Assistant Prof. Yoshiyuki Shibukawa for the expert technical advice and Prof. Tatsuya Ichinohe, Prof. Takashi Suzuki, Prof. Yuzuru Kaneko and Prof. Tatsuya Ishikawa for the valuable comments on this manuscript.

References

[1] B. Bromm, J. Lorenz, E. Scharein, in: J. Kimura, H. Shibasaki (Eds.), Recent Advance in Clinical Neurophysiology, Elsevier, Amsterdam, 1996, pp. 328–335.

[2] R. Kakigi, et al., Pain-related magnetic fields folloeing CO_2 laser stimulation in man, Neurosci. Lett. 192 (1995) 45–48.

[3] S. Watanabe, et al., Pain processing by magnetoencephalography in the human brain, Brain Topogr. 10 (1998) 255–264.

[4] R. Hari, et al., Neuromagnetic localization of cortical activity evoked by painful dental stimulation in man, Neurosci. Lett. 42 (1983) 77–82.

[5] R. Kakigi, et al., Pain-related magnetic fields folloeing CO_2 laser stimulation: magnetoencephalographic studies, Electroencephalogr. Clin. Neurophysiol. (Suppl. 47) (1996) 111–120.

[6] L.C. Mathisen, et al., Effect of ketamine, an NMDA receptor inhibitor, in acute and chronic orofacial pain, Pain 61 (1995) 215–220.

[7] T. Rabben, I. Øye, Interindividual differences in the analgesic response to ketamine in chronic orofacial pain, Eur. J. Pain 5 (2001) 233–240.

[8] E.C. Huskisson, Measurment of pain, Lancet 2 (1974) 1127–1131.

[9] M. Hämäläinen, et al., Magnetoencephalography-theory, instrumentation, and applications to noninvasive studies of the working human brain, Rev. Mod. Phys. 65 (1993) 413–497.

[10] N. Nishitani, R. Hari, Temporal dynamics of cortical representation for action, Proc. Natl. Acad. Sci. U. S. A. 18 (2000) 913–918.

[11] K.L. Casey, et al., Comparison of human cerebral activation pattern during cutaneous warmth, heat pain, and deep cold pain, J. Neurophysiol. 76 (1996) 5715–5781.

[12] R.C. Coghill, et al., Pain intensity processing within the human brain: a bilateral, distributed mechanism, J. Neurophysiol. 82 (1999) 1934–1943.

[13] N.A. Anis, et al., The dissociative anaesthetics, ketamine and phencyclidine, selectively reduce excitation of central mammalian neurons by N-methylaspartate, Br. J. Pharmacol. 79 (1983) 565–575.

[14] H. Monyer, et al., Heteromeric NMDA receptors: molecular and functional distinction of subtypes, Science 256 (1992) 1217–1221.

[15] C. Stannard, G.E. Porter, Ketamine hydrochloride in the treatment of phantom limb pain, Pain 54 (1993) 227–230.

[16] L. Roytblat, et al., Postoperative pain: the effect of low-dose ketamine in addition to general anesthesia, Anesth. Analg. 77 (1993) 1161–1165.

International Congress Series 1270 (2004) 126–129

ELSEVIER

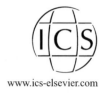

www.ics-elsevier.com

Estimation of the cortical connectivity during a finger-tapping movement with multimodal integration of EEG and fMRI recordings

Fabio Babiloni[a,*], Claudio Babiloni[a,b], Filippo Carducci[a,c], Paolo Maria Rossini[b,c,d], Alessandra Basilisco[a], Laura Astolfi[a,e], Febo Cincotti[f], Lei Ding[g], Y. Ni[g], J. Cheng[g], K. Christine[g], J. Sweeney[g], B. He[g,h]

[a] Department of Human Physiology and Pharmacology, University of Rome "La Sapienza", P.le A. Moro 5, 00185 Rome, Italy
[b] AFaR and CRCCS Ospedale Fatebenefratelli, Isola Tiberina, Rome, Italy
[c] IRCCS "San Giovanni di Dio" Istituto Sacro Cuore di Gesù, Brescia, Italy
[d] Cattedra di Neurologia, Università Campus Bio-Medico, Rome, Italy
[e] Department of Informatics and Systems, University "La Sapienza", Rome, Italy
[f] IRCCS Fondazione "Santa Lucia", Rome, Italy
[g] University of Illinois, Chicago, USA
[h] University of Minnesota, Minneapolis, USA

Abstract. In this paper, advanced methods for the estimation of cortical connectivity from combined high-resolution electroencephalography (EEG) and functional magnetic resonance imaging (fMRI) data are presented. We used a computational approach to the estimation of cortical connectivity by computing the Directed Transfer Function (DTF), a technique used to estimate the direction of the information flow between signals gathered from EEG sensors. The proposed method was able to depict the direction of the information flows between the cortical regions of interest, since it is directional in nature. An application of these technique to the real high-resolution EEG and fMRI signals gathered during visual finger-tapping movements in three normal healthy subjects is also provided. © 2004 Elsevier B.V. All rights reserved.

Keywords: Linear inverse source estimate; EEG and fMRI integration; Directed Transfer Function

1. Introduction

Nowadays, there are several brain-imaging devices that are able to return images of the functional activity of the cerebral cortex, based on the hemodynamic, metabolic or

* Corresponding author. Tel.: +39-649910317; fax: +39-6499103917.
E-mail address: Fabio.Babiloni@uniroma1.it (F. Babiloni).

0531-5131/ © 2004 Elsevier B.V. All rights reserved.
doi:10.1016/j.ics.2004.04.022

neurolectromagnetic measurements. However, static images of brain regions activated during particular tasks do not convey a sufficient amount of information with respect to the central issue of how these regions communicated one to each other. Different approaches for the estimate of the cortical connectivity have been already used in literature with hemodynamic or metabolic measurements, electroencephalography (EEG) scalp potentials and magnetoencephalographic fields [1–3]. Here, we would like to present a computational approach to the estimation of cortical connectivity by using the Directed Transfer Function (DTF), a technique used to estimate the direction of the information flow between signals gathered from EEG sensors [4]. We applied this technology to the high-resolution EEG data gathered during a finger-tapping movement in healthy subjects.

2. Methods

Three normal right-handed human subjects were requested to perform fast repetitive finger movements which were cued by visual stimuli. Ten to fifteen blocks of 2-Hz thumb oppositions for both hands were recorded, with each 30-s blocks of finger movement and rest. Event-related potential (ERP) data were recorded with 96 electrodes and submitted to the artifact removal processing. Six hundreds of ERP trials of 600 ms of duration were acquired. The Magnetic Resonance Images of each subject's head were also acquired. The time-varying spectral values of the estimated cortical activity in the theta (4–7 Hz), alpha (8–12 Hz), beta (13–30 Hz) and gamma (30–45 Hz) frequency bands were also computed in each ROI employed. We divided the analysis period of the analyzed ERP recordings in two phases. The first one, labeled as "PRE", marks the 300 ms before the occurrence of the electromyographic (EMG) trigger of the finger extension before the tap, and it is intended as a generic preparation period. The second phase includes the 300 ms after the EMG trigger up to the end of ERP recording of a single trial and it is intended to give results about the arrival of the somatosensory feedback, and it will labeled "POST" in the following. We maintained the same nomenclature of PRE and POST on the cortical signals estimated at the cortical level.

The Directed Transfer Function (DTF) technique [4] is a full multivariate spectral measure, used to determine the directional influences between any given pair of channels in a multivariate data set. It is computed on a Multivariate Autoregressive model (MVAR) that simultaneously models the whole set of signals. It is based on the concept of Granger causality, according to which an observed time series $b(n)$ can be said to cause another series $y(n)$ if the prediction error for $y(n)$ at the present time is reduced by the knowledge of $b(n)$'s past measurements. This kind of relation is not reciprocal, thus allowing to determine the direction of information flow between channels. We used the DTF approach on the cortical signals estimated from high-resolution EEG recordings, by using realistic head models and a cortical reconstruction with on average of 5000 dipoles uniformly disposed along such cortical surface. The estimation of the cortical activity is obtained by the application of the linear inverse procedure. The solution space can be further reduced by using information deriving from hemodynamic measures (i.e. fMRI-BOLD phenomenon) recorded during the same task

[5]. The connectivity pattern in the different frequency bands between the different cortical regions has been summarized by using appropriate indexes representing the total flow from and toward the selected cortical area. In particular, we defined the total inflow in a particular cortical region the sum of the statistical significant connections (with their values) from all the other cortical regions toward the select area. The total inflow for each ROI is represented by a sphere centered on the cortical region, whose radius is linearly related to the magnitude of all the incoming statistically significant links from the other regions. Such information depicts the ROI as target of functional connections from the other ROIs. Same conventions are used to represent the total outflow from a cortical region toward the others, generated by the sum of the all the statistical significant links obtained by the application of the DTF to the cortical waveforms (with their values).

3. Results

Fig. 1 shows the outflow patterns in all the ROIs obtained for the PRE and POST periods for the subject #1 analyzed, in the alpha frequency band. The figure summarizes the behaviour of each ROI as a source of the information flow towards other ROIs, by adding all the value of the links departing from the particular ROI to all the others. These information are represented with the size of a sphere, centred on the particular ROI analyzed. The larger the sphere, the higher the value of outflow departing from such ROI. The ROIs that are very active as sinks, i.e. that are target of the information flow from other ROIs, are generally stable with respect to the PRE and POST periods. In fact, in all the three subjects examined the major sinks ROIs are located in the parieto-occipital areas (including the B.As 19 and 7 of both sides) and in the premotor and the prefrontal ones, including the areas 8, 9, and 6-F2 of both sides. The most active ROI acting as a source in the PRE and POST period are located in the right parietal (B.A. 5), and primary right motor area (B.A. 4).

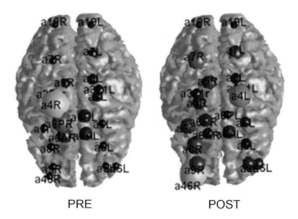

PRE   POST

Fig. 1. Shows the outflow patterns in all the ROIs obtained for the PRE and POST periods for the subject #1 analyzed, in the alpha frequency band.

4. Discussion

The described technology has been applied to the ERP data gathered during a visual guided finger-tapping movements. The main results obtained with the multimodal integration of ERP and fMRI data are related to the activity of a network involving the right frontoparietal cortical structures. The flow of the connections moves from the parietal and premotor areas toward the right and left prefrontal ones. These results were also corroborated by the inflow–outflow analysis, that illustrates how the ROIs located at the parietal (B.A.5) and premotor areas (B.As 6-F2, 6-F4, 6-F7) could be the source of an activity that spreads and reaches virtually all the other ROIs considered, from the occipital (B.A. 19) to the prefrontal (B.A. 9) of both sides. No dramatic variations of the pattern of the inflow–outflow was noted in the time period before and after the EMG onset (the PRE and POST periods). Rather, the same connectivity patterns during these two phases increase or decrease just the strength of the connections.

References

[1] C. Buchel, K.J. Friston, Modulation of connectivity in visual pathways by attention: cortical interactions evaluated with structural equation modelling and fMRI, Cereb. Cortex 7 (8) (1997) 768–778.
[2] A. Gevins, Dynamic functional topography of cognitive task, Brain Topogr. 2 (1989) 37–56.
[3] M. Taniguchi, et al., Movement-related desynchronization of the cerebral cortex studied with spatially filtered magnetoencephalography, NeuroImage 12 (3) (2000) 298–306.
[4] M. Kaminski, et al., Evaluating causal relations in neural systems: granger causality, directed transfer function and statistical assessment of significance, Biol. Cybern. 85 (2001) 145–157.
[5] A. Dale, et al., Dynamic statistical parametric mapping: combining fMRI and MEG for high-resolution imaging of cortical activity, Neuron 26 (2000) 55–67.

International Congress Series 1270 (2004) 130–133

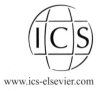

www.ics-elsevier.com

Artefact elimination in spatiotemporal cortical dipole layer imaging with parametric projection filter

Junichi Hori[a,*], Bin He[b]

[a] Department of Biocybernetics, Niigata University, 8050 Ikarashi 2-nocho, Niigata-shi, Niigata, 950-2181, Japan
[b] Department of Biomedical Engineering, University of Minnesota, Minneapolis, MN, USA

Abstract. We explore suitable spatiotemporal filters for inverse estimation of an equivalent cortical dipole layer (DL) distribution from the scalp electroencephalogram (EEG) for imaging of brain electric sources. We have previously developed the parametric projection filter (PPF)-based cortical dipole layer imaging technique, which allows estimating cortical dipole layer inverse solutions in the presence of noise covariance. We have expanded the PPF to the time-varying filter in order to handle the spatiotemporally varying nature of brain electrical activity. The present simulation results indicate that the estimation error is reduced substantially by taking the spatiotemporal properties of the noise into consideration, such as eye-blink artefacts, and the proposed time-variant PPF method provides enhanced performance in rejecting time-varying noise. © 2004 Elsevier B.V. All rights reserved.

Keywords: High-resolution EEG; Inverse problem; Spatiotemporal inverse filter; Equivalent dipole sources; Parametric projection filter; Eye-blink artefact elimination

1. Introduction

It is important to obtain spatiotemporal information regarding brain electrical activity from noninvasive electromagnetic measurements. Because of inherit high temporal resolution of electroencephalogram (EEG) measurements, high resolution EEG imaging, which aims at improving the spatial resolution of the EEG modalities, has received considerable attention in the past decades. Such EEG imaging modalities would facilitate noninvasive localization of foci of epileptic discharges in the brain, and the characterization of rapidly changing patterns of brain activation.

A number of efforts have been made to achieve high resolution EEG imaging. Among them and of interest is the spatial enhancement approach, which attempts to devolve the low-pass spatial filtering effect of volume conduction of the head (for review, see Ref. [1]). The cortical dipole layer (DL) imaging technique, which attempts to estimate the cortical dipole distribution from the scalp potentials, is one of the spatial enhancement techniques.

---

* Corresponding author. Tel.: +81-25-262-6733; fax: +81-25-262-7010.
E-mail address: hori@bc.niigata-u.ac.jp (J. Hori).

0531-5131/ © 2004 Elsevier B.V. All rights reserved.
doi:10.1016/j.ics.2004.05.149

In this approach, an equivalent dipole source layer is used to model brain electrical activity and has been shown to provide enhanced performance in imaging brain electrical sources as compared with the smeared scalp EEG [2–4].

The inverse problem of EEG is ill posed, and in general a regularization procedure is needed in order to obtain stable inverse solutions. We have previously developed the parametric projection filter (PPF)-based cortical dipole layer imaging technique, which allows estimating cortical dipole layer inverse solutions in the presence of noise covariance [3,5]. Our previous results indicate that the results of the PPF provide better approximation to the original dipole layer distribution than that of traditional inverse techniques in the case of low correlation between signal and noise distributions.

In the present study, we have expanded the PPF inverse spatial filter to the time-varying filter in order to handle the spatiotemporally varying nature of brain electrical activity. Concretely, the noise covariance and the regularization parameter of the PPF are supposed to be time-variant in order to eliminate the influence of the background noise and eye-blink artefact.

2. Methods

2.1. Spatiotemporal dipole layer source imaging

The observation system of brain electrical activity on the scalp shall be defined by the following equation:

$$g_k = A f_k + n_k \qquad (k = 1, \ldots, K) \tag{1}$$

where f_k is the equivalent source distribution of a dipole layer (DL), n_k is the additive noise and g_k is the scalp-recorded potentials. Subscript k indicates the time instant. A denotes the transfer matrix from the equivalent source to the scalp potentials.

It is important to estimate the origins from the scalp-recorded EEG, and to image the sources that generate the observed EEG. The inverse process shall be defined by

$$f_{0k} = B_k g_k \tag{2}$$

where B_k is the spatiotemporal restoration filter and f_{0k} is the estimated source distribution of the DL. If the statistical information of the noise or signal are known or estimated for accuracy, the restorative ability of the restoration filter B_k should be improved by using not only the transfer function but also signal and noise information.

In the present simulation study, the head volume conductor is approximated by the inhomogeneous three concentric sphere model [6]. This head model takes the variation in conductivity of different tissues, such as the scalp, the skull and the brain, into consideration. An equivalent DL is assumed within the brain sphere being concentric to the cortical surface. Radial current dipoles are uniformly distributed over the spherical DL to simulate brain electrical sources accounting for the scalp potentials. The electrical sources inside the DL sphere are equivalently represented by the DL surrounding the sources, regardless of the number or the direction of the dipole sources [2–4]. The transfer function from the DL to the scalp potentials is obtained by considering the geometry of the model and physical relationship between the quantities involved. The strength of the DL is estimated from the noise-contaminated scalp potentials.

2.2. Time-varying parametric projection filter

When the statistical information of noise is presented, the projection filter can be applied to the inverse problem. Suppose Q_k, the noise covariance, which can be derived from the expectation over noise $\{n\}$ ensemble, $E[n\ n^*]$. n^* is the transpose of n. The parametric projection filter (PPF) [3,5] is derived by

$$B_k = A^*(AA^* + \gamma_k Q_k)^{-1}. \tag{3}$$

with γ_k a small positive number known as the regularization parameter. The PPF, using the free parameter, can improve the restorative ability from the projection filter, which provides the orthogonal projection of the original signal onto the range of the restoration filter that minimizes the expectation over the noise component in the restored signal. We have applied the time-invariant version of the PPF to the cortical dipole layer source imaging [3] and cortical potential imaging [5]. The time-variant PPF (tPPF) can also be applied to the spatiotemporal inverse problem described by Eq. (2) [7].

We have developed a criterion for determining the optimum parameter. One possibility is to use the following cost function:

$$J(\gamma_k) = E_n \left\| f_{0k} - B_k(A f_{0k} + n_k) \right\|^2 \tag{4}$$

where f_{0k} is the restored DL distribution using an initial value for γ_k, which should be relatively large to reduce the effect of additive noise on the coefficients. Furthermore, we use the recursive procedure that renewing the DL distribution f_{0k} provides the optimum approximation of parameter γ_k.

If there is no spontaneous artefact in the series of EEG measurements, the noise covariance Q_k should be constant and it may be estimated from data that are known to be source free, such as prestimulus data in evoked potentials in a clinical situation [8]. If there are some artefacts, such as eye blink, Q_k should be adaptive to the spatial distribution of the artefacts in order to suppress them. The eye blink covariance is substituted by the voluntary wink data. The eye-blink artefacts may be eliminated by using two types of noise covariance

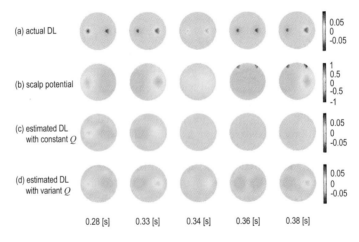

Fig. 1. Cortical DL imaging of two radial dipoles. (a) Actual DL distribution. (b) Scalp potential contaminated with artefact and noise. (c) Estimated result with constant Q_k. (d) Estimated result with time-variant Q_k.

in the tPPF according to the signal conditions with or without artefacts. The time interval of eye blink is estimated by the correlation coefficient between each scalp potential distribution and the eye-blink template measured by voluntary wink data in advance.

3. Results

A DL with 1280 radial dipoles at a radius of 0.8 was used [6]. Fig. 1(a) shows one example of the actual DL distribution of two radial dipoles at several time points. The dipole sources were located at the eccentricity of 0.7 with the angle of $\pi/3$. The strength of each dipole is changed with sinusoid in time (10 and 30 Hz). The scalp potential was contaminated with two kinds of additive noise [Fig.1(b)]. One is the time invariant background noise expressed by Gaussian white noise. The other is the time variant noise of eye-blink artefacts, which appear as spike-like shapes at the upper parts of the eyes. As shown in Fig. 1(d), the DL distribution obtained by the tPPF shows two areas of well-localized activity similar to the actual DL source distribution and the artefacts were eliminated. The RE between the actual and estimated DL distributions was reduced by the tPPF in every time instant. Especially, the RE during the period with the artefact was dramatically reduced.

4. Conclusion

We have developed a time-varying noise covariance incorporated inverse filter for cortical imaging, and showed its applicability in suppressing rapidly changing artefacts. The present simulation results suggest that the estimation error is reduced substantially by taking the spatiotemporal properties of the noise into consideration, such as eye-blink artefacts. Further investigations on other applications of this new method should be addressed in the future.

Acknowledgements

This work was supported in part by a Grant-In-Aid for Scientific Research from the Japanese Society for the Promotion of Science No. 13480291, Grant for Promotion of Niigata University Research Projects, NIH 1RO1EB00178, and NSF BES-0411898.

References

[1] B. He, Brain electric source imaging—scalp Laplacian mapping and cortical imaging, Crit. Rev. BME 27 (1999) 149–188.
[2] A.M. Dale, M.I. Sereno, Improved localization of cortical activity by combining EEG and MEG with MRI cortical surface reconstruction: a linear approach, J. Cogn. Neurosci. 5 (1993) 162–176.
[3] J. Hori, B. He, Equivalent dipole source imaging of brain electric activity by means of parametric projection filter, Ann. Biomed. Eng. 29 (2001) 436–445.
[4] B. He, D. Yao, J. Lian, High resolution EEG: on the cortical equivalent dipole layer imaging, Clin. Neurophysiol. 113 (2002) 227–235.
[5] J. Hori, B. He, EEG cortical potential imaging of brain electrical activity by means of parametric projection filters, IEICE Trans. Inf. Syst. E86-D (2003) 1909–1920.
[6] Y. Wang, B. He, A computer simulation study of cortical imaging from scalp potentials, IEEE Trans. Biomed. Eng. 45 (1998) 724–735.
[7] J. Hori, M. Aiba, B. He, Spatio-temporal dipole source imaging of brain electrical activity by means of time-varying parametric projection filter, IEEE Trans. Biomed. Eng. 51 (2004) 768–777.
[8] K. Sekihara, B. Scholz, Average-intensity reconstruction and Weiner reconstruction of bioelectric current distribution based on its estimated covariance matrix, IEEE Trans. Biomed. Eng. 42 (1995) 149–157.

International Congress Series 1270 (2004) 134–137

ELSEVIER

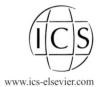

www.ics-elsevier.com

Monitoring of eye movement and its use for artifact elimination

N. Hironaga[a,b,*], K. Haruhana[a], L.C. Liu[a],
P.B.C. Fenwick[a], A.A. Ioannides[a,b]

[a] Laboratory for Human Brain Dynamics, Brain Science Institute, RIKEN, Japan
[b] Department of Brain Science and Engineering, Kyushu Institute of Technology, Japan

Abstract. Electrical activity of the human eye generates the electrooculogram (EOG) and contributes to the magneto-encephalographic (MEG) signal. The EOG and MEG signals around each eye are usually modeled by an equivalent current dipole (ECD). Direct information about the gaze position from the eye tracking system (ETS) can be used to simulate the MEG signal. Eye movement-related time courses can also be obtained from decompositions of the MEG signal, using either independent component analysis (ICA) or principal component analysis (PCA). We compared actual measurements with estimated values for eye movements, MEG signals and with ICA/PCA components. These comparisons are used to explore advantages and limitations of each method as it is used separately and in combinations. © 2004 Elsevier B.V. All rights reserved.

Keywords: Eye movement; Eye tracking system; Noise elimination; MEG; Component analysis

1. Introduction

It is necessary to identify and eliminate signal artefacts when one uses magneto-encephalographic (MEG) or EEG. Subjects are usually asked to fixate on a target during measurements. Off-line regression analysis can use the EOG signal to remove eye movement-related artefacts. Since the EOG also detects brain and muscle activity, a regression method will inevitably eliminate meaningful brain activity [1]. Identification of artefacts based on abstract signal component separation has been tried [independent component analysis (ICA)/principal component analysis (PCA)] [2,3]. Finally, one or more equivalent current dipole (ECD) can be used in a spatio-temporal fit of the data [4]. The last two methods eliminate the need to attach electrodes on the subject, which tends to increase noise in the MEG signal. We have studied each method and their combinations, using as reference estimates of gaze position derived from eye tracking system (ETS). We show here results for saccade, smooth pursuit and small eye movements during fixation.

---

* Corresponding author. Riken Brain Science Institute, Human Brain Dynamics, 2-1, Hirosawa 351-0198, Wako-shi, Saitama, Japan. Tel.: +81-48-467-9737; fax: +81-48-467-5973.
E-mail address: hironaga@brain.riken.go.jp (N. Hironaga).

0531-5131/ © 2004 Elsevier B.V. All rights reserved.
doi:10.1016/j.ics.2004.04.038

2. Methods

Two tasks for main eye movement and one task for small saccade during fixating were performed. MEG measurement was performed using the CTF whole head system, and the sampling rate was 625 Hz. Two EOG electrodes, vertical and horizontal, were attached to each subject. Eye tracking data were recorded, together with the MEG signals, and an off-line process was used to correct the time delay. The main eye movement task used a 10° range for the visual angle. Before the start of the experiment, we calibrate the EOG by controlling recordings of the screen visual angle and the change of the EOG. In the first task, the subject used saccades to follow the target stimulus as its location was changed between three points on a horizontal line (left, right and centre of the screen). In the second task, the subject tracked the target as it moved smoothly along the same horizontal line. For the third task, the subject was required to fixate on a small fixation cross placed at the centre of the screen. In this paper, we focus on changes generated by eye movement only, so we do not model blinks or discuss the influence of luminance change. The room was therefore completely dark (except for the task-related stimuli on the monitor) to limit changes in eye potential generated by background luminance. For electrical potential modelling of the eye, the main factors are retina, pigment epithelium and photoreceptors. The main contribution comes from retina and pigment epithelium. The retina covers 3/4 of the inner posterior wall area of the eyeball and although the geometry is largely symmetric, the potential on the retina is asymmetrical because the density of rods is not uniform [5]. The asymmetry of other factors can be assumed to be small and therefore ignored. Ideally, the computation of the EOG and MEG signal generated by these electrical elements should model the conductivity anisotropies accurately. Furthermore, in the case of EEG, the whole brain is covered by skull, but this is not true for the eyes. Although precise values for the conductivities of the eye compartments are not known, conductivity is not a primary issue for MEG calculations as we employ the widely used spherical head model for MEG. After accurate coregistration based on the 3D camera, the centre for each eye is estimated based on MRI. The dipole centres were shifting between 0.6 and 0.7 cm to posterior once the geometric centre of the eyeballs was determined from the subject's MRI. Next, we address the forward calculation. In general, DC removal eliminates an absolute reference for the magnetic field value and, hence, the actual current dipole moments must be derived from changes in the MEG data. To estimate the moment strength, we use one MEG recording for calibration. Before the calculation of DC removal, third gradient formation, LP filter for 20 Hz and notch filter for 50 Hz and its harmonic were applied. The LP filter setting was set at 20 Hz so that electrical muscle activity was eliminated, leaving just the slow saccadic eye movement. In any case, no information was available at higher frequencies from the ETS because its sampling rate was 60 Hz. The ECD parameters are estimated by a least square fit using the difference in magnetic field generated by the left and right model dipoles. The fit uses 15 channels in the frontal area, which best captures the MEG signal generated by eye movement. The rotational vectors are estimated from gaze position obtained from the eye tracker. The second approximation we employed was that when the eye moves left or right, the angle of rotation was the same for both eyes during slow eye movement.

3. Result

Fig. 1A shows the signal of a frontal MEG channel together with its estimate from a forward solution using ECD based on eye tracker data. The two signals coincide over most of the time range during both saccade (not shown) and smooth pursuit. Possible causes of differences are instability in the eye tracking system and cortical and/or muscular high frequency contribution. Fig. 1B shows the ICA, Eye Tracker and EOG-based signals. The three signals correlate well. However, signals based on ICA still keep the small amplitude of oscillation while the eye tracker-based signal and EOG signal correlate accurately. It is unlikely that these oscillations are due to small saccades. One may speculate that the cause of this oscillation is rhythmical activity of the brain, mainly alpha activity. It is reasonable to consider that ETS detects only eye movement, whereas EOG and MEG detect eye movement, muscle movement and brain activity where the signal-to-noise ratio of the EOG is higher than MEG. Use of statistics on separate, single trial [6] and channel data could provide further improvement by identifying and removing some of the other components. Our next discussion is small saccade. During long runs, large EEG/EOG drifts are generated by electronics and changes in the skin conductance. Hence, we concentrated on small, horizontal eye movement of the EOG and horizontal movement from gaze positions over short periods. Fig. 2A compares the EOG and ETS-derived time courses. It shows enough consistency to suggest that each method detects small eye movement, but with rather coarse accuracy. Some peaks seen in the ETS-derived signal are not clearly seen in the EOG. In our modelling, we have assumed that the two eyes track together. While this assumption is reasonable for slow movements, it is known that during fixation both binocular and monocular small saccades are present [7]. To investigate these phenomena further, it is necessary to monitor each eye separately and at higher sampling rates. We have computed the MEG signal for small saccades from the ETS during short time periods when the EOG and ETS-derived signal agree fairly well. These computations suggest that small eye movements during fixation generate a detectable magnetic field, but its amplitude is considerably weaker than the amplitude background brain activity, notably the alpha rhythm.

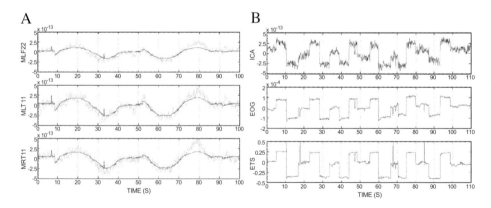

Fig. 1. (A) Forward calculation (solid line) and raw MEG signals (dotted line). (B) Comparison of three signals, each LP filtered below 5 Hz; ICA (top), EOG (middle) and ETS (bottom).

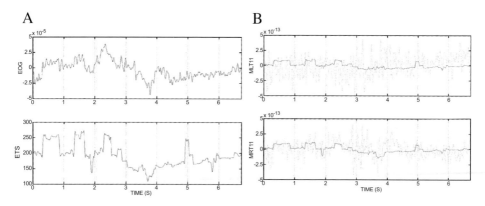

Fig. 2. Comparison of small saccade during fixation. (A) EOG horizontal and gaze horizontal. (B) MEG raw (dotted line) and simulated MEG signal (solid line).

4. Conclusion and discussion

The advantage of using an eye tracking system is that it makes it possible to extract only the component related to the eye movement. Using this signal, we can distinguish the saccade signal from possible myographic and brain activity. To begin with the accuracy and stability of eye tracking systems is highly subject-dependent. PCA and ICA are good methods for signal separation because they work well for eliminating the "spiky signals," e.g. blinks and cardiac activity, but it is difficult to extract the signal only from eye movement using these methods for long recordings and many channels. In general, restricting the subject's behaviour by requiring fixation on a target during measurement is the most reliable and well-tested way to avoid eye movement artefacts. However, even for the best subjects there are always some small eye movements during fixation. The influence of these small eye movements to the overall MEG signal is relatively small, and can be safely ignored, except for cases when reconstructions of activity from very weak generators fairly close to the eyes are attempted. However, since fixation is a dynamic process and these small saccades may have a functional role [8], their understanding may be necessary for detailed investigation of the human visual system. In summary, the method described here offers a partial solution, but further investigation is necessary for establishing any or some combination as routine tools for accurate eye movement monitoring and noise elimination.

References

[1] T. Meier, et al., Electroencephalogr. Clin. Neurophysiol. 108 (6) (1998) 526–535.
[2] A.J. Bell, T.J. Sejnowski, Neural Comput. 7 (6) (1995) 1129–1159.
[3] A. Hyvarinen, IEEE Trans. Neural Netw. 10 (3) (1999) 626–634.
[4] P. Berg, M. Scherg, Electroencephalogr. Clin. Neurophysiol. 79 (1991) 36–44.
[5] T. Katila, et al., J. Appl. Phys. 52 (3) (1981).
[6] C. Jackson, M. Sherratt, Electroencephalogr. Clin. Neurophysiol. 115 (2004) 227–237.
[7] R. Enbert, R. Kliegl, in: J. Hyona, R. Radach, H. Deubel (Eds.), The Minds' Eyes: Cognitive and Applied Aspects of Eye movements, Elsevier, Oxford, 2003, pp. 103–117.
[8] S. Martinez-Conde, S.L. Macknik, D.H. Hubel, Nat. Rev., Neurosci. 5 (2004) 229–240.

International Congress Series 1270 (2004) 138–141

www.ics-elsevier.com

Wavelet-based hemodynamic analyzing method in event-related fMRI with statistical processing

Sayaka Imaeda[a,*], Syoji Kobashi[a], Yuri T. Kitamura[b],
Katsuya Kondo[a], Yutaka Hata[a], Toshio Yanagida[b]

[a] Graduate School of Engineering, University of Hyogo, 2167 Shosha, Himeji, Hyogo 671-2201, Japan
[b] Graduate School of Frontier Biosciences, Osaka University, Japan

Abstract. Investigating the shape and time to peak (hemodynamic response [HR] delay) of the HR introduces a new facet of research on human brain function. This paper proposes a novel method for analyzing event-related functional magnetic resonance images (ER-fMRI). The method is based on wavelet transform. The principal feature of the method is that it can detect an activation area and estimate the HRF simultaneously. To evaluate the proposed method, experiments were done on phantom data and human subjects. The results showed that the method could detect the activation area equivalent to and more than SPM99. Then, examination of variability of HR delay among the activation areas suggests that HR delay at the motor area is significantly faster than that at the visual area. © 2004 Published by Elsevier B.V.

Keywords: fMRI; Wavelength transform; HR delay

1. Introduction

In order to detect an activated region with functional magnetic resonance imaging (fMRI), several methods have been proposed, such as statistical parametric mapping (SPM) [1], principal component analysis (PCA) [2] or analysis of variance (ANOVA). Recently, concerns about the shape of hemodynamic response function (HRF) or hemodynamic response (HR) delays have increased. However, these methods could not detect the shape of HRF or measure HR delays simultaneously. By detecting HR in detail, we may be able to clarify a brain function based on differences of sex or disease [3].

This paper proposes an analysis method for detecting an activated region and measuring HR delays simultaneously with event-related (ER-) fMRI data using wavelet transform, called hemodynamic response analysis using wavelet transform; HAW. The method defines the time from start of a task to a peak of a blood oxygenation level dependent (BOLD) signal as a HR delay. To evaluate the performance of the proposed method, we

* Corresponding author. Tel.: +81-792-67-4989; fax: +81-792-67-4989.
E-mail address: imaeda@comp.eng.himeji-tech.ac.jp (S. Imaeda).

0531-5131/ © 2004 Published by Elsevier B.V.
doi:10.1016/j.ics.2004.05.056

examine receiver operating characteristic curves (ROC curves) of SPM99 and the proposed method. The ROC curves are generated by applying both methods to phantom data.

2. Subjects and materials

Subjects recruited in this study were four healthy male volunteers (the mean age ± standard deviation (S.D.): 24.5 ± 2.9 years old). All subjects were right-handed, which was confirmed by using the Edinburgh inventory test for handedness [4]. They all gave informed consent according to the guidelines approved by the local ethical committee of our institute.

MR images were obtained using a 1.5-T MRI scanner (SIGNA CV/i, GE Medical systems, Milwaukee, WI). High-resolution, axial, T1-weighted structural MR images were obtained for anatomical reference with a 256×256 voxel matrix covering 260×260 mm, 20 axial slices and 5 mm slice thickness. Echo planar imaging (EPI) was used to acquire data sensitive to the BOLD signal at a repetition time (TR) of 2000 ms and an echo time (TE) of 40 ms. The spatial resolution was set by a 64×64 voxel matrix covering 260×260 mm with 5 mm slice thickness.

Motor area and visual area activation experiments were conducted using two kinds of paradigm design: hand-gripping task and visual stimulus. In the case of the hand-gripping task, the subjects were instructed to rapidly open and close their hands for 2 s at the jittering time from 20 to 30 s. In the case of visual stimulus, 10-Hz visual checkerboard reversal stimuli were presented for 2 s; subjects looked at the screen during the examination.

3. Method

Consider a time-course signal, $MR_{xyz}(t)$, at a voxel with a coordinate value of (x,y,z). Our method provides a degree of activation by estimating a signal change using continuous wavelet transform (CWT). The CWT is applied to the time-course signal of each voxel in the ER-fMRI data. The degree of activation is computed by:

$$\mu(a,b) = \Sigma\psi(a,b,t)S_{xyz}(t), \tag{1}$$

where $\psi(a,b,t)$ represents a mother wavelet function, a and b do the scaling parameter and the time parameter, respectively. $S_{xyz}(t)$ is the signal change computed by:

$$S_{xyz}(t) = \frac{MR_{xyz}(t) - \overline{MR_{xyz}(t)}}{\overline{MR_{xyz}(t)}}, \tag{2}$$

where $\overline{MR_{xyz}(t)}$ is a mean of $MR_{xyz}(t)$.

The wavelet coefficient depends on the variances of the time-course signal $S_{xyz}(t)$ and the mother wavelet $\psi(a,b,t)$. To suppress the inferences, we normalize the obtained $\mu(a,b)$ by:

$$\lambda(a,b) = \frac{\mu(a,b)}{\sqrt{\Sigma\left(\psi(a,b,t) - \overline{\psi(a,b,t)}\right)^2}\sqrt{\Sigma\left(S_{xyz}(t) - \overline{S_{xyz}(t)}\right)^2}}. \tag{3}$$

We then define a local maximum $\lambda(a_{max},b_{max})$ as the degree of activation at the voxel of interest. Also, a_{max} is a shape parameter of HRF and b_{max} is the HR delay. The above procedures are applied to all voxels.

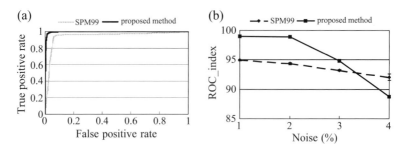

Fig. 1. (a) Comparison of the ROC curves of SPM99 and the proposed method. (b) Comparison of the area under the ROC curve of SPM99 and the proposed method.

To achieve the significance test, the method hypothesizes the population of the local maximum $\lambda(a_{max}, b_{max})$ by approximating a Gaussian distribution using least squares approximation. Using the hypothesized population, the method determines whether the voxel of interest is significantly activated or not using a statistical test with Bonferroni's multiple comparison.

4. Results and discussion

We examined ROC curves of SPM99 and the proposed method to evaluate the performance of these methods. The ROC curves were generated by applying the methods to phantom data. The phantom data were generated by using HRF defined in SPM99 and Gaussian noise. The signal-changing rate of HRF was 3.0%. Fig. 1(a) shows a comparison of the ROC curves of SPM99 and the proposed method using phantom data with the noise rate of 2.0%. In this figure, an area under the ROC curve (ROC_index) was 98.9% with the proposed method and 94.2% with SPM99. It shows that the proposed method could detect an activated region with a higher accuracy than SPM99. Fig. 1(b) shows a comparison of the ROC_index. It shows that the proposed method is effective below the noise rate of the same grade as the signal-changing rate of HRF.

For all subjects, the proposed method successfully detected an activated region and measured HR delay. In the case of hand-gripping tasks, we detected motor area (Brodmann area, BA 4) as an activated region. In the case of visual stimulus, we detected visual area (BA 17) as an activated region. Fig. 2(a) and (b) shows the results of activated regions of the right hand-gripping task, and Fig. 2(c) and (d) shows the results of activated regions of

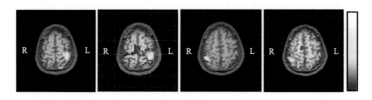

Fig. 2. (a) and (b): activated region maps on right hand-gripping task, (c) and (d): activated region maps on left hand-gripping task for Subject 1. (a) and (c) were our method ($P<0.05$, corrected). (b) and (d) were using SPM99 ($P<0.05$, corrected).

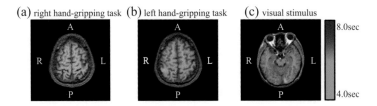

Fig. 3. HR delay on right hand, left hand-gripping tasks and visual stimulus for subject 1.

the left hand-gripping task. Fig. 2(a) and (c) shows the degree of activation maps obtained using our method with statistical significance $P < 0.05$ corrected, whereas Fig. 2(b) and (d) shows the same data analyzed using SPM99 with $P < 0.05$ corrected. In these images, the red–white scale represents the degree of activation and the whiter pixel denotes a higher degree of activation. This shows that the proposed method detected activated regions that were equivalent to SPM99.

Fig. 3 shows HR delay maps obtained by the proposed method of right hand and left hand-gripping tasks and visual stimulus for subject 1. In these images, the green–blue scale represents the delay of HR and the bluer pixel denotes slower HR delay. In these figures, the proposed method detected HR delay of 5.48 ± 0.48 s (the mean HR delay $\pm$ S.D.) at the motor area (BA 4) and 7.65 ± 0.28 s at the visual area (BA 17). These results suggest that HR delay of the visual area is significantly slower than that of the motor area ($P < 0.01$, corrected).

5. Conclusion

This paper has proposed an analysis method for detecting activated regions and measuring HR delays simultaneously with event-related fMRI data using wavelet transform. In the experiments using phantom data, the proposed method could detect an activated region with higher accuracy than SPM99. By investigating the differences of HR delays among activation areas using the proposed method, we found that HR delay of the visual area is significantly slower than that of the motor area. In the future, we will investigate the variability of HR delays among activation areas, between sexes or among ages.

Acknowledgements

This research was supported in part by the Ishikawa Hospital Grant and the Berkeley Initiative in Soft Computing (BISC) program of the University of California at Berkeley, USA.

References

[1] K.J. Frinston, et al., Statistical parametric maps in functional imaging: a general linear approach, Human Brain Mapping 2 (1995) 189–210.
[2] W. Backfriender, et al., Quantification of intensity variations in functional MR images using rotated principal components, Physics in Medicine and Biology 41 (1996) 1425–1438.
[3] L.M. Carusone, et al., Hemodynamic response changes in cerebrovascular disease: implications for functional MR imaging, American Journal of Neuroradiology 23 (2002) 1222–1228.
[4] R.C. Oldfield, The assessment and analysis of handedness: the Edinburgh inventory, Neuropsychologia 9 (1971) 97–113.

ELSEVIER

International Congress Series 1270 (2004) 142–145

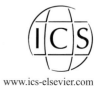

www.ics-elsevier.com

Effects of repetitive transcranial magnetic stimulation on acute pain

Yohei Tamura[a,b,*], Yoshikazu Ugawa[c], Ryusuke Kakigi[a]

[a] Department of Integrative Physiology, National Institute for Physiological Sciences, Japan
[b] Department of Neurology, Jikei University School of Medicine, Japan
[c] Department of Neurology, Division of Neuroscience, Graduate School of Medicine, University of Tokyo, Japan

Abstract. The present study aimed to investigate the efficacy of repetitive transcranial magnetic stimulation (rTMS) on acute pain. We studied effects of 1-Hz rTMS over the primary motor cortex on acute pain induced by capsaicin and by Tm:YAG laser stimulation. rTMS significantly suppressed the subjective pain induced by capsaicin, whereas it aggravated the subjective pain induced by laser stimulation. We found opposite effects of rTMS on C-fiber-mediated pain (suppression) and Adelta-fiber-mediated pain (facilitation). The results provide evidence that the motor cortex plays an important role in the modulation of acute pain perception, and may reflect the distinct biological significance of first and second pain. © 2004 Elsevier B.V. All rights reserved.

Keywords: Acute pain; Repetitive transcranial magnetic stimulation; Capsaicin; Tm:YAG laser; Motor cortex

1. Introduction

Repetitive transcranial magnetic stimulation (rTMS) over the primary motor cortex (M1) was reported to attenuate subjective pain, and has been used to manage chronic pain. These attempts at pain relief are based on the finding that extradural, motor cortex stimulation alleviated chronic pain. These indicate a relationship between the motor cortex and the pain perception system. To clarify the mechanisms underlying this relationship, we investigated the effects of rTMS over M1 on acute pain. Since noxious signals ascend to the central nervous system through the primary afferent Adelta-fibers and C-fibers, we elicited acute pain by intradermal capsaicin injection and also by applying Tm:YAG laser stimulation. Capsaicin is known to induce acute pain mediated by C-fibers. We observed the time course of subjective pain with and without rTMS application and examined the difference in regional cerebral blood flow (rCBF), using single-photon emission computed tomography (SPECT). In contrast, Tm:YAG laser stimulation activates both Adelta- and C-nociceptors. Since the evoked responses at 150–400 ms after the laser stimulation are

---

* Corresponding author. Department of Integrative Physiology, National Institute for Physiological Sciences, Myodaiji, Okazaki 444-8585, Japan. Tel.: +81-564-55-7779; fax: +81-564-52-7913.
E-mail address: ytamura@nips.ac.jp (Y. Tamura).

considered to be mediated by Adelta-fibers, we investigated changes in Tm:YAG laser evoked potentials (LEPs) and the subjective rating of pricking pain after rTMS over M1.

2. Methods

Informed consent to participate in the study was obtained from all participants beforehand. All subjects were completely blinded to the anticipated effects of rTMS (e.g. pain alteration).

2.1. SPECT experiment: effects on acute pain induced by capsaicin

First, we examined the effects of rTMS on subjective pain induced by capsaicin in seven healthy subjects, aged 23–31 (mean 28) years. Acute pain was evoked by intradermal injection of 250 μg capsaicin in the 20-μl vehicle to the right volar forearm. Pain was assessed on a 0–10 visual analogue scale immediately after the capsaicin injection and the ratings were obtained every minute until 10 min after the injection. Three different sessions, real rTMS over M1, realistic sham stimulation, and control condition without either stimulation, were performed in each subject. Magnetic stimulation was applied with a figure-of eight coil connected to a Magstim Rapid Stimulator (The Magstim, Dyfed, UK), and the intensity of the stimuli was adjusted to 1.3 times the motor threshold for the active right FDI muscle, which was lower than the threshold for the relaxed FDI muscle in all subjects. One minute after the capsaicin administration, 300 stimuli were applied at 1 Hz over the left M1 for 5 min. The time courses of the pain ratings were compared among three conditions. Second, to demonstrate the brain region associated with pain alteration, SPECT measurements were performed in 10 healthy volunteers (24–35, mean 28 years) under two conditions: one was the control condition, in which the subjects only received a capsaicin injection; the other was the rTMS condition, in which 120, 1-Hz rTMS was delivered to the right M1 after capsaicin injection. In both conditions, the subjects received capsaicin injections to the left volar forearm. Technetium-99m ethyl cysteinate dimer (740 MBq) was used as a radiotracer. Voxel-based analysis was performed with SPM99 (Wellcome Department of Cognitive Neurology, London, UK) to reveal the condition effects between the rTMS and control conditions. Furthermore, to examine whether or not the resulting foci were activated or deactivated in relation to pain alteration, we conducted a region-of-interest analysis and investigated the correlation between pain rating reduction and rCBF changes in those regions.

2.2. LEP experiment: effects on acute pain induced by Tm:YAG laser stimulation

We examined the changes in subjective pain and LEPs before and after rTMS over M1 in 13 healthy volunteers, aged 24–39 (mean 30) years. We compared the results obtained under three different conditions: real rTMS, realistic sham stimulation and a control condition with no stimulation. The rTMS sessions comprised five runs of recordings at different times: (1) before rTMS, (2) immediately, (3) 10 min, (4) 20 min and (5) 30 min after rTMS. A Tm:YAG laser system (BLM1000S, Baasel Lasertech, Starnberg, Germany) was used for pain stimulation and the laser pulses were applied to the radial part of the dorsal surface of the right hand at the intensity adjusted to approximately 1.5 times the pain threshold. Electroencephalograms were recorded with an Ag/AgCl disk electrode placed over Cz and the responses were referenced to the linked earlobes level (A1 + A2). Fifteen epochs were measured for each LEP run. In the rTMS session, 600 magnetic stimuli were applied at 1 Hz over the left M1 and the intensity was adjusted to 90% of the motor threshold for the rest FDI muscle. For the indices of LEP, we analysed the N2-P2 components, which are generated after the N1 component, because N2-P2 components can be measured with high reproducibility.

3. Results

3.1. SPECT experiment

Fig. 1 shows the time course of the pain ratings in each condition (Fig. 1a, b) and the voxels with significant, relative rCBF differences between rTMS and control conditions (Fig. 1c). It was found that rTMS significantly suppressed the subjective pain rating. Correlation analyses for the resulting regions showed a significant relationship between the pain rating reduction and rCBF changes in right BA9 and right BA24.

3.2. LEP experiment

Fig. 2 shows the LEP waveforms obtained from two representative subjects and the time courses of the change in pain ratings and the LEP parameters. As was demonstrated, both the pain ratings and N2-P2 amplitudes decreased after the stimulation period in the

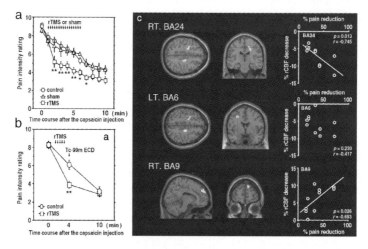

Fig. 1. (a, b) Time courses of subjective pain ratings in three different conditions (a), and in SPECT experiment (b). Ratings were significantly lower in the rTMS condition than in the other conditions. *$P<0.05$, **$P<0.01$. (c) Regions with significant rCBF changes following rTMS over the right M1 as compared with the control condition. An rCBF increase was observed in right BA24 (upper) and left BA6 (middle), while rCBF decrease was observed in right BA9 (lower). Particularly, rCBF in right BA24 and that in right BA9 significantly correlated with pain reduction induced by rTMS. Height threshold, $Z=3.09$, $P=0.001$; extent threshold, $P=0.05$, corrected. (Modified from Tamura et al. [1]).

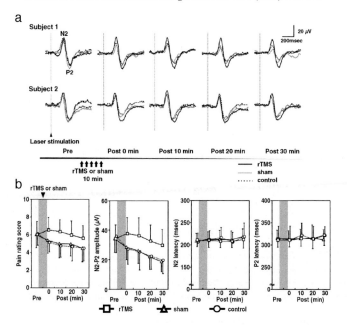

Fig. 2. Time courses of the LEP waveforms obtained from two representative subjects and each LEP parameter in three conditions. Significant differences were found in both subjective pain ratings and N2-P2 amplitudes between the rTMS and the other two conditions. Modified from Tamura et al. [2].

sham and control conditions, whereas they showed a transient increase followed by a decrease in the rTMS condition.

4. Discussion

We found opposite effects of rTMS on C-fiber-mediated pain (suppression) and Adelta-fiber pain (facilitation). The results provide evidence that the motor cortex plays an important role in the modulation of acute pain perception. Since the distinct biological significance of first and second pain has been described [3], it is likely that rTMS over M1 modulates C-fiber-mediated pain and Adelta-fiber pain in a different manner. rTMS is expected to be one of the treatments applicable to relieve both acute and chronic pain and our results may contribute to the potential therapeutic use of rTMS for pain relief.

References

[1] Y. Tamura, et al., Effects of 1-Hz repetitive transcranial magnetic stimulation on acute pain induced by capsaicin, Pain 107 (2004) 107–115.

[2] Y. Tamura, et al., Facilitation of Aδ-fiber-mediated acute pain by repetitive transcranial magnetic stimulation, Neurology (in press).

[3] M. Ploner, et al., Cotical representation of first and second pain sensation in humans, Proc. Natl. Acad. Sci. U.S.A. 99 (2002) 12444–12448.

International Congress Series 1270 (2004) 146–148

ELSEVIER

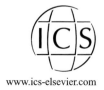

www.ics-elsevier.com

The late response in the soleus muscle evoked by transcranial magnetic stimulation at the foramen magnum level

Kotoe Sakihara[a,*], Aya Ihara[a,b], Yuko Takahashi[a],
Syunnsuke Koreeda[a], Ai Sakagami[a], Masayuki Hirata[a,c],
Shiro Yorifuji[a]

[a]Department of Functional Diagnostic Science Medicine, Graduate School of Medicine,
Osaka University, 1-7, Suita, 565-0879, Yamadaoka, Osaka, Japan
[b]Department of Integrative Physiology, National Institute for Physiological Science, Okazaki, Japan
[c]Department of Neurosurgery, Graduate School of Medicine, Osaka University, Osaka, Japan

Abstract. In healthy subjects, we studied the late electromyographic response elicited by transcranial magnetic stimulation (TMS) applied at the level of the foramen magnum in the left soleus muscle in an upright and supine posture. The late response at the latency of approximately 40 ms was constantly elicited during both postures. It was elicited during planter flexion, but not dorsi flexion. Additionally, no response appeared in the relaxed muscle. Those behaviours are the same as that of the long-loop reflex (LLR). We believe that the late response may be a long-loop reflex. © 2004 Elsevier B.V. All rights reserved.

Keywords: Magnetic stimulation; Foramen magnum; Soleus muscle; Late response

1. Introduction

Transcranial magnetic stimulation (TMS) at the foramen magnum activates descending tracts and elicits an early neural response with an onset latency of about 25 ms in the lower limb [1–3]. TMS at the level of foramen magnum also activates the ascending tracts and evokes a late response in patients with myoclonic epilepsy [3]. This late response is the cortical long-loop reflex (LLR). However, in healthy subjects, a late response evoked by TMS at the foramen magnum has not been reported to date.

2. Subjects and methods

Ten healthy volunteers (two males and eight females, aged 22 to 53 years) participated in the present study. Subjects adopted standing or supine postures to contract the soleus

---

* Corresponding author. Tel./fax: +81-6-6879-2583.
E-mail address: sakihara@sahs.med.osaka-u.ac.jp (K. Sakihara).

0531-5131/ © 2004 Elsevier B.V. All rights reserved.
doi:10.1016/j.ics.2004.05.085

A: Standing

B: Supine

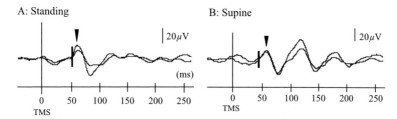

Fig. 1. (A) Standing posture. (B) Supine posture. The late response was evoked both posture.

muscle. A double cone coil (MAGSTIM 200 magnetic stimulator, The Magstim Company, UK) was placed over the inion. Stimulating intensity was set at 10% less than the threshold for the activation of motor tracts when the motor cortex was stimulated magnetically. EMG activity was recorded in the left soleus muscle using a narrow band-pass filter, 2–20 Hz. Thirty responses were averaged.

3. Results

The late response at the onset latency of approximately 40 ms was elicited constantly in the left soleus muscle in a standing (Fig. 1A) and supine posture (Fig. 1B). The late response was evoked only during planter flexion, but not dorsi flexion in the standing posture (Fig. 2). It was not elicited in the relaxed muscle and no response was detected in the tibialis anterior muscle (antagonist) (data not shown).

4. Discussion

TMS at the foramen magnum could constantly elicit the EMG response at the latency of approximately 40 ms in the soleus muscle. We believe the late response may be a long-loop reflex. Berardelli et al. [4] reported that long latency reflex in the triceps surae muscle is obtained and facilitated by planter flexion, while they are suppressed or inhibited by ankle dorsi flexion. Moreover, the long-loop reflex cannot be elicited in the relaxed muscle [3]. The behaviours of long-loop reflex were the same as that of late response in the present study.

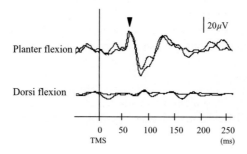

Fig. 2. The late response was not elicited by dorsi flexion, but by planter flexion in the standing posture.

References

[1] Y. Ugawa, et al., Percutaneouselectrical stimulation of corticospinal pathway at the level of the pyramidal decussation in humans, Ann. Neurol. 29 (1991) 418–427.
[2] Y. Ugawa, et al., Magnetic stimulation of corticospinal pathways at the foramen magnum level in humans, Ann. Neurol. 36 (1994) 618–624.
[3] Y. Ugawa, Magnetic stimulation of the descending and ascending tracts at the foramen magnum level, Electroencephalogr. Clin. Neurophysiol. 105 (1997) 128–131.
[4] A. Berardelli, et al., Stretch reflexes of triceps surae in normal man, J. Neurosurg. Psychiatry 45 (1982) 513–525.

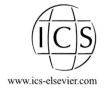
ELSEVIER

Event-Related Potential due to vocalization of a single syllable in Down syndrome

Noriko Yazawa[a], Hiroaki Shoji[a], Atsuko Gunji[b], Hisaki Ozaki[a],*

[a]Laboratory of Physiology, Ibaraki University, 2-1-1 Bunkyo, Mito, Ibaraki 310-8512, Japan
[b]Department of Integrative Physiology, National Institute for Physiological Sciences, Okazaki, Japan

Abstract. Event-Related Potential (ERP) due to vocalization of a single syllable was recorded in normal adults and in persons with Down syndrome, and their cerebral processes during single syllable vocalization were studied. EEGs were recorded from 20 locations on the scalp including Broca's and Wernicke's areas. EMG of orbicularis oris muscle and subject's voice through a microphone were also monitored during the EEG measurement, and were averaged after rectification. From EEGs averaged before and after vocalizing a Japanese syllable, /u/ or /mu/, we recognized Vocalization-Related Cortical Potential (VRCP) with Bereitschaftpotential (BP) before vocalization contains. Significant difference of BP due to vocalization of a vowel syllable (/u/) was not observed between subject groups. For vocalizing a Consonant–Vowel (CV) syllable (/mu/), however, BP amplitude in Down syndromes was significantly larger than normal adults. Therefore, the increased BP in Down syndromes might be brought by their enhanced effort and expectation to vocalize CV syllable. VRCP after the onset of vocalization may contain not only motor component related to control of vocalization organ but also auditory response to one's own voice as an auditory feedback. As people with Down syndrome vocalize louder voice with longer duration, motor and auditory components might be increased respectively and remain longer. Therefore, enhanced VRCP after the onset of vocalization in Down syndrome might be associated with inflamed cortical activation. © 2004 Elsevier B.V. All rights reserved.

Keywords: Down syndrome; Vocalization-Related Cortical Potential (VRCP); Vocalization of a vowel syllable; Vocalization of a Consonant–Vowel (CV) syllable

1. Introduction

Many studies revealed unclear pronunciation in children with Down syndrome even though they already attained school age. Such difficulty in vocalization might be due to their poor auditory information processing and/or insufficient operation of vocalizing organs. Because processing of auditory information as well as control of vocal organs are done within the brain, recent neuroimaging approach in people with Down syndrome will

---

* Corresponding author. Tel.: +81-29-228-8292.
E-mail address: ozaki@mx.ibaraki.ac.jp (H. Ozaki).

0531-5131/ © 2004 Elsevier B.V. All rights reserved.
doi:10.1016/j.ics.2004.04.095

extend the findings obtained through behavioural data. McAdam and Whitaker [1] reported an anterior negativity prior to speech onset as a Bereitschaftpotential (BP), and such negative potential prior to vocalization was referred as a Vocalization-Related Cortical Potential (VRCP). VRCP involves not only Motor-Related Cortical Potential (MRCP) but also Auditory-Evoked Potential (AEP) [2–4]. Therefore, VRCP might be suitable to reveal auditory monitoring of spoken sounds as well as preparatory processes for articulation in Down syndrome. In this study, we recorded VRCP due to vocalization of a vowel syllable or a consonant–vowel syllable, and examined cerebral process associated with single syllable vocalization in Down syndrome.

2. Methods

Six subjects with Down syndrome (four males and two females; 14–17 years) and seven normal adults (one male and six females; 18–19 years) participated in this study. Their mother tongue was Japanese and all subjects were right-handed. Prior to the experiment, we obtained their informed consent to participate in the experiment. Subjects seated on the chair and were asked to fixate a small circle 1.0 m away in front of the subjects. A single syllable /u/ or /mu/ with female voice was delivered in 60 dB SPL in each 4.0-s interval, and subjects were asked to repeat it. Before the experiment, subjects had practiced to vocalize a syllable with their bodies relaxed.

EEGs were recorded from 20 locations on the scalp including Broca's and Wernicke's areas with the linked earlobe as a reference. The equidistant point from F3, T3, F7 and C3 was designated as an electrode position of Broca's area (BL). For Wernicke's area (WL), the electrode was set at the equidistant point from C3, T5, T3 and P3. EEGs were also recorded from homologous locations of Broca (BR) and Wernicke (WR) in the right hemisphere. Simultaneously, vertical and horizontal EOGs and EMG from the upper orbicularis oris muscle were monitored. To pick up vocalized sound, a microphone was placed 5.0 cm from the lip of the subject.

All signals were digitized at a sampling rate of 500 Hz by SCAN systems (NeuroScan). After DC-30 Hz band-pass filtering, artefact-free EEGs were averaged before and after vocalization in each condition (/u/ or /mu/). EMG and vocalized sound were low-pass filtered at 100 Hz and averaged after rectification. All averaged data were baseline corrected within 2000 to 1500 ms before the onset of vocalization, and calculated the grand averaged waveforms. For the amplitude of VRCP, statistical *t*-test was done between subject groups (normal adults vs. subjects with Down syndrome) and also between vocalized syllables (/u/ vs. /mu/).

3. Results and discussion

3.1. Preparatory process for vocalization

Early component of MRCP, starting in 1500–1000 ms and lasting to 400–500 ms before voluntary movement, is designated as BP. BP is concerned with cortical preparatory process of voluntary movement [5] and starts in earlier period by more difficult movement task than easy one [6]. In this study, MRCP due to vocalization shifted gradually toward negativity in 1000 ms prior to the vocalization onset in both subject groups. Its amplitude remarkably increased toward negative direction around 200 ms before the vocalization onset. Amplitude of VRCP in each EEG recording site was statistically examined by t-test in each sampling point between subject groups. Significant difference of BP due to vocalization of /u/ was not observed between subject groups (Fig. 1). For vocalizing /mu/, however, BP amplitude in subjects with Down syndrome was significantly larger than normal adults during the time period of 1346–956 ms prior to the vocalization onset. BPs due to different syllable vocalization were also compared within the same group, and it turned out that amplitude of BP due to /mu/-vocalization was larger than BP due to /u/-vocalization in subjects with Down syndrome, but not in normal adults. To pronounce CV syllable (/mu/), control of facial muscle, larynx and diaphragm will be needed. However, vocalization of vowel syllable (/u/) might be possible without facial muscle contracture. Therefore, the increased BP in subjects with Down syndrome might be brought by their enhanced effort and expectation to prepare vocalization of /mu/.

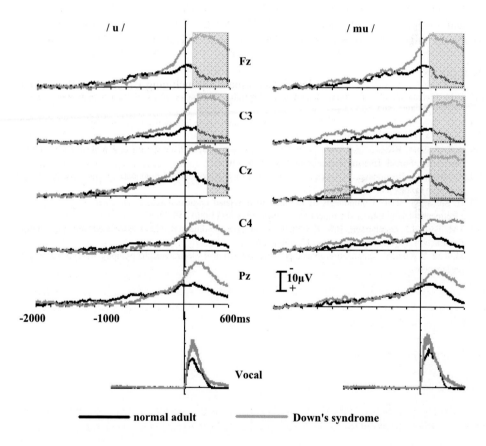

Fig. 1. Grand averaged waveforms of VRCP in the normal adult (black line) and the Down syndrome (gray line). Significant difference between VRCPs of subject groups was observed during time period indicated by gray shadow.

3.2. VRCP and auditory feedback of vocalized sound

The negative potential of VRCP kept increasing after the onset of vocalization and reached the negative peak during vocalization. VRCP after the onset of vocalization in subjects with Down syndrome was characterized by the sustained negativity with high amplitude. The amplitude of VRCP in each EEG recording site was statistically examined by *t*-test between subject groups in each sampling point. Whatever the vocalized syllable was /u/ or /mu/, amplitude of VRCP in subjects with Down syndrome was significantly larger than that in normal adults (Fig. 1). VRCP after the onset of vocalization was also compared between vocalized syllables within the same subject group, and significant difference was not observed in both subject groups.

VRCP after the onset of vocalization may contain not only motor component related to control of vocalization organ but also auditory response to one's own voice as an auditory feedback [7]. In addition, AEP component declines under the condition where vocalized voice is masked by noise [4]. As people with Down syndrome vocalize louder voice with longer duration, increased motor and auditory components might be brought about and remain longer. Therefore, enhanced VRCP after the onset of vocalization in Down syndrome might be associated with inflamed cortical activation.

References

[1] D.M. McAdam, H.A. Whitaker, Electroencephalographic localization in the normal human brain, Science 175 (1971) 499–502.
[2] A.B. Wohlert, M.A. Laeson, Cerebral averaged potentials preceding oral movement, Speech Hearing Research 34 (1991) 1387–1396.
[3] A.B. Wohlert, Event-related brain potentials preceding speech and nonspeech oral movement of varying complexity, Speech Hearing Research 36 (1993) 287–905.
[4] A. Gunji, M. Hoshiyama, R. Kakigi, Identification of auditory evoked potentials of one's voice, Clinical Neurophysiology 111 (2000) 214–219.
[5] H. Shibasaki, et al., Components of the movement-related cortical potential and their scalp topography, Electroencephalography and Clinical Neurophysiology 49 (1980) 213–226.
[6] J.M. Ford, L. Macpherson, B.S. Kopell, Differences in readiness potential associated with push-botton construction, Psychophysiology 9 (1972) 564–567.
[7] M. Kita, Y. Kikuchi, Vocalization-related potential (1), Clinical Electroencephalography 36 (1994) 259–293 (in Japanese).

Language-related brain regions during "shiritori" task (Japanese capping verses): a spatial filtered MEG analysis

Masakiyo Yamamoto[a,*], Satoshi Ukai[a], Shunsuke Kawaguchi[a], Ryouhei Ishii[a], Asao Ogawa[a], Yuko Mizuno-Matsumoto[a], Norihiko Fujita[b], Toshiki Yoshimine[c], Kazuhiro Shinosaki[d], Masatoshi Takeda[a]

[a] Department of Psychiatry and Behavioral Science, Osaka University Graduate School of Medicine D-3, 2-2, Yamada-oka, Suita, Osaka 565-0871, Japan
[b] Department of Radiology, Osaka University Graduate School of Medicine, Osaka, Japan
[c] Department of Neurosurgery, Osaka University Graduate School of Medicine, Osaka, Japan
[d] Department of Neuropsychiatry, Wakayama Medical University, Wakayama, Japan

Abstract. There is a Japanese traditional word game, "shiritori" (capping verses), analogous to English word generation. "Shiritori" task is characterized by demanding a subject to detect the phonetic factor of words as well as to generate words, and is expected to activate brain regions related to phonological processing, such as Wernicke's area. The aim of this study is to visualize neural activated brain regions during performance of a "shiritori" task using a MEG neuroimaging technique, Synthetic Aperture Magnetometry (SAM). Eight healthy right-handed, native Japanese speakers were studied. They gave their informed consents. Subjects were instructed to play "shiritori" by themselves silently during the "shiritori" task. In 8–25 Hz band, neural activated regions (corresponding to event-related desynchronization) were estimated in language-related brain regions with left-side dominancy: dorsolateral prefrontal cortex (DLPFC), post-inferior frontal gyrus (IFG), primary motor cortex, post-superior temporal gyrus (STG), visual cortex, inferior parietal lobule. The results suggest that the "shiritori" task requires neural activations in Wernicke's area more strongly when compared with verbal fluency paradigm and that this task can be used for assessing pathophysiology of diseases with dysfunction of Wernicke's area such as schizophrenia. © 2004 Elsevier B.V. All rights reserved.

Keywords: Shiritori; Verbal fluency; Dorsolateral prefrontal cortex; Wernicke's area; MEG

1. Introduction

In order to investigate the neural basis of language, neuroimaging studies have employed various language tasks, such as verbal fluency paradigms. Among them, word

---

* Corresponding author. Tel.: +81-6-6879-3051; fax: +81-6-6879-3059.
E-mail address: yamamasa@psy.med.osaka-u.ac.jp (M. Yamamoto).

0531-5131/ © 2004 Elsevier B.V. All rights reserved.
doi:10.1016/j.ics.2004.05.051

generation to a letter is most often employed. Word generation tasks were reported to activate several brain regions with left-side dominancy, especially left dorsolateral prefrontal cortex (DLPFC) and inferior frontal gyrus (IFG) [1–3].

There is a Japanese traditional word game, "shiritori" (capping verses), which is analogous to English word generation. In a "shiritori", when a person says a noun, another person has to generate a noun whose first syllable is coincident with the end syllable of the former noun. Therefore, a "shiritori" task is characterized by demanding a subject to detect the phonetic factor of words as well as to generate words and is expected to activate brain regions related to phonological processing, such as Wernicke's area.

Among neuroimaging techniques, fMRI, PET and SPECT are often used, however, they cannot directly prove neural activities but merely detect hemodynamic responses while MEG can directly prove them. Using MEG signals, a novel spatial filtering technique, Synthetic Aperture Magnetometry (SAM) can estimate three-dimensional neural activities in a prescribed frequency band in a brain. The aim of this study is to examine language-related brain regions during performance of a "shiritori" task using SAM.

2. Material and methods

Eight healthy native speaking Japanese (men and women, mean age 27 years) were studied. They were all right-handed according to the Edinburgh Handedness Inventory [4]. Prior to the experiments, consent in writing was given by all the subjects.

Subjects were instructed to play shiritori by themselves silently, generating as many nouns and as quickly as possible during the task period and to concentrate their breathings during the rest period. They were required to keep their eyes open in both periods. A trial consisted of a 20-s task and successive 20-s rest periods. Eight trials were performed. Before and after the MEG recordings, the subjects were confirmed to be able to generate 10 or more nouns for 20 s. A 64-channel whole-head MEG system equipped with third-order SQUID gradiometers (CTF Systems) was used. MEG signals were digitally recorded at a sampling rate of 250 Hz, and filtered online with 80 Hz low-pass filter and 60, 120, and 180 Hz notch filters.

The tomographic distributions of neural activations were determined using SAM. SAM is a spatial filter, in which adaptive signal processing techniques in the space are applied to MEG [5,6]. Using SAM, three-dimensional images (current source density (CSD) mapping) of MEG signal sources can be estimated, and a statistical parametric map (SPM) can be produced using voxel-to-voxel comparison by the Student's t-test of the images taken in control and active state [7]. Functional images related to the anatomical structure can be obtained by superimposing SPM on MR images.

MEG signals were filtered through a band-pass of 8–25 Hz and submitted to SAM. SPM images were produced regarding the control periods (20 s × 8 trials) as rest and the active periods (20 s × 8 trials) as task state. Then, images of cortical regions in which CSD significantly increased or decreased were examined with a 5 mm voxel resolution.

3. Results

All eight subjects showed localized significant event-related desynchronization (ERD) in six brain regions related to language processing: DLPFC, post-IFG, primary motor

Table 1
Neural activated regions (asterisks) per subject

Subject no.	Sex	Left						Right					
		DLPFC	IFG	M1	p-STG	Visual C	IPL	DLPFC	IFG	M1	p-STG	Visual C	IPL
1	F	*			*		*	*		*			
2	M			*	*	*	*			*		*	*
3	F	*	*	*				*		*			
4	M	*			*	*	*	*		*			
5	M		*	*	*	*						*	
6	M		*	*	*	*		*					
7	M	*				*		*			*		
8	M	*	*		*			*					
Total		5/8	4/8	4/8	6/8	5/8	3/8	3/8	3/8	2/8	2/8	3/8	1/8
		total 27						total 14					

DLPFC, dorsolateral prefrontal cortex; IFG, inferior frontal gyrus; M1, primary motor cortex; STG, superior temporal gyrus; visual C, visual cortex; IPL, inferior parietal lobule.

cortex (M1), post-superior temporal gyrus (STG), visual cortex, inferior parietal lobe (Table 1). The SAM tomographic images in a subject are shown in Fig. 1.

Brain regions with significant ERD were highly lateralized with almost twice the number of regions in the left hemisphere than in the right hemisphere (27 vs. 14). In all subjects except Subject 7, the number of brain regions with significant ERD showed left-side dominancy. Left post-STG showed the largest numbers of subjects with significant

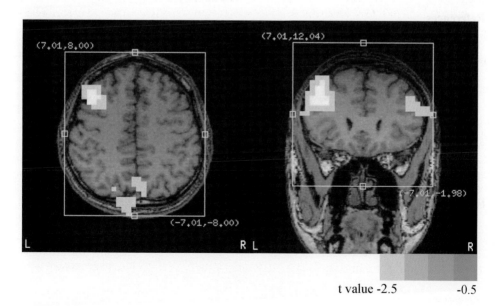

Fig. 1. The SAM images of Subject 7. Bilateral DLPFC and left visual cortex were activated. Gray color shows significant neural activated regions where current source density during the "shiritori" task is significantly smaller than the control period. The color is lighter, the t-statistic is larger.

ERD (six out of eight subjects). In five of eight subjects, significant ERD in the left DLPFC and visual cortex were found, respectively.

4. Discussion

In this study, MEG SAM analysis showed localized neural activations in the brain regions related to language processing in the "shiritori" task. When neural activation is elicited in a region, synchronization between neural cells in a frequency band decreases and makes CSD estimated by SAM to decrease while neural activation is elicited [8–10]. Neural activated brain regions and their left-side dominancy are consistent with previous reports using verbal fluency paradigm.

Left post-STG (Wernicke's area) was activated in the most subjects during the "shiritori" task. Left post-STG might subserve phonological processing related with repeating the letter of the previous noun in the "shiritori" task. Neural activations in left DLPFC is also estimated and is considered to reflect evocation of verbal working memory necessary for this language-related task.

Since most Japanese people are used to playing "shiritori" and can play it even from about 3 years of age, the "shiritori" task is a useful language task for the wide range of diseases with cognitive impairment as well as healthy subjects for Japanese. In addition, this study have shown that the "shiritori" task requires neural activations in Wernicke's area more strongly when compared with verbal fluency paradigm, suggesting that this task can be used for assessing pathophysiology of diseases with dysfunction of Wernicke's area such as schizophrenia.

References

[1] C.D. Frith, et al., A PET study of word finding, Neuropsychologia 29 (12) (1991) 1137–1148.
[2] C.A. Cuenod, et al., Functional MRI during word generation, using conventional equipment: a potential tool for language localization in the clinical environment, Neurology 45 (10) (1995 Oct) 1821–1827.
[3] S.E. Petersen, et al., Positron emission tomographic studies of the cortical anatomy of single-word processing, Nature 331 (6157) (1988 Feb 18) 585–589.
[4] R. Oldfield, Neuropsychologia 9 (1971) 97–113.
[5] B. Widrow, S.D. Stearns, Analysis of adaptive beamformers, Adaptive Signal Processing, Prentice-Hall, Upper Saddle River, 1985, pp. 409–455.
[6] S.E. Robinson, D. Cheyne, J. Jpn. Biomag. Bioelectromag. Soc. 10 (1997) 180–183.
[7] K.J. Friston, et al., Hum. Brain Mapp. 1 (1994) 214–220.
[8] R. Ishii, et al., NeuroReport 10 (1999) 675–679.
[9] R. Ishii, et al., NeuroReport 11 (2000) 3283–3287.
[10] S. Ukai, et al., MEG functional neuroimaging of schizophrenic patients and comparison subjects during word generation, in: K. Miyoshi, C.M. Shapiro, M. Gaviria, et al. (Eds.), Contemporary Neuropsychiatry, Springer-Verlag, Tokyo, 2001, pp. 39–45.

International Congress Series 1270 (2004) 157–160

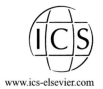

ELSEVIER

www.ics-elsevier.com

Estimation of equivalent current dipoles and the analysis of synthetic aperture magnetmetry on auditory evoked magnetic responses

Hiroshi Nishimura*, Nakagami Tetsuhiro, Yasuhiro Osaki, Takeshi Kubo

Department of Otolaryngology and Sensory Organ Surgery, Osaka University School of Medicine, 2-2 Yamadaoka, Suita, Osaka 565-0871, Japan

Abstract. We have been studying auditory evoked magnetic fields and dipole analysis. Today synthetic aperture magnetometry (SAM) was applied to the data of auditory evoked responses. Auditory evoked N100 potentials originate in actions of the auditory cortices. The magnetic recordings of this 100-ms response are the major studies. We acquired auditory evoked magnetic fields (AEF) with a whole head array of 64-channel SQUID sensors and averaged whole hundred trials then estimated equivalent current dipoles (ECD) at 100-ms latencies. We analyzed the AEF data from whole channels with dual-state SAM analyze of pseudo-Student's T statistics around 100 ms between each frequency band (α: 8–13 Hz, β: 13–25 Hz, γ: 25–50 Hz). The resulting ECDs and SAM images are plotted/superimposed into own MR images. SAM images were estimated around the locations of the ECDs in the auditory cortices of the temporal lobes. Synchronization of the electrical activations around 100 ms was observed in all frequency bands. Synchronization of source power revealed by SAM and ECD analyses showed compatible temporal information. The novel technique SAM appears useful for cortical activation in processing perceptual information. © 2004 Elsevier B.V. All rights reserved.

Keywords: Magnetoencephalography; Auditory cortex; Synthetic aperture magnetmetry (SAM); Auditory evoked magnetic fields (AEF); Equivalent current dipoles (ECD); Auditory M100 responses

1. Introduction

Auditory evoked potentials (AEP) have been recorded in EEG, and the responses in various latencies are recognized such as ABR, MLR, and SVR. The most prominent peak of negative AEP occurs approximately 100 ms after the sound onset and is called N1 or N100. The magnetic homologue of N100 is called M100, which is the magnetic record of the same neuro-electric activity. We have been studying these auditory evoked magnetic fields and dipole analysis [1]. However, dipole coordinate stands for a point of centre of

* Corresponding author. Tel.: +81-6-6879-3951; fax: +81-6-6879-3959.
E-mail address: hnishimura@ent.med.osaka-u.ac.jp (H. Nishimura).

0531-5131/ © 2004 Elsevier B.V. All rights reserved.
doi:10.1016/j.ics.2004.05.012

gravity of the volumetric extent and dipole source modelling is inverse solution of a time-point of magnetic fields.

Recently, synthetic aperture magnetometry (SAM) developed as a novel spatial filtering technique based on the nonlinear constrained minimum-variance beamformer. This technique overcomes the nonuniqueness of generalized inverse solutions, such as the minimum norm, and thereby permits unambiguous three-dimensional source mapping during task performance. SAM can estimate source changes as a function of time for any arbitrary voxel or power changes subjected to statistical analysis [2–5]. Compared with equivalent current dipoles (ECD) analysis, SAM can identify the volume of activation rather than the centre of gravity by using a spatial filtering method to identify separate volumes of tissue that are active for specific time periods in the MEG waveform. Now we applied synthetic aperture magnetmetry to the data of auditory evoked responses.

2. Method

A normal hearing volunteer participated in this study. He was right-handed, with no history of otologic or neurological disorders. The magnetic brain activities evoked by auditory stimulations were recorded with 64-channel MEG Whole-Cortex System (CTF Systems, Canada). The relative position of the subject's head to that of the MEG sensors was determined using three head localization coils attached at nasion and preauricular points. The anatomical magnetic resonance images were obtained for the subject using a SIEMENS 1.5 Tesla MRI scanner with three fiducial markers.

A frequency modulated toneburst was presented 100 times with intensity of 60 dB nHL to the right ear with an interstimulous interval randomized from 6.0 to 6.5 s. Auditory stimuli were generated by a magnetically silent piezoelectric loud speaker EARTONE®3A and delivered through short tube.

The MEG signals were digitized with 16 bit AD converter at 625 samples per second. Each trial was on-line filtered with 60 Hz notch filters and with low-pass filters under 200 Hz and with offset removal on prestimulous baseline. One hundred stimulus-evoked events of 4 s, including 2 s pretrigger baselines, were recorded.

The 100 trials were averaged and the auditory evoked magnetic wave forms emerged. Two dipoles model was applied to analyze the auditory evoked field at the most prominent peak near the 100-ms latency, solving the inverse problem on least-mean-squared error method.

SAM operates on unaveraged MEG data and requires simultaneous acquisition of signals from an array of sensors. Source images are generated by applying SAM to each

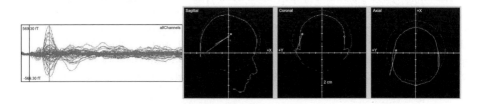

Fig. 1. MEG channels and ECD estimation.

voxel in the region of interest (ROI). The covariance matrices were generated within the α (8–13 Hz) and β (13–25 Hz) and γ (25–50 Hz) frequency bands. A volumetric image of root-mean-squared source activity with 5 mm voxel resolution in generated for time intervals of − 70 to 0 ms and 70 to 140 ms relative to trigger onset as control and active states, respectively. We used a statistical resampling method termed the "jackknife" in order to determine the trial-by-trial variability of the MEG. Then dual-state static SAM

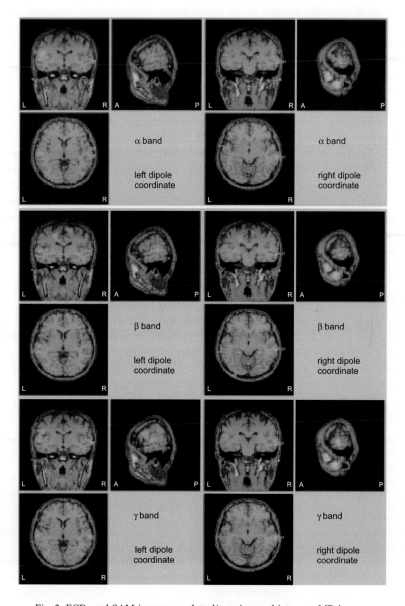

Fig. 2. ECDs and SAM images are plotted/superimposed into own MR images.

statistical parametric images were computed using the multiple covariance files. A statistical parametric image was computed with a pseudo-Student's T parametric method, on a voxel-by-voxel basis, from the difference in cortical power for the two states, relative to their noise variance.

3. Result

The original magnetic records of all MEG sensor channels were averaged for dipole estimation. A prominent N1 peak was clearly recorded approximately 100 ms. Equivalent current dipoles were estimated with two-dipole model. The dipoles were located in both temporal areas (Fig. 1).

The resulting ECDs and SAM images are plotted/superimposed into own MR images. Only voxels displaying significant power changes are displayed on the individual MRI. The images are shown in three-dimensional view that contains the left/right dipole coordinates (Fig. 2). Therefore, the SAM areas consisting of voxels displaying strong signal change were evaluated relative to ECD results for auditory stimulation.

The SAM statistical imaging for α band revealed predominant statistical power on the contralateral superior temporal lobe to auditory stimuli. The significant areas of SAM statistical imaging are located around the dipole coordinates. In β band, strong SAM signal was detected in the left superior temporal lobe and it corresponded to the dipole location of left hemisphere. Similar areas are activates as well as in α band, and stronger synchronization was observed than in α band. SAM areas in γ band appeared more posterior than dipole points and the areas of α and β band. The significant areas of SAM statistical imaging are not detected in right hemisphere within γ band.

4. Discussion

SAM images were estimated around the locations of the ECDs in the auditory cortices of the temporal lobes. Synchronization of the electrical activations around M100 ms was observed in all frequency bands. Synchronization of source power revealed by SAM and ECD analyses showed compatible temporal information. The novel technique, SAM, appears useful for cortical activation in processing perceptual information.

References

[1] H. Nishimura, et al., Different Processing between Auditory Evoked Magnetic Off- and On-Responses in the Auditory Cortex, in: T. Yoshimoto, M. Kotani, S. Kuriki, H. Karibe, N. Nakasato (Eds.), Recent Advances in Biomagnetism, Tohoku Univ. Press, Sendai, pp. 302–305.
[2] S.E. Robinson, D. Cheyne, Functional imaging of language cortex by MEG, J. Jpn. Biomagn. Bioelectromagn. Soc. 10 (1997) 180–183.
[3] R. Ishii, et al., Medial prefrontal cortex generates frontal midline theta rhythm, NeuroReport 10 (1999) 675–679.
[4] M. Taniguchi, et al., Movement-related desynchronization of the cerebral cortex studied with spatially filtered magnetoencephalography, NeuroImage 12 (3) (2000) 298–306.
[5] S.E. Robinson, D. Cheyne, W.W. Sutherling, Magnetoencephalographic imaging of interictal spikes, NeuroImage 7 (1998) 663.

International Congress Series 1270 (2004) 161–164

ELSEVIER

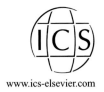

www.ics-elsevier.com

Variations of N100m responses in auditory evoked magnetic field

Yuko Suzuka[a,*], Masanori Higuchi[b], Natsuko Hatsusaka[b],
Shinji Kawashima[c], Kanako Yamada[a], Koichi Tomoda[a]

[a] Department of Otolaryngology, Kanazawa Medical University, 1-1 Daigaku, Uchinada,
Ishikawa 920-0293, Japan
[b] Applied Electronics Laboratory, Kanazawa Institute of Technology, Japan
[c] Ishikawa Sunrise Industries Creation Organization,
Collaboration of Regional Entities for the Advancement of Technological Excellence, Japan

Abstract. The purpose of this study was to investigate the interaction of the auditory pathway at the level of the primary auditory cortex by magnetoencephalography (MEG). Auditory evoked magnetic fields have been investigated from the beginning of MEG studies. We examined auditory responses in healthy 13 subjects, 6 males and 7 females. The responses were averaged by 100 stimulus presentations of each measurement. We could find clear response peaks, such as N100m and P200m in 12 subjects. Especially in N100m, it revealed that there were some patterns and it was not simple to determine contralateral dominancy or hyperactivity of the right auditory cortex over the left, and there were some differences with previous studies. In this measurement, we could classify them into three major groups using the isofield contour map and peak amplitude of N100m. The explanation of individual variation requires further investigations of binaural integration and interaural differentiation. © 2004 Elsevier B.V. All rights reserved.

Keywords: Magnetoencephalography; Tone-burst stimulus; Auditory evoked magnetic field; N100m

1. Introduction

The purpose of this study was to investigate the interaction of the auditory pathway at the level of the primary auditory cortex. Auditory evoked magnetic fields have been investigated from the beginning of magnetoencephalography (MEG) studies. The auditory evoked magnetic field contains the responses of P50m, N100m and P200m that occurred in the primary auditory cortex. We discussed the N100m response in certain conditions, which differed from previous studies.

2. Subjects and methods

Thirteen neurologically normal subjects, six males and seven females aged 23–50, participated in this study. Informed consent was obtained from each subject

---

* Corresponding author. Tel.: +81-76-286-2211; fax: +81-76-286-5566.
E-mail address: suzie-nt@kanazawa-med.ac.jp (Y. Suzuka).

0531-5131/ © 2004 Elsevier B.V. All rights reserved.
doi:10.1016/j.ics.2004.04.049

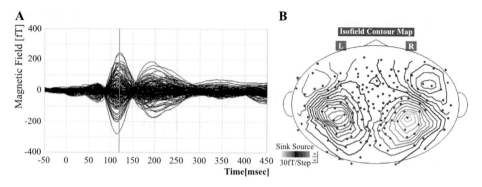

Fig. 1. An example data (both ears' stimuli) of the first group. A: Waveforms, B: isofield contour map.

before the experiment. All subjects were right-handed and had no hearing disturbance.

MEG signals were recorded in a magnetically shielded room using a 320-channel whole-head MEG system, which consists of 160 channels for magnetometers and 160 channels for 50 mm base-lined, co-axial gradiometers, developed by Kanazawa Institute of Technology [1]. Subjects lay down on the bed and inserted their heads into the helmet-shaped sensing part. They were instructed to keep their eyes open and to fix their eyes on a certain point to minimize their eyes' movements.

The auditory stimuli were 1 kHz short tone burst of 50 ms duration with an interstimulus interval of about 1 s, delivered to the right ear, left ear and both ears, respectively, through plastic tubes attached to earplugs. The responses were filtered with 0.1–200 Hz passband by analog filters, sampled with 1 kHz and averaged by 100 stimulus presentations of each measurement. The analysis period was 100 ms before to 500 ms after stimulus onset.

3. Results

We could find clear response peaks such as N100m and P200m, in 12 subjects. Especially in N100m, it revealed that there were some patterns and it was not simple to determine contralateral dominancy or hyperactivity of the right auditory cortex over the

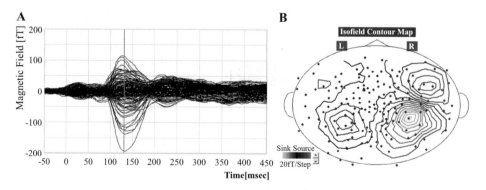

Fig. 2. An example data (right ear's stimuli) of the second group. A: Waveforms, B: isofield contour map.

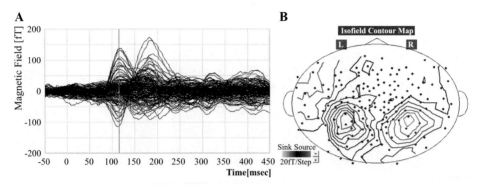

Fig. 3. An example data (left ear's stimuli) of the third group. A: Waveforms, B: isofield contour map.

left. Some results were not compatible with previous studies. In this measurement, we could classify them into three major groups using the isofield contour map and peak amplitude of the N100m.

The first group has contralateral dominancy and slightly hyperactivity of the right hemisphere in both ears' stimuli. In this group, N100m responses were observed dominantly in the left hemisphere by the right ear's stimuli, and dominantly in the right hemisphere by the left ear's stimuli. When stimuli were added to both ears, N100m responses were slightly dominant in the right hemisphere as shown in Fig. 1. Five subjects were included in this group.

The second group has right hemisphere dominancy even by the right ear's stimuli. In this group, N100m responses were observed dominantly in the right hemisphere by the left ear's stimuli. However, in the left hemisphere, they were not dominant even by the right ear's stimuli, as shown in Fig. 2. When the stimuli were added to both ears, N100m responses were dominant in the right hemisphere. So, it is very clear that the right hemisphere is more active than the left hemisphere. Six subjects were included in this group.

The third group's left hemisphere is dominant even by the left ear's stimuli. In this group, N100m responses were observed dominantly in the left hemisphere over the right hemisphere by the right ear's stimuli. However, in the right hemisphere they were not

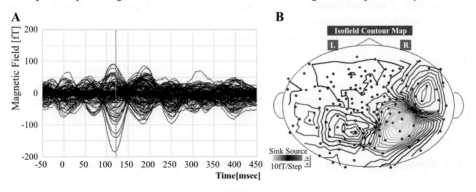

Fig. 4. Extremely right hemisphere dominant data (right ear's stimuli) in the second group. A: Waveforms, B: isofield contour map.

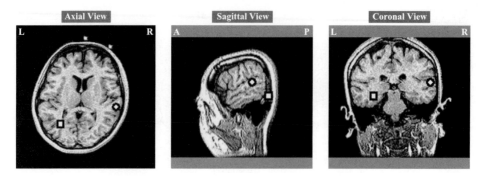

Fig. 5. Dipole fitting of the extreme data, as shown in Fig. 4.

dominant even by the left ear's stimuli, as shown in Fig. 3. When stimuli were added to both ears, they were observed dominantly in the left hemisphere. So, this means that the left hemisphere is more active than the right hemisphere. One subject was included in this group.

As a quite special case in the second group, one subject showed N100m responses hardly appear in the left hemisphere even by the right ear's stimuli, as shown in Fig. 4. The subject was a 24-year-old female with no history of ear disease nor deafness. The pure-tone audiometric and the ABR tests were normal. The equilibrium test was also normal. Furthermore, there were not any abnormal findings MRI morphologically and PET metabolically in the brain. The dipole localization in the right hemisphere was supposed to exist in the auditory cortex in the right temporal lobe. But, the dipole in the left hemisphere was located out of the auditory cortex, as shown in Fig. 5.

4. Discussion

We have discussed hemisphere asymmetry by stimuli like vowel and non-speech [2] and the presence of an anatomical difference of myelination [3]. In the extreme case of the second group, there are some speculations, including that there are none or less f activated neurons in the left hemisphere with any stimuli in N100m, due to synchronization of activated neurons in the recording and orientation of dipole direction.

Therefore, it was not simple to determine contralateral dominancy or hyperactivity of the right auditory cortex over the left. The explanation of individual variation requires further investigations of binaural integration and interaural differentiation.

Acknowledgements

This study was carried out as part of the Cooperative Link of Unique Science and Technology for Economy Revitalization "Ishikawa Hi-tech Sensing Cluster" supported by MEXT Japan.

References

[1] M. Higuchi, et al., Development of a 320 channel MEG system for deep source measurements, Journal of Japan Biomagnetism and Bioelectromagnetics Society 16 (1) (2003) 96–97 (in Japanese).
[2] L. Gootjes, et al., Left-hemisphere dominancy for processing if vowels, NeuroReport 10 (1999) 2987–2991.
[3] V.B. Penhune, et al., Interhemispheric anatomical differences in human primary auditory cortex, Cerebral Cortex 6 (1996) 661–672.

International Congress Series 1270 (2004) 165–168

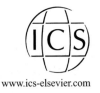

www.ics-elsevier.com

ELSEVIER

Change of auditory evoked magnetic field in a half-sleep state

Natsuko Hatsusaka*, Masanori Higuchi

Applied Electronics Laboratory, Kanazawa Institute of Technology, 3 Amaike, Kanazawa, Ishikawa 920-1331, Japan

Abstract. Although many studies have reported auditory evoked magnetic fields in a wakeful state, it is not clear how the auditory evoked magnetic field is affected by a half-sleep state. We investigated change in the auditory evoked magnetic field in a half-sleep state. Eight normal hearing subjects (five men, three women) participated in this study. In order to make a half-sleep state, the measurement was started about 1 h after having lunch. Auditory stimulation was 1000 Hz tone bursts and was delivered to the right ear through an air tube attached to an earplug. The responses were averaged by 100 stimuli. A significant response was observed after the N1m response in a half-sleep state. This response was estimated to come from the deep area. We speculate that it has some relation to the theta rhythm activities and is synchronized with auditory stimulation. © 2004 Elsevier B.V. All rights reserved.

Keywords: MEG; Half-sleep; Auditory evoked magnetic field; N1m; P2m; Theta rhythm activities

1. Introduction

There have been many studies of the auditory evoked magnetic field. Most of the studies show that N1m and P2m responses are typically observed in a wakeful state. The magnetic fields of these responses are distributed in the superior temporal cortex. From these fields, the sources are estimated in the primary auditory cortex. However, it is not clear how the auditory evoked magnetic field is affected by a half-sleep state. In this study, we measured the auditory evoked magnetic fields in wakeful and half-sleep states and investigated the difference between both states.

2. Methods

Eight subjects (five men, three women) with normal hearing ability participated in this study. Informed consent was obtained from each subject before the experiment.

Auditory stimulation was 1000 Hz tone bursts 50 ms in duration with an interstimulus interval of 1000 ms, delivered to the right ear through an air tube attached to an earplug.

* Corresponding author. Tel.: +81-76-229-8071; fax: +81-76-229-8072.
E-mail address: hatusaka@ishikawa-sp.com (N. Hatsusaka).

0531-5131/ © 2004 Elsevier B.V. All rights reserved.
doi:10.1016/j.ics.2004.05.005

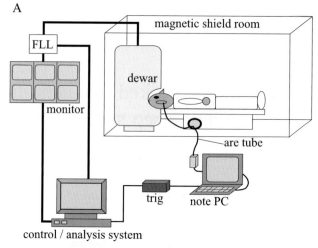

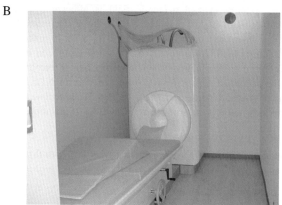

Fig. 1. Block diagram of the experimental setup (A) and photograph of the 320-channel, whole-head MEG system (B).

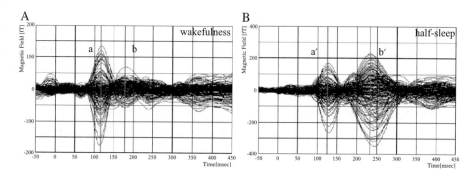

Fig. 2. Example of auditory magnetic fields in wakeful state (A) and half-sleep state (B).

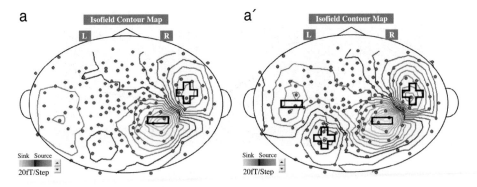

Fig. 3. Isofield contour maps for the first peaks in wakefulness and half-sleep. a and a′ correspond to Fig. 2.

Auditory evoked signals were averaged by 100 stimuli. In order to make a half-sleep state, the measurement was started about 1 h after having lunch.

As Fig. 1 shows, magnetic signals were recorded in a magnetically shielded room using a 320-channel, whole-head MEG system developed by the Kanazawa Institute of Technology [1]. Subjects lay down on the bed and were instructed to stare at a fixed point. After the measurements, we asked the subjects about their sleepiness during the measurements.

3. Results

We found two significant peaks in both wakeful and half-sleep states, as shown in Fig. 2. Especially the second peak observed in a half-sleep state had very large amplitude. We confirmed that this peak was not an artefact caused by eye movement. Fig. 3 shows the isofield contour maps of the first peaks and Fig. 4 shows the second peaks. Map a′ was almost the same as map a, which shows a typical field pattern of N1m response. This means that the source of N1m response does not change by sleepiness. On the other hand, map b′ was clearly different from map b, which shows the reversed pattern of N1m response. Considering the field pattern, the source of map b′ seems to be deeper than the

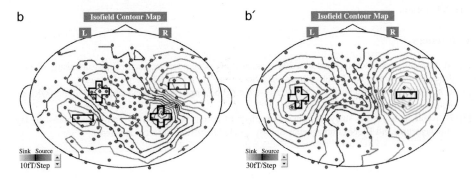

Fig. 4. Isofield contour maps for the second peaks in wakefulness and half-sleep. b and b′ correspond to Fig. 2.

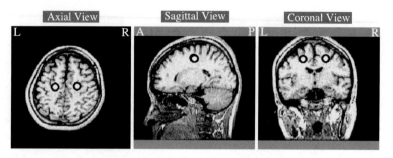

Fig. 5. Dipole estimation of the significant response observed after the N1m response in a half-sleep state.

hearing cortex. Actually, the dipole sources were estimated in the vicinity of the cingulate gyrus as shown in Fig. 5. We obtained similar results from five of the subjects.

4. Discussion

Portas et al. [2] reported that the N1 response of the auditory evoked potential was not influenced by sleep. In our study, the N1m response also did not change by sleepiness.

We observed a significant response after the N1m response in a half-sleep state. The sources were estimated in the deeper area than the auditory cortex. Asada et al. [3] reported that the current sources of the theta rhythm activities observed sleeping conditions were estimated in the deep brain area. Their study suggests the significant response in our study of some relation to the theta rhythm activities. Generally, the theta rhythm activities are spontaneous, and are not generated with regularity. Therefore, the components of the activities should be uniformly distributed in a recording window by means of an averaging process. However, our results showed that they were not distributed uniformly and significantly observed at certain latency. This means the theta rhythm activities were synchronized with auditory stimuli.

Acknowledgements

This study was carried out as part of the Cooperative Link of Unique Science and Technology for Economy Revitalization "Ishikawa Hi-tech Sensing Cluster" supported by MEXT Japan.

References

[1] M. Higuchi, et al., Development of a 320 channel MEG system for deep source measurements, Journal of Japan Biomagnetism and Bioelectromagnetics Society 16 (1) (2003) 96–97 (in Japanese).
[2] C.M. Portas, et al., Auditory processing across the sleep–wake cycle: simultaneous EEG and fMRI monitoring in humans, Neuron 28 (2000) 991–999.
[3] H. Asada, et al., MEG study of frontal theta rhythms during mental activity and sleep, Journal of Japan Biomagnetism and Bioelectromagnetics Society 13 (1) (2000) 134–135 (in Japanese).

ELSEVIER

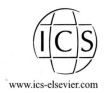

www.ics-elsevier.com

Magnetoencephalographic study of human auditory steady-state responses to binaural beat

Shotaro Karino[a,*], Masato Yumoto[b], Kenji Itoh[c], Akira Uno[d], Maki Matsuda[e], Keiko Yamakawa[c], Sotaro Sekimoto[c], Yuu Kaneko[f], Kimitaka Kaga[a]

[a] Department of Otolaryngology Head and Neck Surgery, Faculty of Medicine, University of Tokyo, 7-3-1 Hongo, Bunkyo, Tokyo 113-8655, Japan
[b] Department of Laboratory Medicine, Faculty of Medicine, University of Tokyo, Japan
[c] Department of Cognitive Neuroscience, Faculty of Medicine, University of Tokyo, Japan
[d] National Institute of Mental Health, National Center of Neurology and Psychiatry, Japan
[e] Tokyo National University of Fine Arts and Music, Japan
[f] Department of Neurosurgery, National Center Hospital for Mental, Nervous and Muscular Disorders, National Center of Neurology and Psychiatry, Japan

Abstract. Presentation of one sinusoid to each ear with a small difference of frequency elicits subjective fluctuations called binaural beat (BB). BB is a classic example of binaural interaction and provides a typical demonstration that the discharges of the auditory nerve fibers preserve information on the phase of the acoustic stimuli. Neural spikes tend to occur at a particular phase of the sinusoidal waveform (phase locking). The central auditory system utilizes the information of interaural phase difference (IPD) with continuous and periodical oscillation. The apparent beat frequency heard is equal to the IPD provided. In order to confirm the cortical representation of fluctuation of BB, we recorded the magnetic field of the auditory steady-state response (SSR) evoked by BBs in six normal-hearing right-handed subjects. Periodical responses with small amplitude were recorded around the bilateral temporal areas by a wholescalp neuromagnetometer under presentation of slow BB (4 and 6.66 Hz). Spectral analysis detected peaks of the BB frequency in the channels of bilateral temporal areas. These results suggested that activity of cerebral cortex, especially auditory cortex, can be synchronized with slow BB and have capacity for preserving the information of IPD. © 2004 Elsevier B.V. All rights reserved.

Keywords: Binaural beat; MEG; Steady-state response; Interaural phase difference

1. Introduction

Presentation of one sinusoid to each ear with a small difference of frequency (Δf) provides an orderly and continuously changing interaural relative phase through one cycle of Δf. When Δf is smaller, a single auditory image moves toward the leading ear to which a

---

* Corresponding author. Tel.: +81-3-5800-8665; fax: +81-3-3814-9486.
E-mail address: karinos-tky@umin.ac.jp (S. Karino).

tone of higher frequency is presented [1,2]. As Δf is increased, subjective periodic fluctuations called binaural beats (BBs) are elicited at a rate equal to Δf. Perrott and Nelson [3] have reported that, when the frequency of sinusoidal tone presented unilaterally to one ear is 250 Hz, BBs are detected when Δf at the other ear is between about 2 and 30 Hz. BBs demonstrate that the discharges of the auditory nerve fibers preserve information on the phase of the acoustic stimuli. Neural spikes tend to occur at a particular phase of the sinusoidal waveform (phase locking) and the central auditory system has capacity for preserving temporal information (frequency coding). In most mammals, phase locking becomes progressively less precise at frequencies above 1 kHz, and it disappears completely at approximately 4–5 kHz [4]. BBs are essentially a low-frequency phenomenon and are heard most distinctly for frequencies between 300 and 600 Hz [5]. Perception of BBs depends on detecting the continuously changing IPD. The goal of this study is to demonstrate the cortical representation of fluctuation of BBs by magnetoencephalography (MEG) and to confirm that IPD is coded in the human auditory cortex.

2. Material and methods

2.1. Subjects

Six normal-hearing, right-handed subjects (four males, two females; ages 24–57 years; mean ± S.D. age of 40.3 ± 11.5 years) participated in this study. Subjects had no history of otological and neurotological disorders and had normal audiological status.

2.2. Stimulation

Continuous pure tones were played on an Apple personal computer via MOTU 828 (Mark of the Unicorn, Massachusetts, USA) audio interface and led to foam insert earphones through plastic tubes. As frequency of BB, 4 and 6.66 Hz were employed, and the combination of pure tone of 240 and 244 Hz, 240 and 246.66 Hz, 480 and 484 Hz, and 480 and 486.66 Hz were presented to elicit BB. Measurement under control condition with binaural presentation of same pure tones (240 or 480 Hz) was also performed to elucidate the characteristics of response evoked by BB. Triggers for averaging had an interval of four BB cycles to display periodical fluctuation of signals evoked by four BBs.

2.3. Recording

Neuromagnetic cortical signals were recorded with a wholescalp neuromagnetometer (Vectorview; Neuromag, Helsinki, Finland), which has 204 first-order planar gradiometers. During the recordings, the subjects were seated under the helmet-shaped dewar in a magnetically shielded room. The position of the head under the helmet was determined by attaching four coils to the head surface and measuring the coil positions with respect to landmarks on the skull with a three-dimensional (3-D) digitizer; the coil locations in the magnetometer coordinate system were determined by leading current through the coils and measuring the corresponding magnetic fields. The recording passband was 1.0–200 Hz, and the data were digitized at 600 Hz. The averaged signals were low-pass filtered at 40 Hz.

2.4. Data analysis

To obtain steady-state responses, 1000–2000 epochs synchronized with BBs were averaged. The analysis period of four BB cycles was used to display periodical fluctuation of signals evoked by BBs.

Fast Fourier transform (FFT) spectra were calculated across 8192 samples of the continuously recorded MEG signals, and the FFT window was moved in steps of 4096 samples; this procedure resulted in frequency resolution of 0.074 Hz. In order to explore the channels in which MEG signals were synchronized to BB, first, we extracted the channels whose amplitude of just BB frequency (4 or 6.66 Hz) was maximum in the range of 2 Hz width (3–5 and 5.66–7.66 Hz). Then, the channel with maximum amplitude of BB frequency in each hemisphere was selected.

3. Results

Steady-state responses with dominant amplitudes in bilateral temporal areas were observed in all the subjects. In some channels of these regions, four peaks were clearly recognized in the time window which corresponds to four cycles of BBs (Fig. 1a). Spectral analysis detected evident peaks of the frequency of BB (4 or 6.66 Hz) in several channels of the bilateral temporal areas (Fig. 1b).

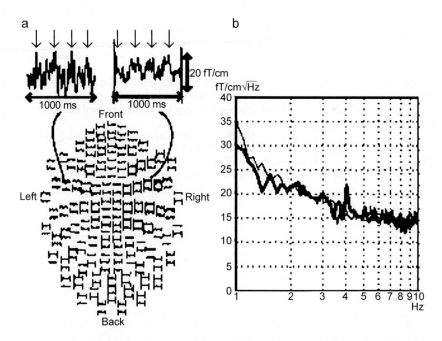

Fig. 1. (a) Typical waveforms of steady-state fields of one subject. Four peaks (arrows) during analysis time of 1000 ms were clearly demonstrated in bilateral temporal areas under the presentation of 240 Hz tone to the left ear and 244 Hz tone to the right ear (BB of 4 Hz). (b) FFT spectra in demonstrative channel of one subject under the presentation of 240 Hz tone to the left ear and 244 Hz tone to the right ear (thick line) and the presentation of 240 Hz tone to both ears (thin line). An evident peak of 4 Hz was confirmed in case of BB.

4. Discussion

BBs provide a classic example of binaural interaction, considered to result from neural interaction in the central auditory pathway that receives input from both ears. Some papers reported that the central auditory system utilizes the information of continuously changing IPD when BBs are presented to mammals. Kuwada et al. [2] found that the responses of cat inferior colliculus neurons are phase-locked to the frequency of BBs. Reale and Brugge [6] studied the interaural phase difference sensitivity of single neurons in the primary auditory cortex of the anesthetized cat. Approximately 26% of the cells that showed sensitivity to static changes in IPD also showed sensitivity to dynamically changing IPD created by BBs. The discharges were highly periodic and tightly synchronized to a particular phase of the BB cycle. Malone et al. [7] revealed the responses to dynamic IPD in the auditory cortex of awake macaques. In our study, periodical steady-state responses with small amplitude were evoked by slow BB, especially around the bilateral temporal areas. Spectral analysis detected peaks of the BB frequency. These results suggested that activity of human cerebral cortex, especially auditory cortex, can be synchronized with slow BB and have capacity for preserving the information of IPD.

References

[1] D.R. Perrott, A.D. Musicant, Rotating tones and binaural beats, J. Acoust. Soc. Am. 61 (5) (1977) 1288–1292.
[2] S. Kuwada, T.C. Yin, R.E. Wickesberg, Response of cat inferior colliculus neurons to binaural beat stimuli: possible mechanisms for sound localization, Science 206 (4418) (1979) 586–588.
[3] D.R. Perrott, M.A. Nelson, Limits for the detection of binaural beats, J. Acoust. Soc. Am. 46 (6) (1969) 1477–1481.
[4] J.E. Rose, et al., Patterns of activity in single auditory nerve fibres of the squirrel monkey, in: A.V.S. de Reuck, J. Knight (Eds.), Hearing Mechanisms in Vertebrates, Churchill, London, 1968, pp. 144–168.
[5] J.C.R. Licklider, J.C. Webster, J.M. Hedlun, On the frequency limits of the binaural beats, J. Acoust. Soc. Am. 22 (1950) 468–473.
[6] R.A. Reale, J.F. Brugge, Auditory cortical neurons are sensitive to static and continuously changing interaural phase cues, J. Neurophysiol. 64 (4) (1990) 1247–1260.
[7] B.J. Malone, B.H. Scott, M.N. Semple, Context-dependent adaptive coding of interaural phase disparity in the auditory cortex of awake macaques, J. Neurosci. 22 (11) (2002) 4625–4638.

International Congress Series 1270 (2004) 173–176

ELSEVIER

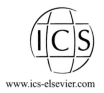

www.ics-elsevier.com

Spatiotemporal neuromagnetic activities during pitch processing in musicians

M. Yumoto[a,*], K. Itoh[b], A. Uno[c], M. Matsuda[d], S. Karino[e], O. Saitoh[f], Y. Kaneko[g], K. Nakahara[a], K. Kaga[e]

[a] Department of Clinical Laboratory, Faculty of Medicine, University of Tokyo,
7-3-1 Hongo, Bunkyo, Tokyo 113-8655, Japan
[b] Department of Speech and Cognitive Science, Faculty of Medicine, University of Tokyo, Tokyo, Japan
[c] National Institute of Mental Health, National Center of Neurology and Psychiatry, Chiba, Japan
[d] Department of Musicology, Tokyo National University of Fine Arts and Music, Tokyo, Japan
[e] Department of Otolaryngology, Faculty of Medicine, University of Tokyo, Tokyo, Japan
[f] Department of Psychiatry, National Center of Neurology and Psychiatry, Tokyo, Japan
[g] Department of Neurosurgery, National Center of Neurology and Psychiatry, Tokyo, Japan

Abstract. Although the spatial distribution of neural subsystems involved in music processing has been elucidated by recent neuroimaging studies, little is known about the temporal profile of such neural activities. In this study, spatiotemporal neuromagnetic activities during pitch processing in a musical context were investigated using a cross-modal pitch-matching task, which required subjects to find infrequent pitch errors implanted in heard performance while sight-reading its musical score. Eight right-handed musicians and eight right-handed non-musicians participated in this study. Neuromagnetic responses to each tone onset were recorded using VectorView™ (Neuromag, Helsinki, Finland). The source localization was estimated by minimum current estimates (MCE) algorithm and was verified by a multiple-current-dipole model. Although every subject showed magnetic components, M50, M100 and M200 in both erroneous and correct conditions, significant amplitude difference between these two conditions was detected only in musicians. Incongruent condition activated spatiotemporally distributed brain regions, including not only superior temporal gyrus but also other areas; the middle temporal, inferior temporal, inferior frontal, dorsolateral prefrontal cortex, inferior parietal lobule and sensorimotor cortex were activated in musicians. On the contrary, activated areas were limited in the vicinity of the auditory cortex in both conditions in non-musicians. Our findings suggest musicians' multiple strategies of pitch processing. © 2004 Elsevier B.V. All rights reserved.

Keywords: Magnetoencephalography (MEG); Minimum current estimate (MCE); Music; Pitch; Score sight-reading

* Corresponding author. Tel.: +81-3-3815-5411; fax: +81-3-5689-0495.
E-mail address: yumoto-tky@umin.ac.jp (M. Yumoto).

0531-5131/ © 2004 Elsevier B.V. All rights reserved.
doi:10.1016/j.ics.2004.05.046

1. Introduction

As letters of the alphabet have auditory (phonemic) and visual (graphemic) modalities [1], a musical score also has these modalities for trained musicians [2]. Although such multimodal integration of music processing has been studied [3], little is known about its temporal profile [4]. In this study, a spatiotemporal aspect of the functional neuroanatomy of music processing was investigated by applying cross-modal tonal violation technique [5] to the neuromagnetic measurement.

2. Materials and methods

2.1. Subjects

Eight right-handed musicians (aged 22–28 years, 4 females and 4 males) and eight right-handed non-musicians (aged 21–35 years, 5 females and 3 males) participated in this study. All the subjects gave written informed consent prior to the experiments, and the procedure used in this study had been approved by the Ethics Committee of the University of Tokyo.

2.2. Stimulation and task

Tone series were presented both visually and auditorily to the subjects. To exclude the contamination of long-term memory and emotion, we used unfamiliar atonal melodies of computer-generated oboe tones between musical C4 (262 Hz) and B4 (494 Hz) in semitone steps. Auditory stimuli were played on an Apple personal computer via MOTU 828 (Mark of the Unicorn, Massachusetts, USA) audio interface and were presented binaurally through ER-3A (Etymotic Research, Illinois, USA) foam insert earphones at a comfortable listening level.

Subjects were instructed to sight-read the score projected onto the screen in front of them while listening to the melody, and to detect infrequent (probability = 13.2%) performance errors without overt response. The errors implanted in each trial were all melodic in this study. Pitch errors perturbed a written note by raising or lowering it a diatonic interval randomly in equal probability.

2.3. Measurement

The brain's neuromagnetic signals were recorded using VectorView™ (Neuromag, Helsinki, Finland), which has 102 magnetometers and 204 planar first-order gradiometers at 102 measurement sites on a helmet-shaped surface that covers the entire scalp. In this study, all magnetometers were inactivated. The passband of the MEG recordings was 1.0–200 Hz and the data were digitized at 600 Hz. Horizontal and vertical electro-oculograms (EOG; passband 0.03–100 Hz) and electroencephalograms (EEG; passband 0.3–100 Hz) were recorded simultaneously in order to measure eye position and scalp potential distribution, respectively.

2.4. Data analysis

Brain evoked magnetic fields to correct (congruent) and erroneous (incongruent) tones were selectively averaged off-line. All the trials with MEG gradients greater than

3000 fT/cm were excluded. Approximately 1–4 noisy channels were also excluded from further analysis. The averaged signals were low-pass filtered at 45 Hz prior to analyses. Amplitudes of the activity in both conditions were compared by repeated measures ANOVA. Localization of the activity was analyzed by minimum current estimates (MCE) [6] and multiple-current-dipole model. Source localization results were superimposed onto 3D-reconstructed MR images and evaluated neuroanatomically.

3. Results

Every subject showed three prominent magnetic components, M50, M100 and M200 evoked at latencies of approximately 50, 100 and 200 ms from each tone onset in both hemispheres. In musicians, the waveforms of evoked responses in congruent and

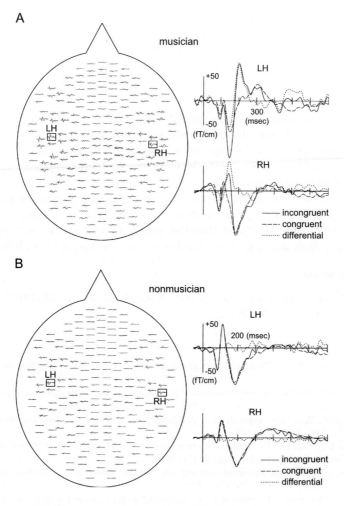

Fig. 1. Evoked magnetic fields in a representative musician (A) and those in a representative non-musician (B) (LH and RH represent selected channels in the left and in the right hemisphere, respectively).

Table 1
Activated brain areas detected by both MCE and multidipole modelling

Group	Condition	Left hemisphere	Right hemisphere
Musicians	Congruent	AC, mT	AC, mT, FG
	Incongruent	AC, mT, FG, dlPFC, iPL, SM, FO	AC, mT, FG, dlPFC, iPL, FO
Non-musicians	Congruent	AC	AC
	Incongruent	AC	AC

Abbreviations: AC, auditory cortex; mT, middle temporal cortex; FG, fusiform gyrus; dlPFC, dorsolateral prefrontal cortex; iPL, inferior parietal lobule; SM, sensorimotor cortex; FO, frontal operculum.

incongruent conditions were significantly different ($p < 0.01$). On the contrary, differences between the two conditions in non-musicians were not significant (Fig. 1).

In musicians, although activities were limited within the temporal lobe in the congruent condition, incongruent condition revealed spatiotemporally distributed brain regions, including not only superior temporal gyrus but also other areas; middle temporal, inferior temporal, inferior frontal, dorsolateral prefrontal cortex, inferior parietal lobule and sensorimotor cortex were activated. In non-musicians, activated areas were limited to the vicinity of the auditory cortex in both conditions (Table 1).

4. Discussion

Both subject groups showed consistent auditory evoked magnetic fields that were time-locked with each tone onset, however, only musicians showed additional activities in incongruent conditions. Considering that reading music induces auditory imagery in trained musicians [2], violation to the imagery expected from notation may modulate perception of incongruent tones. This interpretation by sensory encoding of the pitch information explains only a part of the incongruent activities detected in this study. Musicians may have other types of strategies to encode the pitch information, such as verbal encoding (naming), visual encoding (notation) and motor encoding (playing instruments) [7]. Activated brain areas detected in this study may agree with this postulate.

Acknowledgements

This work was supported in part by JSPS Scientific Research, 12610163, 13680926, 13877400, 15300209 and 15500312.

References

[1] T. Raij, K. Uutela, R. Hari, Audiovisual integration of letters in the human brain, Neuron 28 (2) (2000) 617–625.
[2] W. Brodsky, et al., Auditory imagery from musical notation in expert musicians, Percept. Psychophys. 65 (4) (2003) 602–612.
[3] J. Sergent, et al., Distributed neural network underlying musical sight-reading and keyboard performance, Science 257 (5066) (1992) 106–109.
[4] T.C. Gunter, B.H. Schmidt, M. Besson, Let's face the music: a behavioral and electrophysiological exploration of score reading, Psychophysiology 40 (5) (2003) 742–751.
[5] L.M. Parsons, Exploring the functional neuroanatomy of music performance, perception, and comprehension, Ann. N.Y. Acad. Sci. 930 (2001) 211–231.
[6] K. Uutela, M. Hamalainen, E. Somersalo, Visualization of magnetoencephalographic data using minimum current estimates, Neuroimage 10 (2) (1999) 173–180.
[7] M. Mikumo, Motor encoding strategy for pitches of melodies, Music Percept. 12 (2) (1994) 175–197.

International Congress Series 1270 (2004) 177–180

www.ics-elsevier.com

ELSEVIER

Prolonged interhemispheric neural conduction time evaluated by auditory-evoked magnetic signal and cognitive deterioration in elderly subjects with unstable gait and dizzy sensation

Hiroshi Oe[a],*, Akihiko Kandori[b], Tsuyoshi Miyashita[b],
Kuniomi Ogata[b], Naoaki Yamada[c], Keiji Tsukada[d],
Kotaro Miyashita[a], Saburo Sakoda[e], Hiroaki Naritomi[a]

[a] Department of Cerebrovascular Medicine, National Cardiovascular Center, 5-7-1 Fujishiro-dai,
Suita, Osaka 565-8565, Japan
[b] Central Research Laboratory, Hitachi Ltd., Tokyo, Japan
[c] Department of Radiology, National Cardiovascular Center, Osaka, Japan
[d] Okayama University, Okayama, Japan
[e] Department of Neurology, Osaka University, Osaka, Japan

Abstract. Magnetoencephalography (MEG) studies have showed that the latency of auditory-evoked neuronal action peak (N100m peak) detected at the temporal cortex ipsilateral to the auditory stimulation is delayed as compared with that detected at the contralateral side. Our recent auditory evoked magnetic fields (AEFs) study has indicated that auditory impulses, originated from the unilateral ear, first arrive at the contralateral temporal cortex and later reach the ipsilateral temporal cortex through interhemispheric neural connections, thus leading to the delay of ipsilateral N100m peak latency. Such a conduction pathway of auditory impulses makes it possible to measure interhemispheric neural conduction time (INCT). We measured INCT in 33 elderly patients (72 ± 10 years of age) complaining of unstable gait and dizzy sensation to study its relationship with cognitive function. Cognitive function was estimated with mini-mental state examination (MMSE) scores. The patients were classified into two groups, such as Group A with normal cognitive function (MMSE score ≥ 24, $n = 23$) and Group B with cognitive dysfunction (MMSE score ≤ 23, $n = 10$). INCT was significantly longer in Group B (50.5 ± 14.7 ms) than in Group (15.6 ± 13.9 ms, $p < 0.05$). In the entire patient group, INCT was prolonged negatively correlating with MMSE scores ($r = -0.84$, $p < 0.001$). The results of the present study suggest that the impairment of cognitive function may be closely related with the prolongation of

* Corresponding author. Tel.: +81-6-6833-5012; fax: +81-6-6872-7486.
E-mail address: hirooe@hsp.ncvc.go.jp (H. Oe).

0531-5131/ © 2004 Elsevier B.V. All rights reserved.
doi:10.1016/j.ics.2004.05.090

INCT. The measurement of INCT with AEFs may be useful for early detection of cognitive impairment in elderly patients with dizziness who may later develop dementia. © 2004 Elsevier B.V. All rights reserved.

Keywords: Auditory evoked magnetic fields; N100m peak latency; Cognitive deterioration; Mini-mental state examination; Dizziness

1. Introduction

Auditory impulses, originating from the unilateral ear, reach the temporal auditory cortex bilaterally [1], although detailed neural pathways are unknown. MEG studies have indicated that the latency of auditory-evoked neuronal action peak (N100m peak) detected at the temporal cortex ipsilateral to the auditory stimulation is always delayed as compared with that detected at the contralateral side [2]. Regarding this phenomenon, our recent MEG study has suggested that auditory impulses originating from the unilateral ear first arrive at the contralateral temporal cortex and later reach the ipsilateral temporal cortex through interhemispheric neural connections, thus leading to the delay of ipsilateral N100m peak latency [3]. Such a conduction manner of auditory impulses enables us to measure interhemispheric neural conduction time (INCT) with MEG. We estimated the INCT, using MEG, in elderly patients with unstable gait and dizziness and studied its relationship with cognitive function.

2. Subjects and methods

2.1. Subjects

Thirty-three patients (18 males and 15 females, 72 ± 10 years of age) complaining of unstable gait and dizzy sensation, who had otherwise no focal neurological abnormality, were subjected. We excluded patients with auditory impairments at 30 dB or less in 1000 Hz pure tone audiograms or abnormal findings in otorhinologic examinations, caloric test and auditory brain stem response.

2.2. Methods

MEG studies were performed using a superconducting quantum interference device (SQUID) system (MC-6400, Hitachi) with 64 co-axial gradiometer (8×8 matrix) in a two-dimensional plane. Auditory stimuli with 90 dB normal hearing level in intensity and 1 kHz tone burst were provided in the right ear, and N100m peak latency was measured at both temporal cortices (Fig. 1). Cognitive function was estimated by measurement of the mini-mental state examination (MMSE) score. The patients were classified into two groups, according to MMSE scores as follows: Group A with normal cognitive function (MMSE scores ≥ 24) and Group B with cognitive dysfunction (MMSE scores ≤ 23). The INCT (ms) was calculated from the

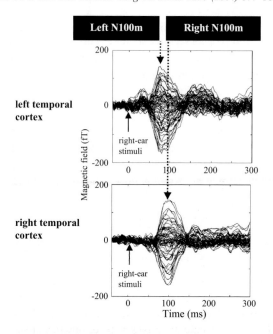

Fig. 1. Left N100m and right N100m peak latencies in a patient (right-ear stimuli). Interhemispheric neural conduction time (INCT) (ms)=right N100m peak latency − left N100m peak latency.

right and left N100m peak latencies. The INCT was compared between the two groups.

3. Results

MMSE scores were normal in 23 patients (Group A: MMSE score 24–30; 71 ± 12 years of age) and reduced in 10 patients (Group B: MMSE score 19–23; 73 ± 6 years of age). The ages in the two groups were the same. With the right ear stimuli, the N100m peak latency at the left temporal cortex was almost the same in Group A (92.8 ± 15.3 ms) and Group B (93.9 ± 13.9 ms), whereas the N100m peak latency at the right temporal

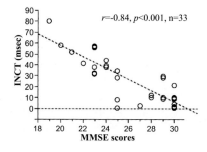

Fig. 2. The relationship between MMSE scores and interhemispheric neural conduction time (INCT) in 33 patients (right ear stimuli).

cortex was significantly longer in Group B (143.3 ± 13.7 ms) than in Group A (109.3 ± 16.7 ms, $p < 0.01$). The INCT was significantly longer in Group B (50.5 ± 14.7 ms) than in Group A (15.6 ± 13.9 ms, $p < 0.05$). When analyzed in the entire patient group, there was a significantly negative correlation between MMSE scores and INCT ($r = -0.84$, $p < 0.001$) (Fig. 2).

4. Discussion

Cognitive function takes place under rapid interactions of multiple cerebral regions interconnected with neurons. The results of the present study suggest that cognitive function may deteriorate correlating with the prolongation of INCT in elderly patients with unstable gait and dizziness. The INCT may represent the time required for the inter-regional neural process to perform cognitive function. Dizziness is related with gait unstableness that is known to be a predictor of non-Alzheimer's dementia. The measurement of INCT with AEFs may be useful for early detection of cognitive impairment in elderly patients with unstable gait and dizziness who may later develop dementia.

Acknowledgements

This study was supported by a Grant-in-Aid for Scientific Research No. 13072601, supported by the Ministry of Health, Welfare and Labor of Japan.

References

[1] C.M. Hackney, Anatomical features of the auditory pathway from cochlea to cortex, Br. Med. Bull. 43 (1987) 780–801.
[2] C. Pantev, et al., Study of the human auditory cortices using a whole-head magnetometer: left vs. right hemisphere and ipsilateral vs. contralateral sitmulation, Audiol. Neuro-otol. 3 (1998) 183–190.
[3] H. Oe, et al., Interhemispheric connection of auditory nerural pathways assessed by auditory evoked magnetic fields in patients with fronto-temporal lobe infarction, Neurosci. Res. 44 (2002) 483–488.

International Congress Series 1270 (2004) 181–183

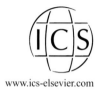

www.ics-elsevier.com

Animated gradient magnetic field topography

Akira Hashizume*

Department of Neurosurgery, Hiroshima University, Kasumi-1-2-3, Hiroshima 734-8551, Japan

Abstract. It is difficult to comprehend extents and dynamic changes of biomagnetic brain activities from electrically equivalent current dipole (ECD) estimation. The author proposed animated gradient magnetic field topography to solve this. Neuromag System with 102 orthogonal paired planar type gradiometers was used. Measured data at 102 sensor points were projected over subjects' individual brain surfaces and gradient magnetic field topographies were calculated after interpolation among projected sensor points. Furthermore, hundreds or thousands of consecutive topographies were packed as motion picture experts group (MPEG) files. Information provided by this method was helpful to imagine actual brain activities as compared with conventional ECD estimation. © 2004 Elsevier B.V. All rights reserved.

Keywords: MEG; MPEG; Topography

1. Introduction

Magnetoencephalography (MEG) is one of the powerful tools to reveal brain functions and electrically equivalent current dipole (ECD) estimation is usually executed to display locations of brain activities. However, the information of estimated ECDs shows only centers and electric moments of target brain activities. To know extents or dynamic changes of brain activities, the author proposed another method in this proceeding.

2. Methods

A whole head type magnetometer, Neuromag System (Neuromag, Helsinki, Finland) was used. This magnetometer has 102 orthogonal paired planar type gradiometers [1], which return maximum signals if electric sources exist just below the coils [2]. This unique property somewhat resembles that of bipolar lead in electroencephalography. The author calculated sensor values as

$$S = \sqrt{(\partial Bz/\partial x)^2 + (\partial Bz/\partial y)^2}$$

where S is sensor value and $\partial Bz/\partial x$ and $\partial Bz/\partial y$ are signals from orthogonal paired gradiometers at arbitrary time point. Then S at 102 points were projected over subjects'

* Tel./fax: +81-82-257-5227.
E-mail address: hdrtj718@ybb.ne.jp (A. Hashizume).

0531-5131/ © 2004 Elsevier B.V. All rights reserved.
doi:10.1016/j.ics.2004.05.049

individual brain surfaces in direction normal to each coil plane [3]. After interpolation among projected sensor points, gradient magnetic field topographies at arbitrary time point were computed as image data object. Furthermore, consecutive hundreds or thousands of these image data objects were packed as uncompressed audio-video interleaved (AVI) files and compressed as motion picture experts group (MPEG) files with a freeware TMPGenc [4]. Except for the last compressing step, the author programmed all steps using MATLAB (MathWorks, Natick, USA) and Delphi (Borland Software, Scott Valley, USA).

3. Results

MPEG files were screened at the meeting held on April 13, 2004, however, in this proceeding, only one frame of an auditory evoked field by 1 kHz pure tone is demonstrated (Fig. 1).

4. Discussion

This animated gradient magnetic field topography provides not precise, but rough information of actual brain activities because any biomagnetic inverse problems were not

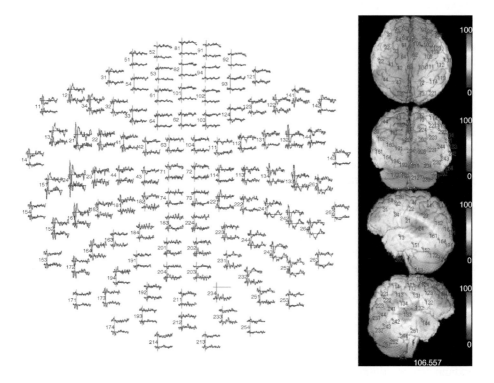

Fig. 1. Waveforms and gradient magnetic field topography of auditory evoked field by 1 kHz pure tone at 106 ms from stimulus (red lines in waveforms). The unit of color-coded scale bar is femtotesla/centimetre [fT/cm]. These images were packed consecutively as motion picture experts group (MPEG) files.

solved. However, this method is quite helpful to imagine extents or dynamic changes of brain activities, which are difficult in conventional ECD estimation.

References

[1] Neuromag, Neuromag System™ User's Manual: Hardware 1999, pp. 18–22.
[2] M. Hämäläinen, et al., Magnetoencephalography-theory, instrumentation, and applications to noninvasive studies of the working human brain, Rev. Mod. Phys. 65 (2) (1993) 413–498.
[3] A. Hashizume, et al., Development of magnetoencephalography—magnetic resonance imaging integration software, Neurol. Med.-Chir. (Tokyo) 42 (2002) 455–457.
[4] http://www.tmpgenc.net/j_main.html (in Japanese).

International Congress Series 1270 (2004) 184–187

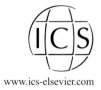

www.ics-elsevier.com

Estimation of encoding of pictorial stimuli from visually evoked magnetic fields

Klevest Gjini*, Takashi Maeno, Keiji Iramina, Shoogo Ueno

Department of Biomedical Engineering, University of Tokyo, 7-3-1 Hongo, Bunkyo, Tokyo 113-0033, Japan

Abstract. Magnetic fields were recorded from human subjects during the performance of a 1-back recognition short-term memory task with pictorial stimuli using a whole-head neuromagnetometer. In the memory condition the subjects were required to respond to the same stimuli and memorize the presented pictures for a short period of time, in control condition to respond to all stimuli and not memorize the picture. Magnetic event-related fields (MEFs) were computed and analyzed to reveal information about the encoding process of pictorial stimuli in short-term memory. Based on comparative MEFs analysis between conditions and behavioral response times, the encoding process for pictorial stimuli in this particular memory task was estimated at an interval with peaking activity around 500–550 ms from the stimulus presentation onset. Equivalent current dipoles (ECDs) were fitted to localize the brain sources related to visual information processing and the encoding process. A dipole located in the left anterior medial temporal lobe was estimated as an important source underlying encoding activity. © 2004 Elsevier B.V. All rights reserved.

Keywords: Encoding; Magnetic event-related fields; Pictorial stimuli; Equivalent current dipole

1. Introduction

Pictorial stimuli constitute an important part of our daily contact with surrounding environment through the visual sensory system. We sporadically focus our attention on different natural scenes, and presumably during this time a process of perception, comparison (same as those we already have memorized or different), and encoding strengthened by a rehearsal process in case of attentional learning, is going on. Our knowledge on neural correlates and timing of encoding processes in the brain derives mainly from lesion, neurophysiological, behavioral and recently, functional brain imaging studies. Effects of lesions and removals of important temporal lobe structures (either part or not part of limbic system) in monkeys on visual recognition and performance on short-term memory tasks have been evaluated in lesion studies [1–3], showing the importance of these structures in visual memory processes. Several studies using functional magnetic resonance imaging fMRI [4,5], positron emission tomography PET [6] and single-photon emission computer tomography SPECT [7] have revealed the activation of the medial temporal lobe during successful encoding of pictorial scenes. The present study uses magnetoencephalog-

* Corresponding author. Tel.: +81-3-5841-3389; fax: +81-3-5689-7215.
E-mail address: gjini@medes.m.u-tokyo.ac.jp (K. Gjini).

0531-5131/ © 2004 Elsevier B.V. All rights reserved.
doi:10.1016/j.ics.2004.05.061

raphy as a noninvasive technique to localize the neural correlates of the encoding process in human subjects.

2. Materials and methods

Four healthy subjects with normal or corrected-to-normal vision volunteered in this study; aged 24–31 years. Subjects gave their informed consent to participate in this study, approved by the Ethics Committee of the Faculty of Medicine, University of Tokyo.

The 1-back recognition short-term memory task consisted in the presentation of colored pictures every 4 s for a period of 1s each. The subjects had to compare the presented stimulus with the previous one and after decision reacted with motor response in case of the "same" state. After the decision or response a short-term maintenance of new stimulus was required for usage during next comparison. In the memory condition subjects were instructed to give a motor response in the case of "same" decision (the proportion between "DIFFERENT" and "same" was 80% to 20%). The mentioned proportion between different and same stimuli was chosen to reduce the motor inhibitory response in the trials where the decision "different" is not followed by a motor response. Beside the memory condition, the same sequence was used in a "control" condition, where subjects gave a motor response after perceiving each stimulus. Stimuli consisted in colored visual scenes from seaside projected on the center of a screen situated inside the electromagnetically shielded room.

Magnetic fields were recorded using a 204-channel whole-head device. Data from 4 subjects were acquired using a 0.1–200 Hz analog bandpass filter and 600 Hz sampling rate. On-line averaging was used to obtain the average visually evoked magnetic fields for two conditions, memory ("DIFFERENT" state averages not containing motor response) and control (the same sequence of trials, all containing motor response). Eye blink activity was monitored. Average magnetic data were digitally filtered to a 1–40 Hz frequency band. More than 100 trials were averaged and analyzed for both conditions.

The equivalent current dipoles (ECDs) fitting procedure was based on a spherical conductor model. The radius and center of this sphere was determined by fitting it onto the surface points of the cortex from subject's MRI data. First a rough selection of sensor area was used for ECDs fitting with a 1.7 ms step based on nonlinear least-squares search [8]. From these results and visual observation of flux contour maps, later localized selection of channels was made for more accurate fitting. Acceptance was made for dipoles with goodness-of-fitting larger than 80% in general; and a small value of confidence volume also, in particular cases.

3. Results

All subjects performed the tasks well (the percentage of exact responses was 94.3 ± 3.6% (mean ± S.D.) in memory condition, and 98.6 ± 1.1% (mean ± S.D.) in the control condition). The timing of motor response in memory condition was used for the evaluation of the timing of the encoding process. Average response time was 550 ± 120 ms (mean ± S.D.) for memory condition and 305 ± 70 ms (mean ± S.D.) for motor condition.

According to a simple behavioral assumption on how a subject could perform the 1-back short-term memory task, the subject who is always concentrated on the screen at first should perceive the most recently presented stimulus, followed by a "same-different" decision as

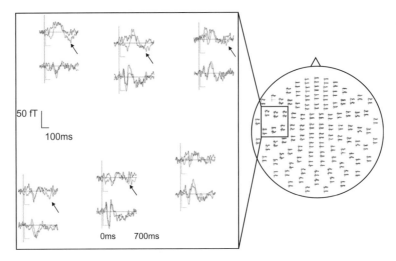

Fig. 1. Magnetic event-related fields (MEFs) waveforms at a set of channels selected from the left anterior part of sensor array. Waveforms are shown in red for memory condition and blue for control condition. Note the difference peaking around 500–550 ms (pointed by black arrows). Data from subject 1 are shown.

compared with the previous one, give a response (only when required, 20% of trials), and encode it in memory as is necessary to remember it after the short period of delay for the next judgement. Based on the knowledge of the average response time in memory condition we

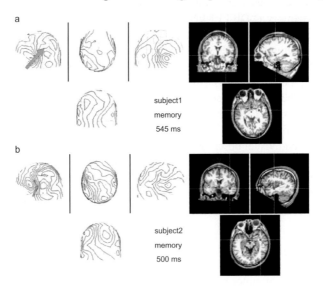

Fig. 2. Magnetic flux contour maps for memory condition at time points shown on each image (20 fT contour step). Data from three subjects are presented. Magnetic flux contour lines in blue (flux in), in red (flux out). A set of channels at the left anterior part of sensor array was selected and data from these selected channels were used in dipole fitting procedure. Positions of fitted dipoles were projected to subject's MRI data (images on the right). Fitted dipoles in the left anterior medial temporal lobe were considered to represent an important source of the activity during encoding of presented pictorial stimuli. Data from two subjects are shown.

could estimate a possible time interval when encoding of the new picture takes place in this particular task; activity which peaked around 500–550 ms after the stimulus presentation (Fig. 1).

As the duration of stimulus presentation was 1 s, the process of maintenance of these stimuli is unlikely to start until 1000 ms related to stimulus onset. The flux contour maps during the above-mentioned interval related to encoding of stimuli were very similar in all subjects (four out of four subjects). The estimated dipoles were projected to subject's individual MRI data in three cases. Results of the dipole fitting procedure are shown in Fig. 2, pointing out the activation of left anterior medial temporal lobe related to encoding process of pictures in memory condition. In control condition (simple motor reaction task) dipolar sources were localized in the occipital visual areas and contralateral motor cortex (subjects were instructed to press a button with their right index finger after perceiving each stimulus).

4. Discussion

In this study, easy to be performed 1-back short-term memory tasks with complex colored pictorial stimuli were chosen, with the hope of insuring a comfortable environment for good performance, and as good as possible concordance regarding to the timing of all involved processes in different trials in case of well-attended performance. This could increase the accuracy of making assumptions about the timing of such memory processes as encoding. The usage of more complicated n-back tasks could be well-indicated when the analysis of the process of short-term maintenance of different stimuli is the main purpose. As data were analyzed in the time domain, the basic approach was to use for dipole fitting a certain interval when the encoding could have a major impact in these data. The process of maintenance of visual stimuli in memory is unlike to be mixed with encoding during this interval, because visual stimuli were on the screen for a period of 1 s each. Beside the estimated activity in the left hemisphere, another dipolar source was estimated in the posterior part of the right temporal gyrus in two out of four subjects during the presumable interval for encoding of pictures, which could represent an additional area of activation during this interval.

References

[1] L. Malkova, M. Mishkin, One-trial memory for object-place associations after separate lesions of hippocampus and posterior parahippocampal region in the monkey, J. Neurosci. 23 (5) (2003 Mar 1) 1956–1965.

[2] M. Meunier, et al., Effects on visual recognition of combined and separate ablations of the entorhinal and perirhinal cortex in rhesus monkeys, J. Neurosci. 13 (12) (1993 Dec) 5418–5432.

[3] E.A. Murray, M. Mishkin, Visual recognition in monkeys following rhinal cortical ablations combined with either amygdalectomy or hippocampectomy, J. Neurosci. 6 (7) (1986 Jul) 1991–2003.

[4] S.A. Rombouts, et al., Parametric fMRI analysis of visual encoding in the human medial temporal lobe, Hippocampus 9 (6) (1999) 637–643.

[5] C.E. Stern, et al., The hippocampal formation participates in novel picture encoding: evidence from functional magnetic resonance imaging, Proc. Natl. Acad. Sci. U. S. A. 93 (1996) 8660–8665.

[6] S. Kohler, et al., Episodic encoding and recognition of pictures and words: role of the human medial temporal lobes, Acta Psychol. (Amst) 105 (2–3) (2000 Dec) 159–179.

[7] D. Montaldi, et al., Associative encoding of pictures activates the medial temporal lobes, Hum. Brain Mapp. 6 (2) (1998) 85–104.

[8] M. Hamalainen, et al., Magnetoencephalography—theory, instrumentation, and applications to noninvasive studies of the working human brain, Rev. Mod. Phys. 65 (1993) 1–93.

International Congress Series 1270 (2004) 188–191

ELSEVIER

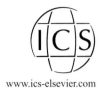

www.ics-elsevier.com

A study of the visual evoked magnetic field related to memory function by using a 320-channel MEG system

Masanori Higuchi*, Natsuko Hatsusaka

Applied Electronics Laboratory, Kanazawa Institute of Technology, 3 Amaike, Kanazawa, Ishikawa 920-1331, Japan

Abstract. We are studying how to find the early stages of dementia, such as Alzheimer's disease (AD), by using a MEG system. In relation to brain functions and dementia, memory defects are characterized as the most obvious signs of dementia. In a preliminary study, we tried to measure the visual evoked magnetic field related to memory function by using a simple memory task. In the memory task measurement, the subject memorized one figure for a few seconds, and then counted the number of memorized figures that appeared in the sequence of figures presented randomly. Evoked responses by visual stimuli were averaged for each condition. We compared the results of the control and memory task and identified the components, which seem to be related to memory functions. © 2004 Elsevier B.V. All rights reserved.

Keywords: MEG; Alzheimer's disease; Memory function; Visual evoked magnetic field

1. Introduction

We are studying how to find the early stages of dementia, such as Alzheimer's disease (AD), by using a MEG system. Although there are some studies about AD by means of MEG [1,2], most of them deal with primitive responses, such as N1m of auditory evoked response. In relation to brain functions and dementia, memory defects are characterized as the most obvious signs of dementia. Considering these points, we have developed a 320-channel, whole-head MEG system, which has the potential to detect magnetic field signals from the cerebral cortex and deep brain areas. In a preliminary study, we tried to measure the visual evoked magnetic field related to a memory function by using a simple memory task. We compared the results of the

* Corresponding author. Tel.: +81-76-229-8071; fax: +81-76-229-8072.
E-mail address: higuchi@ael.kanazawa-it.ac.jp (M. Higuchi).

0531-5131/ © 2004 Elsevier B.V. All rights reserved.
doi:10.1016/j.ics.2004.05.001

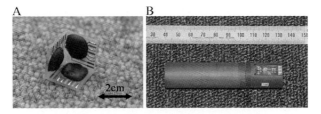

Fig. 1. Vector magnetometer (A) and gradiometer (B) of the 320-channel MEG system.

control and memory task, and identified the components that seem to be related to a memory function.

2. Material and methods

2.1. MEG system

We have developed a new type of 320-channel, whole-head MEG system, which has the potential to detect magnetic field signals from the cerebral cortex and deep brain areas. Conventional MEG systems, however, have usually adopted gradiometers with which it is very difficult to detect magnetic field signals in deep brain areas, such as the hippocampus. For deep brain measurement, our MEG system has used magnetometers that are more sensitive to the magnetic field caused by deep sources. In addition, the sensors are arranged to detect three orthogonal components of magnetic fields. This enables advanced signal processing and data analysis. Our MEG system can operate 320 channels, which consists of 160 channels for magnetometers and the rest for 50 mm, base-lined, co-axial gradiometer (Fig. 1) [3].

2.2. Measurements

Three neurologically normal subjects (two males, one female) participated in this study. Visual stimuli were presented to each subject on a screen by projection from outside of a magnetically shielded room. The image size was about 5 cm^2 at a 20-cm distance from the eyes. In the memory task, subjects were instructed to memorize one figure for a few

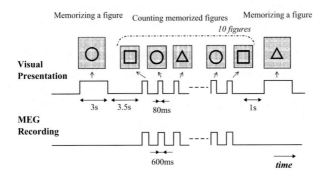

Fig. 2. Time sequence of visual presentation and MEG recording.

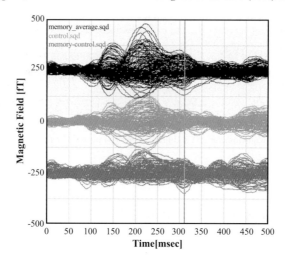

Fig. 3. Averaged MEG signals. Upper: memory task; Middle: control task; Lower: difference waveforms.

seconds, and to count the number of the memorized figure, which appeared in a sequence of figures presented randomly. The figures were three simple symbols (circle, triangle, square). To suppress primary visual evoked responses, we used a gray colour for the background of the figures and reduced the contrast in brightness.

The time sequence of visual presentation and MEG recording is shown in Fig. 2. One figure to memorize was presented for 3 s. After 3.5 s, 10 figures were presented randomly at 1.2-s intervals over a duration of 80 ms. Appearance probability of each symbol was equal to 1/3. Subjects were counting the appearance of the memorized figure among these figures. The correct answer was presented on a screen before the next trial started. This trial was repeated 10 times in one session. In this task, any response equipment was not used. It was carried out only in mind. MEG signals were recorded from 100 ms before to 500 ms after visual onset (passband 0.1–200 Hz, sampling frequency 1 kHz).

3. Results

Fig. 3 shows averaged MEG signals of one subject. The upper waveforms are the results of the memory task, the middle waveforms are the results of the control task and the lower

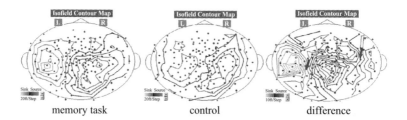

Fig. 4. Isofield contour maps at 300 ms after visual onset. Left: memory task; Middle: control task; Right: difference field.

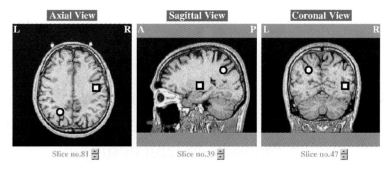

Fig. 5. Current dipole estimation by using the difference field data at 300 ms.

waveforms are the difference between the two tasks. In the control task, visual stimuli were presented randomly without memorization. As the figure shows, significant visual evoked responses were observed from 100 to 250 ms after visual onset in both tasks. We observed a distinct response at about 300 ms in the memory task. This response was not so significant in the control task. Therefore, clear peaks appear at this latency in the difference waveforms. We found similar responses in another subject. Fig. 4 shows isofield contour maps at this latency. These maps suggested that there are two dipole sources related to a memory function. Using the difference field, we applied the dipole fitting procedure. The dipoles were estimated at the right frontal area and the left parietal area as shown in Fig. 5.

4. Discussion

C.L. Grady et al. [4] have reported significant activation in the right prefrontal cortex, including the inferior and middle prefrontal regions, and the right parietal cortex during face recognition by using positron emission tomography. In our study, the results suggest recognition process has some relation to the right frontal cortex and the left parietal cortex. While our results on the source in the right frontal cortex were compatible with their study, those on the left parietal cortex were opposite in hemisphere. We speculate that it was caused by the difference between face and symbol used as visual stimulation.

Acknowledgements

This study was carried out as part of the Cooperative Link of Unique Science and Technology for Economy Revitalization "Ishikawa Hi-tech Sensing Cluster" supported by MEXT Japan.

References

[1] D. Osipova, et al., Cholinergic modulation of spontaneous MEG activity: implications for Alzheimer's disease, Biomag2002 Proceedings, VDE Verlag GmbH, Berlin, 2002, pp. 170–172.
[2] E. Pekkonen, et al., Cholinergic system modulate preattentive auditory processing in ageing and in Alzheimer's disease, Biomag2002 Proceedings, VDE Verlag GmbH, Berlin, 2002, pp. 176–178.
[3] M. Higuchi, et al., Development of a 320 channel MEG system for deep source measurements, Journal of Japan Biomagnetism and Bioelectromagnetics Society 16 (1) (2003) 96–97 (in Japanese).
[4] C.L. Grady, et al., Age-related reductions in human recognition memory due to impaired encoding, Science 269 (5221) (1995) 218–221.

International Congress Series 1270 (2004) 192–196

ELSEVIER

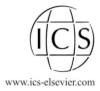

www.ics-elsevier.com

Neuromagnetic analysis of the late phase of readiness field for hand precision movement using magnetoencephalography

Yutaka Watanabe[a,*], Gen-yuki Yamane[a], Shinichi Abe[b], Masanori Takahashi[c], Tatsuya Ishikawa[d]

[a] Department of Oral Medicine, Oral Health Science Center, Tokyo Dental College, Ichikawa General Hospital, 5-11-13 Sugano Ichikawa City, Chiba 272-8513, Japan
[b] Department of Anatomy, Oral Health Science Center, Tokyo Dental College, Chiba 272-8513, Japan
[c] Department of Orthopedic Surgery, Oral Health Science Center, Ichikawa General Hospital, Tokyo Dental College, Chiba 272-8513, Japan
[d] Department of Operative Dentistry, Oral Health Science Center, Tokyo Dental College, Chiba 272-8513, Japan

Abstract. The aim of this study was to elucidate the cortical regulation of precise finger movements using magnetoencephalography (MEG). Magnetic brain signals of the following two tasks were recorded by magnetoencephalography. The first task was to bend the right thumb once as quickly as possible (a simple movement). The second task was to alternately oppose the thumb with the index finger and the middle finger of the right hand (a precise movement). In this study, we confirmed the differences between the two tasks observed in the late phase of the readiness field (RF), especially in the magnetic field 600 ms before the onset of movement. There were obvious differences in parietal aspects and temporal aspects of the left hemisphere. In the dipole estimation, activities of the parietal aspects were in the prefrontal area and in the supplementary motor area (SMA). Activities of the temporal aspect were in the premotor area. In the precise finger movement, it is interesting to note that the prefrontal area and the SMA are active right before the onset of movement. These results indicate that communication of the motor area, the prefrontal area and the SMA before the onset of movement is necessary for precise hand movements. © 2004 Elsevier B.V. All rights reserved.

Keywords: Magnetoencephalography; Precision movement; Readiness field (RF); Prefrontal area; Supplementary motor area

1. Introduction

The brain and hand provide humans with the ability to develop science and culture and have played important roles in manufacturing and expression. Therefore, we investigated to elucidate the cortical regulation of precise finger movements using magnetoencepha-

* Corresponding author. Tel.: +81-47-322-0151x2800; fax: +81-47-324-8577.
E-mail address: ywata@tdc.ac.jp (Y. Watanabe).

0531-5131/ © 2004 Elsevier B.V. All rights reserved.
doi:10.1016/j.ics.2004.04.033

lography (MEG). Magnetic brain signals of the following two tasks were recorded by MEG. The first task was to bend the right thumb once as quickly as possible (a simple movement). The second task was to alternately oppose the thumb with the index finger and the middle finger of the right hand (a precise movement). The purpose of the present study was to clarify the significance of the spatial and temporal progress by comparing and examining activity during the cerebral cortex in the preparatory stage of voluntary movement of the human finger.

2. Subjects and methods

None of the subjects had a history of hand motion problems in terms of subjective or objective symptoms, and they were all right handed as assessed with a modified version of the Edinburgh Inventory [1].

The first task was a simple movement task, i.e. to bend the right thumb once as quickly as possible while the right arm and the right four fingers were fixed in the rest position by a regin splint and bandage. The second task was a precise movement task, to alternately oppose the thumb with the index finger and the middle finger of the right hand under the same conditions. More than 100 single epochs were recorded with a 5-min rest period for each of the two tasks.

Magnetic brain signals were recorded non-invasively with pairs of gradiometers of 306 channels from 102 loci in the cerebral cortex using a MEG (4-D Neuromaging, Vector-view, Helsinki, Finland). All signals were digitized at 401 Hz, and were band pass filtered (0.03–15 Hz for MEG and EOG, and 100–200 Hz for EMG).

The MEG signal was 3000 ms in duration, starting 2500 ms prior to the EMG onset and ending 500 ms after the EMG onset, and was recorded during the two tasks. The onset was determined by the time when the EMG of the right flexor pollicis longus muscles exceeded a certain level (17.5 ± 1.7 mV). One hundred epochs were averaged for each task. Isocontour maps were constructed from the measured data at selected time points by the method of minimum norm estimates [2]. To identify the sources of movement-related magnetic fields, the signals were divided into several periods. During each period, one equivalent current dipole (ECD) was first determined by a least-square search for a subset of channels over the areas where movement-related magnetic fields were visually detected. Only ECDs attaining more than 85% of the goodness-of-fit (gof) and less than 268 mm^3 of 95% confidence-volume were accepted for analysis, in which the entire time period and all the channels were taken into account for computing the parameters of a time-varying multidipole model [2]. The ECDs were then superimposed on the subject's magnetic resonance images (MRIs) to show the source locations with respect to anatomical structure.

3. Results

The magnetic components of brain electromagnetic activity of all five subjects during the two tasks are shown in Fig. 1. These contrasted magnetic waves confirmed the previous differences between the two tasks. In four of the five subjects, it is clear that the precise movement-related activities were distributed widely for 600 ms before the EMG onset; however, the simple movement-related activity occurred in the late stage of the recording window.

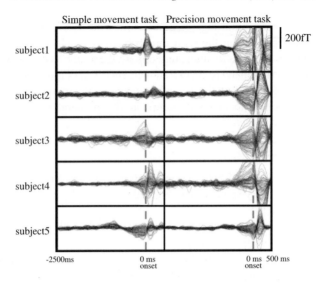

Fig. 1. The component of the finger movement-related magnetic fields of all subjects during the two tasks.

Spatial and temporal aspects of the cortical foci with simple and precise movement-related MEGs are shown in Fig. 2. The MEG signal of 400-ms duration, from the time 400 ms prior to the EMG onset, is plotted in the time sequence, separately at the cortical loci of the prefrontal cortex, the supplementary motor area (SMA), the premotor area and the

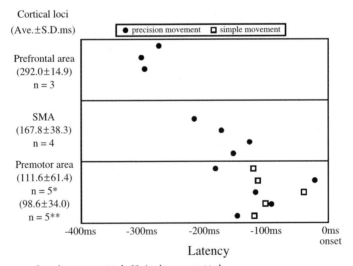

Fig. 2. Spatial and temporal aspects the cortical loci of the current source estimated by simple and precise finger movement-related MEG signals.

motor area. In the two tasks, the ECDs fit the standard and were not estimated after the EMG onset.

In the simple movement, the premotor area or the motor area was activated in the late phase of the time window. The average latency from the EMG onset was obtained at -98.6 ± 34.0 ms ($n = 5$).

In the precise movement, the prefrontal area and the SMA were activated in the early and/or middle phases of the time window. The average latency from the EMG onset was -292.0 ± 14.9 ms ($n = 3$) for the prefrontal cortex, and -167.8 ± 38.3 ms ($n = 4$) for the SMA. The premotor area or the motor area was activated in the late stage of the readiness field (RF) as well as the simple movement. The average latency from the EMG onset was -111.6 ± 61.4 ms ($n = 5$). In the two tasks, the activation loci detected (i.e., prefrontal area, the SMA and the premotor area) were lateralized to only the left hemisphere. Thus, this study showed only the contralateral cortical activation of the movement before the EMG onset.

4. Discussion

In the task of alternately opposing the thumb with the index finger and the middle finger on the same side, the activity of the prefrontal area, the SMA and the premotor area was induced in the preparatory stage of the motion from about 600 ms before the onset of movement. In the next section, we discuss the confirmed activities of the prefrontal area, the SMA and the premotor area.

4.1. Prefrontal area

In three of the five subjects in this study, activities of the prefrontal area were estimated. It has been considered that the prefrontal area regulates spatial recognition and movements, and is involved in higher motor function. The prefrontal area plans a series of movements, executes the movement plan and then assesses whether the movement has been carried out properly or not [3,4].

In this study, the activities in the prefrontal area were not observed by simple movements, but were observed by precise movements before the SMA or the premotor area were activated. These findings suggest that the activities in the prefrontal area are needed for complicated movements, such as precise movements. The prefrontal area carries out higher functions than the SMA or the premotor area.

4.2. Supplementary motor area (SMA)

The SMA is associated closely with spontaneous movements [5], especially activated strongly during memory-based intrinsic movements [6]. In a study for piano players, the amount of blood flow in the posterior side of the SMA increased when the subjects played songs that they had memorized, whereas blood flow in the anterior side of the SMA increased when they played songs which were unfamiliar [7]. In this study, SMA activities were observed in four of the five subjects. These activities were observed from all of them in the anterior area. When compared with the simple movement, alternatively touching the index and middle fingers with the thumb is more complicated.

4.3. Premotor area

The premotor area is a region before the motor area, and is divided into the above-mentioned SMA and the premotor area. The premotor area is involved in induced movements. When compared with the motor area, the ratio of neurons that are active while the motor preparation period for motoneuron becomes higher [8]. In this study, each subject was required to alternatively touch the index and the middle fingers using the thumb as the precise movement. When compared with the simple movement, the integration of spatial and body-part information was clearly required. In the regulation of movement, the premotor area is activated following the excitation of the prefrontal area and the SMA.

4.4. Concerning latency

In most studies, the RF was evoked 1000–2000 ms before the movement onset, although it was only 600 ms in this study. Libet et al. [9] indicated that recognizing the intention to perform a voluntary movement is faster than the movement becoming conscious, and this occurs about 200 ms before the start of the EMG. Furthermore, they concluded that the start of the voluntary movement is performed unconsciously, and that voluntary control of a movement does not indicate the start of a voluntary movement, but rather the selection and control of movements. Hence, in this study, brain activities representing enhanced consciousness for controlling voluntary movements were determined.

References

[1] R.C. Oldfield, The assessment and analysis of handedness: the Edinburgh inventory, Neuropsychologia 9 (1) (1971) 97–113.
[2] M.S. Hamalainen, R.J. Ilmoniemi, Interpreting magnetic fields of the brain: minimum norm estimates, Med. Biol. Eng. Comput. 32 (1) (1994) 35–42.
[3] K. Kubota, S. Funahashi, Direction-specific activities of dorsolateral prefrontal and motor cortex pyramidal tract neurons during visual tracking, J. Neurophysiol. 47 (3) (1982) 362–376.
[4] N. Matsunami, et al., Preferential transcription of HTLV-I LTR in cell-free extracts of human T cells producing HTLV-I viral proteins, Nucleic Acids Res. 14 (12) (1986) 4779–4786.
[5] D. Laplane, et al., Clinical consequences of corticectomies involving the supplementary motor area in man, J. Neurol. Sci. 34 (3) (1977) 301–314.
[6] K. Okano, J. Tanji, Neuronal activities in the primate motor fields of the agranular frontal cortex preceding visually triggered and self-paced movement, Exp. Brain Res. 66 (1) (1987) 155–166.
[7] N. Picard, P.L. Strick, Motor areas of the medial wall: a review of their location and functional activation, Cereb. Cortex 6 (3) (1996) 342–353.
[8] M. Weinrich, S.P. Wise, K.H. Mauritz, A neurophysiological study of the premotor cortex in the rhesus monkey, Brain 107 (Pt 2) (1984) 385–414.
[9] B. Libet, et al., Time of conscious intention to act in relation to onset of cerebral activity (readiness-potential). The unconscious initiation of a freely voluntary act, Brain 106 (Pt 3) (1983) 623–642.

International Congress Series 1270 (2004) 197–200

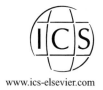

www.ics-elsevier.com

Responses of the gustatory area following electrical stimulation of palatine ridge

Masakazu Tazaki[a,*], Yuki Tazaki[a], Hiroki Bessho[b], Eizou Takeda[b], Yasutomo Yajima[b], Hiroyuki Noma[b]

[a] Department of Physiology, Tokyo Dental College, 1-2-2 Masago, Mihamaku, 261-8502 Chiba, Japan
[b] First Department of Oral and Maxillofacial Surgery, Tokyo Dental College, Japan

Abstract. The topography of the insula and operculum responses to electrical stimulation, applied to the first and third transverse palatine ridge and mucosa of foramen palatinum majus of normal volunteers, was analyzed using a 306-channel, whole-head DC-superconducting quantum interference device (SQUID) magnetoencephalography (MEG). The following order of a location of equivalent current dipoles (ECD) was found: third transverse palatine ridge—Insula, Parietal operculum, SI-Frontal operculum, Parietal operculum-SI or SI. It has been reported that the primary gustatory area is the transition area between the operculum and insula in macaque monkeys and humans, and the neurons in the insular cortex of rats are mechanoreceptive. Stimulus to the oral mucosa, therefore, has the possibility to influence the sense of taste. © 2004 Elsevier B.V. All rights reserved.

Keywords: Insular cortex; Neuromagnetometer; Electrical stimulation; Palatine mucosa

1. Introduction

It had been reported that in the insular cortex, a part of which comprises the primary gustatory area, a vast majority of neurons are mechanoreceptive, responding to mechanical stimulation of the oral tissue and/or lip, and the insular cortex represents the oral cavity in rats [1]. On the other hand, it has been reported that the primary gustatory area is the transition area between the operculum and insula in humans [2]. It has been clinically known that covering the hard palate with a dental plate reduces the sense of taste. However, there is no report about the cause. The purpose of this report is to prove the hypothesis that the primary gustatory area responds to the mechanical stimulation to the oral cavity.

2. Subjects and methods

Five right-handed subjects (four male and one female adult) without any previous neurological problems and disorders in oral sensory function were studied. We obtained

* Corresponding author. Tel.: +81-43-270-3771; fax: +81-43-279-2052.
E-mail address: mtazaki@tdc.ac.jp (M. Tazaki).

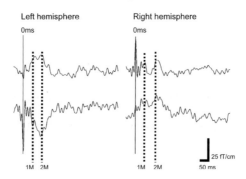

Fig. 1. SEFs following electrical stimulation of the third transverse palatine ridge.

their written informed consent to participate in the experiment, according to the guidelines approved by the Ethics Committee at our institute in accordance with the Declaration of Helsinki.

For electrical stimulation, the EMG-electronic stimulator (SEM-4201, Nihonkohden, Tokyo) was used. A constant current of square pulse waves was stimulated to the right first and third transverse palatine ridge and mucosa of the foramen palatinum majus via a pair of silver ball electrodes. Though the silver ball electrodes were fixed on a plastic splint, the palatine mucosa area of the plastic splint maintained a distance of 1 mm between the mucous membranes. The stimulus amplitude (1–5 mA) was set at two times the minimum strength where it feels stimulus, and adjusted for every experiment. The electric stimulus to the palatine mucosa membrane felt like pressure stimulus. Stimulus frequency and duration was 1 Hz and 0.05 ms.

A 306-channel, whole-head superconducting quantum interference device (SQUID) magnetoencephalography (MEG; Vectorview, Neuromag, Helsinki, Finland) was used for recording magnetic fields. All responses were digitized at a sampling rate of 999 Hz and were bandpass-filtered at 0.1–330 Hz. Four hundred trials were averaged on SEFs for each condition. The analysis window was set to 900 ms between 100 ms before and 800 ms after stimulation. Only equivalent current dipoles (ECDs) attaining more than 80% of the goodness of fit were accepted for further analysis in which the entire time period and all channels were taken into account in computing the parameters of a time-varying multi-

Table 1
Peak latencies for SEFs following electrical stimulation of the palate

| | | Latency (ms ± S.E.) | |
		1M	2M
Contralateral	first transverse palatine ridge	59.1 ± 5.6	140.7 ± 7.7
	third transverse palatine ridge	57.9 ± 8.2	123.7 ± 8.3
	foramen palatinum majus	55.6 ± 5.6	106.9 ± 8.5
Ipsilateral	first transverse palatine ridge	57.2 ± 2.7	122.5 ± 7.2
	third transverse palatine ridge	53.9 ± 5.2	133.5 ± 8.5
	foramen palatinum majus	52.8 ± 2.8	127.4 ± 10.3

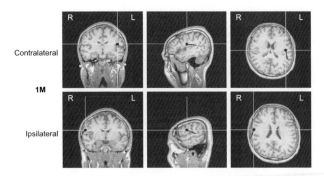

Fig. 2. ECDs of SEFs following electrical stimulation of the third transverse palatine ridge (1M).

dipole model. The ECDs were then overlapped on brain magnetic resonance imaging (MRI) to show the source locations with MEG-MRI coordinate systems.

3. Results and discussion

SEFs were recorded following electrical stimulation on the right transverse palatine ridge. Two peaks were obtained in the SEF's response. We termed them 1M for the earlier in latency and 2M for the later (Fig. 1). In three electrical stimulation points, peak latencies (1M, 2M) were shown (Table 1).

The first and second peak latencies were about 55 and 130 ms, respectively. It has been reported that the first peak latency of tactile stimulation to the tongue, lower lip and upper lip in humans was about 34–36 ms [3]. Our result of first peak latency was later than this. However, our result of first peak latency was about the same as the first sub-peak latency (M1') [3].

The ECD of the first and second peak in the SEF overlapped on each subject's MRI (Figs. 2 and 3). The location of the ECD was the insular cortex and/or the transition area between the primary sensory cortex and operculum (Table 2).

The neuron, which responded to mechanical stimulation of the oral tissue and/or lip in the insula cortex of rats, was recorded [1]. Our result was the same as the result of the

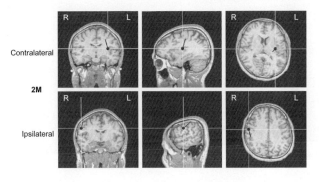

Fig. 3. ECDs of SEFs following electrical stimulation of the third transverse palatine ridge (2M).

Table 2
ECDs of SEFs following electrical stimulation of the third transverse palatine ridge (1M and 2M)

Subject		1M	2M
Sub. 1	Contralateral	Insula	Parietal operculum
	Ipsilateral	Parietal operculum	ND
Sub. 2	Contralateral	SI-Frontal operculum	Insula
	Ipsilateral	SI	SI
Sub. 3	Contralateral	SI-Frontal operculum	SI-Frontal operculum
	Ipsilateral	Parietal operculum-SI	Parietal operculum-SI

ND: no data.

electric physiological experiment of rat [1]. It has also been reported that the primary gustatory area is the transition area between the operculum and insula in macaque monkeys and humans [2]. Though stimulation to the transverse palatine ridge did not evoke a sense of taste, electrical stimulation to the oral mucosa has the possibility to influence a sense of taste.

This result suggests that mechanical stimulation of the hard palate by food and/or the tongue is correlated with the sense of taste.

Acknowledgements

This work was supported by a grant for Scientific Research No. HRC3A02 from the Oral Health Science Center of Tokyo Dental College.

References

[1] H. Ogawa, S. Wang, Representation of the oral cavity in the insular cortex in rat, Jan. J. Physiol. 50 (2000) S154.
[2] T. Kobayakawam, et al., The primary gustatory area in human cerebral cortex studies by magnetoencephalography, Neurosci. Lett. 212 (1996) 155–158.
[3] A. Nakamura, et al., Somatosensory homunculus as drawn by MEG, NeuroImage 7 (1998) 377–386.

International Congress Series 1270 (2004) 201–204

ELSEVIER

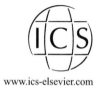

www.ics-elsevier.com

Elucidation of face categorization process by visual top down control task—seeing-as-face task: an MEG study

Y. Kato[a,b,*], M. Kato[a], M. Shintani[c], F. Yoshino[c]

[a] Department of Neuropsyhiatry, School of Medicine, Keio University, Japan
[b] Inokashira Hospital, Tokyo, Japan
[c] Laboratory of Brain Research, Oral Health Science Center, Tokyo Dental College, Japan

Abstract. We measured MEG responses to investigate the processing of face perception using novel "seeing-as-face task", in which visual inputs were identical across two conditions, but subject perceptions differed by visual top down control: one being a non-specific pattern of geographical shapes, the other being a percept of a face. Subtraction between the two conditions revealed a response occurring 120 ms after stimulus onset in right occipital lobe, which were supposed to be the component of face categorization in the two-stage theory of face processing. © 2004 Elsevier B.V. All rights reserved.

Keywords: Neurosciences; Magnetoencephalography (MEG); Visual perception; Cognition; Form perception

1. Introduction

The neural basis of face processing represents one of the most interesting topics in the field of cognitive neuroscience. Neuroimaging studies using PET or functional MRI, and ERP have shown that faces elicit specific brain responses from relatively well-defined areas in the ventral occipitotemporal cortex, called fusiform face area (FFA) [1–3]. Furthermore, the time sequence of cognitive and neural process underlying this ability also has been studied extensively during the past few years and converging evidence from ERP and MEG suggests that an essential stage in the cerebral processing of faces occurs in the FFA 170 ms after stimulus onset [4]. Recently, by using MEG, Liu et al. [5] demonstrated that an earlier component, M100, was associated with the detection of face category, i.e. categorization, which awaits further replication studies. Our novel seeing-as-face task paradigm MEG experiment allowed us to compare the processing of the same visual input having different task-related status.

---

* Corresponding author. Department of Neuropsychiatry, Inokashira Hospital, Kamirenjaku 4-14-1, Mitaka-shi, 181-8531 Tokyo, Japan. Tel.: +81-422-44-5331; fax: +81-422-44-0388.
E-mail address: yutaka-k@db3.so-net.ne.jp (Y. Kato).

0531-5131/ © 2004 Elsevier B.V. All rights reserved.
doi:10.1016/j.ics.2004.05.073

2. Materials and methods

Eleven normal subjects (seven female) participated in this paradigm, with mean age 26.5. 50 images of seeing-as-face visual stimuli were presented four times. These experiments were carried out through two succeeding blocks, before and after instruction. These visual stimuli consist of four ovals and four rectangles (Fig. 1), which are composed to be perceived as upright human face only to pay attention to four oval images, but not perceived as a face to four rectangles. The verbal instruction to pay attention to four oval images could give rise to the top down process in visual perception, resulting in a percept of face.

First experimental block: Pay attention to only rectangles (Non-Face condition).

Second experimental block: Pay attention to only ovals (Face condition).

MEG recordings are taken by Vector View Whole Head 306 ch (Neuromag). In this procedure, Visual evoked magnetic fields (VEF) were recorded with subjects to perform a one-back repetition detection task in which they were required to press a button whenever they saw two identical patterns in a row.

3. Results

3.1. Waveforms

In all subjects, four major components occurred at approximately 90, 120, 170 and 220 ms were identified within the time window of 0–300 ms in the waveforms measured at each condition. Fig. 2 shows the grand average waveforms measured at these two conditions, and subtraction from representative subject 1. Panels A and B depict 306-channel grand average waveforms measured through Face and Non-Face Conditions, respectively. Subtracting waveforms (Panel C) were obtained by subtracting each point of the response measured through Non-Face condition from that through Face condition in every channel separately, which showed three components in all subjects.

3.2. RMS

Fig. 3 shows root mean squares (RMSs) from the 24 channels of the occipital region in Subject 1. Thin-gray and thin-gray-dashed lines denoted Face and Non-Face conditions in the right occipital region, respectively. The most prominent finding was dissociation of

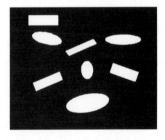

Fig. 1. An example of stimulus.

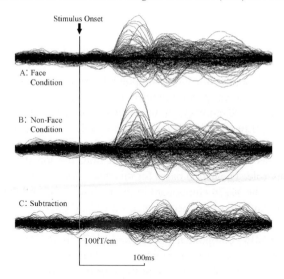

Fig. 2. MEG waveforms of a representative subject.

amplitudes in RMSs around the latency of 120 ms between these two conditions, causing the peak around this latency seen from subtraction waveforms (Black line). Subtractions between the two conditions are shown as black and dark-gray lines, for the right and left occipital channels (24 each), respectively, which were more marked in the right occipital channels.

3.3. Source modeling

ECDs were estimated from averaged data measured under each condition. At latencies of 158–198 ms, ECD was estimated only from averaged data measured in Face condition at the occipito-temporal region. By the integration to MRI data where available, the source location was along the posterior ventral surface of temporal lobe, which corresponded to fusiform gyrus.

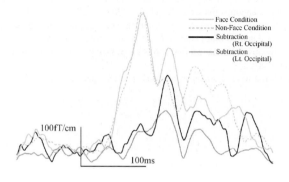

Fig. 3. RMS from 24 channels located at right occipital in each condition.

4. Discussion

In the present study, two MEG components were clearly identified, at latencies of ~ 120 and ~ 170 ms. Response at the latency of ~ 170 ms was consistent with previously reported face identification components in many studies. The component at ~ 120 ms was observed predominantly in the right occipital region and was correspondent to the M100 component which was the stage of face categorization in the previous report by Liu et al. [5]. By using our novel "seeing-as-face task" paradigm, we were able to offset low-level encoding mechanisms by subtracting each other. To perceive four ovals as a face by the verbal instruction, the top down process in visual perception has a key role. The neural bases for this visual top down control remain unclear. As a result, however, the M170 component in the fusiform gyri and the M100 in the right occipital cortex sequentially developed as a result of brain activation eliciting the visual percept of a face.

We observed two MEG components, M100 and M170, in the processing stages of face perception. The nature of our task paradigm, i.e. identical stimuli identical across two conditions, strongly supports the notion that the observed responses are face-specific. In addition, we have provided evidence that task paradigms such as the seeing-as-face task are able to identify neural activity that is inextricably involved in face perception. This implies that the same approach, where comparison is made between neural activations in response to identical inputs under different perceptions, may be extended to other classes of objects. Unfortunately, we cannot run experiments comparable with those reported herein on other stimulus categories, as we have not found MEG markers selective for other categories. When these markers are found in future, some of the limitations inherent in the present study will be resolved and moreover, the task paradigm can be applied to object recognition in a more general sense. Furthermore, this paradigm might also prove useful not only for MEG, but also for the fMRI and PET techniques, which are susceptible to changes in low-level physical features in visual stimuli.

References

[1] G. McCarthy, et al., Face-specific processing in the human fusiform gyrus, J. Cogn. Neurosci. 9 (1997) 605–610.
[2] N. Kanwisher, J. McDermontt, M.M. Chun, The fusiform face area: a module in human extrastriate cortex specialized for face perception, J. Neurosci. 17 (1997) 4302–4311.
[3] T. Allison, et al., Electrophysiological studies of human face perception: I. Potentials generated in occipito-temporal cortex by face and non-face stimuli, Cereb. Cortex 9 (1999) 415–430.
[4] E. Halgren, et al., Cognitive response profile of the human fusiform face area as determined by MEG, Cereb. Cortex 10 (2000) 69–81.
[5] J. Liu, A. Harris, N. Kanwisher, Stages of processing in face perception: an MEG study, Nat. Neurosci. 5 (2002) 910–916.

International Congress Series 1270 (2004) 205–208

ELSEVIER

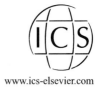

www.ics-elsevier.com

Prefrontal oscillatory activity in auditory oddball paradigm studied with Synthetic Aperture Magnetometry

Ryouhei Ishii[a,*], Wilkin Chau[b], Anthony Herdman[b],
Atsuko Gunji[c], Satoshi Ukai[a], Kazuhiro Shinosaki[d],
Masatoshi Takeda[a], Christo Pantev[e]

[a]*Department of Psychiatry and Behavioral Science, Osaka University Graduate School of Medicine,
D3-, 2-2, Yamadaoka, Suita, Osaka 565-0871, Japan*
[b]*The Rotman Research Institute, Baycrest Centre for Geriatric Care, University of Toronto, Toronto, Canada*
[c]*Department of Integrative Physiology, National Institute for Physiological Sciences, Okazaki, Japan*
[d]*Department of Neuropsychiatry, Wakayama Medical University, Wakayama, Japan*
[e]*Institute of Biomagnetism and Biosignalanalysis, University of Munster, Germany*

Abstract. Previous MEG studies of auditory P300 have identified complex and widespread distributions of equivalent current dipoles in the temporal, parietal and frontal cortices. We recorded the magnetic responses in an auditory oddball task and analyzed these data by using Synthetic Aperture Magnetometry (SAM) and SPM permutation analysis. Twelve normal subjects (aged 27–36 years) participated in this study. MEG data were obtained by using a standard auditory oddball paradigm under the instruction to press the buttons when subjects heard the target stimuli. SAM and SPM permutation analyses were used to visualize the multiple brain regions related to P300 generation within the latencies between 200 and 600 ms during target detection processing. Evoked magnetic fields for target stimuli calculated by simple averaging were peaking at approximately 300 to 400 ms over the various regions on both hemispheres. SAM and SPM permutation analysis showed that the suppressions in the 8–15, 15–30 and 30–60 Hz bands were distributed mainly in the left primary sensorimotor area. The activations in the 4–8 and 8–15 Hz bands were found primarily in the bilateral frontal cortices, including the dorsolateral and medial prefrontal areas. Basar et al. (E. Basar, Brain Function and Oscillations: I. Brain Oscillations: Principles and Approaches, Springer, Berlin, 1998, 1999) reported that, by using an oddball paradigm, prolonged event-related alpha oscillations up to 400 ms were observed. They named this alpha component "functional alpha." We suggested that the distributed alpha and theta activity in the prefrontal cortex is "functional" and engaged in auditory attention and memory updating. © 2004 Elsevier B.V. All rights reserved.

Keywords: P300; Oddball paradigm; MEG; EEG; SAM; SPM; Permutation; Alpha rhythm; Theta rhythm

* Corresponding author. Tel.: +81-6-6879-3051; fax: +81-6-6879-3059.
E-mail address: ishii@psy.med.osaka-u.ac.jp (R. Ishii).

0531-5131/ © 2004 Elsevier B.V. All rights reserved.
doi:10.1016/j.ics.2004.05.008

1. Introduction

Although the neural sources underlying the generation of P300 responses have also been intensively investigated by utilizing several neuroimaging methods, such as EEG, ECoG, intracranial depth recording, MEG, PET and fMRI, the findings of these studies are still inconsistent each other. Previous MEG studies [1] of auditory P300 have identified complex and widespread distributions of equivalent current dipoles in the temporal, parietal and frontal cortices.

The purpose of this study is to visualize the distributed brain activity involved in auditory P300. To accomplish this, we recorded magnetic responses in an auditory oddball task and analyzed these data by using Synthetic Aperture Magnetometry (SAM) [2,3] and SPM permutation analysis [4].

2. Methods

Twelve healthy volunteers (six males, six females, aged 27–36 years, mean age 32 years, one left-handed) participated in the study.

The data were collected using a standard oddball paradigm, in which the tones of either 1 kHz (non-target) or 2 kHz (target) were delivered binaurally at 65 dB HL with the probability of 80% (200 trials) for the non-target and 20% (50 trials) for the target stimuli. The duration of each tone was 500 ms consisting of 10 ms rise/fall time. The order of tone presentation was randomized. Inter-stimulus intervals were also randomized from 2.0 to 4.0 s. All subjects were asked to press the button with their right index fingers as soon as possible when they heard the target tones.

MEG data were obtained using a whole head, helmet-shaped, 151-channel SQUID sensor array (Omega 151, CTF Systems) in a magnetically shielded room. The MEG time series were low-pass filtered at 200 Hz, notch filtered at 60 Hz, and digitized with a sample frequency of 625 Hz.

SAM was used to generate a $16 \times 12 \times 12$ cm volumetric image of root-mean squared (RMS) source activity from the filtered MEG signals with 5 mm voxel resolution. The contribution of the common-mode brain activity was cancelled by subtracting the control state image from the active state image for each voxel, divided by their ensemble standard error, including both the instrumental (SQUID-sensor) and brain noise. For N1m, we selected the time window from 0 ms to 200 ms as an active state and -200 to 0 ms as a control state of non-target response and selected a 1–20 Hz frequency band. For fast components of P300, we selected the time window from 200 to 600 ms of the target responses as an active state and the same time window of the non-target responses as a control state, and selected six frequency bands (4–8, 8–15, 15–30, 30–60, 60–125 and 125–200 Hz). For slow components of P300, we selected the time window from -300 to 600 ms of the target responses as an active state and same time window of the non-target responses as a control state, and selected two frequency bands, 0–1 and 1–4 Hz.

The distributions of the SAM images were transformed to the SPM T1 template space. A nonparametric permutation technique was applied to the normalized SAM results to determine the statistical significance of the results. The omnibus null hypothesis of no activation anywhere in the brain was rejected if at least one t-value was above the critical

Deviant stimuli (50trial)

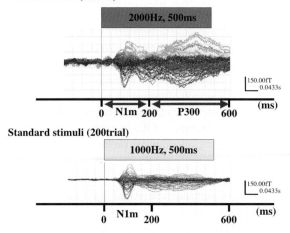

Fig. 1. The average waveforms of one subject.

threshold for $P < 0.05$ determined by a 1024 permutation. The voxel with t-values above this critical 0.05 threshold was considered as a region of activation [4].

3. Results

Fig. 1 depicts the average waveforms of the target and non-target stimuli in one subject. N1m responses were recognized around 100 ms latency in both hemispheres. In all subjects, the contour map at the peak latency of N1m for the target and non-target stimuli on each hemisphere showed a clear dipolar pattern. Between 300 and 400 ms, the large deflections were only observed in response to the target stimuli. There were several peaks in waveforms. The MEG field topography of this late component showed a non-dipolar and complicated pattern at each peak.

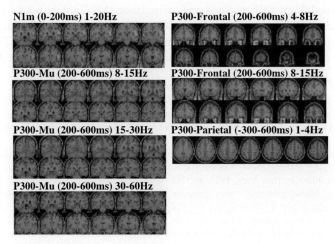

Fig. 2. The SAM–SPM permutation images of pseudo t-value computed by the source current density.

The SAM analysis and permutation tests performed revealed statistically significant source regions of N1m and P300 in several frequency bands ($P>0.05$). Fig. 2 shows the results of SAM analysis and permutation testing in 12 subjects. The current source densities of ERS in an N1m time window (0–200 ms) for 1–20 Hz band are distributed in a superior temporal region on each hemisphere. The current source densities of ERS in a P300 time window (200–600 ms) are distributed for 4–8 and 8–15 Hz bands, in bilateral frontal cortices (left dorsolateral and right medial prefrontal areas) and, for 8–15, 15–30 and 30–60 Hz bands, ERD in the parietal cortex (the vicinity of the bilateral primary sensorimotor areas, left>right). The current source densities of ERS in a whole time window (– 300–600 ms) for 1–4 Hz bands in the right parietal cortex are distributed.

4. Discussion

SAM and SPM permutation analysis showed that the current source densities of N1m for 1–20 Hz band were distributed in the superior temporal region and mu rhythm suppression for 8–15, 15–30, and 30–60 Hz band were distributed in the primary sensorimotor area. We suggest that SAM is a useful analysis method for auditory evoked response and mu rhythm.

We suggest that prefrontal activation at 200–600 ms for 4–8 and 8–15 Hz is related to attentional processing during an oddball task. These oscillatory activities might be different from the slow wave component of P300. Basar [5] reported that by using an oddball paradigm, prolonged event-related alpha oscillations up to 400 ms were observed. They named these alpha components "functional alpha." They also reported that event-related theta oscillations are prolonged and/or have a second time window approximately 300 ms after target stimuli in oddball experiments. They suggested that prolongation of theta is interpreted as being correlated with selective attention. Our results are consistent with these previous studies. We suggest that the parietal slow component for 1–4 Hz is related to sensory integration. This slow wave component might be directly related to the P300 waveform.

In this study, we could not find any temporal cortex or hippocampal activation at 200–600 ms. We observed N1m activity in 0–200 ms, so this absence of temporal activity is not due to the methodology, such as SAM and permutation. MEG might not be good at deep sources. We adopted 500 ms pure tone stimuli and used pseudo t-value calculation subtracting the responses between the deviant stimuli and the standard stimuli at 200–600 ms. Therefore, we could omit an auditory off-response and sustained response in this study.

References

[1] N. Nishitani, et al., The role of the hippocampus in auditory processing studied by event-related electric potentials and magnetic fields in epilepsy patients before and after temporal lobectomy, Brain 122 (1999) 687–707.
[2] S.E. Robinson, D.F. Rose, Current source estimation by spatially filtered MEG, in: M. Hoke, S.N. Eme, Y.C. Okada (Eds.), Biomagnetism: Clinical Aspects. Proceedings of the 8th International Conference on Biomagnetism, Elsevier, New York, 1992, pp. 761–765.
[3] R. Ishii, et al., Medial prefrontal cortex generates frontal midline theta rhythm, NeuroReport 10 (1999) 675–679.
[4] W. Chau, et al., Group analysis for the Synthetic Aperture Magnetometry (SAM) data, Biomag 2002, Proceedings of the 13th International Conference on Biomagnetism, VDE Verlag, Berlin, 2002.
[5] E. Basar, Brain Function and Oscillations: I. Brain Oscillations: Principles and Approaches, Springer, Berlin, 1998.

International Congress Series 1270 (2004) 209–212

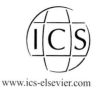

www.ics-elsevier.com

Spatiotemporal imaging of the brain activities during 3-D structure perception from motion

Sunao Iwaki[a,b,*], Giorgio Bonmassar[b], John W. Belliveau[b]

[a] National Institute of Advanced Industrial Science and Technology, USA
[b] NMR Center, Massachusetts General Hospital, USA

Abstract. Here, we used both MEG and fMRI to detect dynamic brain responses to 3-D structure perception from random-dot motion in humans. The visual stimuli consisted of 1000 random dots, which started to move 500 ms after the onset of presentation. The coherence of the motion was controlled from 0 to 100%. A stimulus that is fully coherent had all the dots moving as if they belonged to a rotating spherical surface. On the other hand, the 80, 60, 40, 20, and 0% coherence stimuli contain dots having the same speed as the fully coherent stimuli, but the directions of the 20, 40, 60, 80, and 100% of the dots were randomized, respectively. Neuromagnetic signals were measured with a 306-channel MEG system. More than 60 stimulus-related epochs of 2000 ms, including a 1000 ms pre-stimulus baseline, were recorded and averaged for each condition with a sampling rate of 600 Hz. FMRI experiments were conducted using a 3 Tesla scanner covering the entire brain using blocked design, in which 12 s blocks were presented in pseudo-randomized order. The results of the fMRI analysis were used to impose plausible constraints on the MEG inverse calculation using a "weighted" minimum-norm approach to improve spatial resolution of the spatiotemporal activity estimates. The bilateral occipito-temporal and the intra-parietal regions showed increased neural activity in the fully coherent motion condition around the latencies of 180 ms and 240 ms after the onset of motion, respectively. These results indicate that the bilateral occipito-temporal and intra-parietal regions play an important role in the perception of 3-D structure from random-dot motion. Also, the present study adds further insight into the temporal characteristics of the neural activities in these regions. © 2004 Published by Elsevier B.V.

Keywords: 3-D structure perception from random-dot motion; MEG; fMRI; Spatio-temporal source modeling; Weighted minimum-norm estimate

1. Introduction

Perception of three-dimensional structure from motion requires visual motion to be integrated spatially as well as the recognition of the object shape. Many psycho-

* Corresponding author. NMR Center, Massachusetts General Hospital, Building 149, Room 2301, 13th Street, Charlestown, MA 02129, USA. Tel.: +1-617-726-6584; fax: +1-617-726-7422.
E-mail address: sunao@nmr.mgh.harvard.edu (S. Iwaki).

0531-5131/ © 2004 Published by Elsevier B.V.
doi:10.1016/j.ics.2004.04.036

physical studies have been done to investigate how the visual system extracts the 3-D structure of objects from 2-D motion of random dots (structure-from-motion: SFM).

Recent neuroimaging studies suggest the involvement of the parieto-occipital junction, the superior-occipital gyrus, and the ventral occipito-temporal junction in the perception of 3-D structure from motion [1], though the neural dynamics underlying the reconstruction of a 3-D perception from optic flow is not fully understood.

In this study, we used both the neuromagnetic (magnetoencephalography: MEG) and the hemodynamic (functional MRI: fMRI) measurements to detect the dynamic brain responses to 3-D structure perception from random-dot motion in humans.

2. Methods

2.1. Visual stimuli

The visual stimuli consisted of 1000 random dots, which started to move 500 ms after the onset of presentation. The coherence of the motion was controlled from 0% to 100%. A stimulus that is fully coherent had all the dots moving as if they belonged to a rotating spherical surface with a radius of 10 degrees in visual angle. On the other hand, the 80%, 60%, 40%, 20%, and 0% coherence stimuli contain dots having the same speed as the fully coherent stimuli, but the directions of the 20%, 40%, 60%, 80%, and 100% of the dots were randomized, respectively.

2.2. MEG experiment

Neuromagnetic signals were measured during subjects viewing visual stimuli with a 306-channel MEG system. The stimulus-related epochs of 2000 ms, including a 1000 ms pre-stimulus baseline, were recorded with a pass-band of 0.01–200 Hz and a sampling rate of 600 Hz. More than 60 epochs were averaged for each condition.

2.3. fMRI experiment

The scanning was conducted using a 3 Tesla Siemens Allegra scanner. For functional imaging, the single shot echo-planer imaging sequence was used with the imaging parameters TR 3000 ms, TE 40 ms, FA 90°, 40 axial slices, 3 mm thickness with 0 mm gap, 64 × 64 matrix, and FOV 220 mm, which covered the entire brain. Three to fourteen minutes functional scans were divided into 12 s phases, randomly alternating between different stimulus (coherency) conditions and resting (fixation) periods. Within each phase, motion stimuli were presented every 4 s.

2.4. Data processing

Reconstruction and analysis of the fMRI data were performed using FreeSurfer software. The data were realigned using the first image as a reference and spatially smoothed using Gaussian kernels of 6 mm. A boxcar wave function was applied as a reference function, and a statistical parametric map was generated for each voxel. The results of the fMRI analysis were used to impose plausible constraints on the MEG inverse calculation using a "weighted" minimum-norm approach [2] to improve spatial resolution of the spatio-temporal activity estimates. In this experiment, we introduced fMRI weighting, which was determined by thresholding the fMRI statistical parametric map for each (0%, 20%, 40%, 60%, 80%, and 100% coherence) condition vs. fixation condition, into a linear inverse operator used to map measured MEG signal into estimated neural source distributions [2].

3. Results

Subjects' responses collected during the MEG measurements showed that the perception of 3-D structure (rotating sphere) was dominant only in the 80% and 100% coherence conditions.

Fig. 1 shows fMRI statistical parametric maps for coherent motion ((a) 100%, (b) 80%, and (c) 60% coherence) conditions vs. a random-dot motion (0% coherence) condition in the typical subject. Activation in the bilateral occipital/occipito-temporal and the intra-parietal regions were modulated by the change of motion coherence.

Fig. 2 shows the neural activity distributions for (a) the random-dot motion condition and (b) the fully coherent motion condition estimated using an fMRI-constrained MEG inverse procedure in the typical subject. The bilateral occipito-temporal and the intra-parietal regions showed increased neural activity in the fully coherent motion condition around the latencies of 180 and 240 ms after the onset of motion, respectively.

4. Discussion

The results shown here indicate that the bilateral occipito-temporal and intra-parietal regions play an important role in the perception of 3-D structure from random-dot motion.

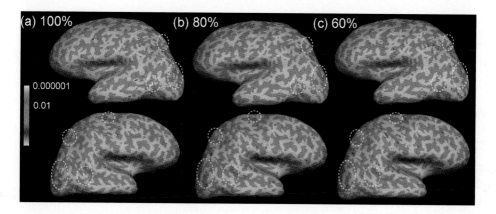

Fig. 1. Results of the fMRI analysis for coherent motion (a) 100%, (b) 80%, and (c) 60% coherence conditions vs. random-dot motion (0% coherence) condition.

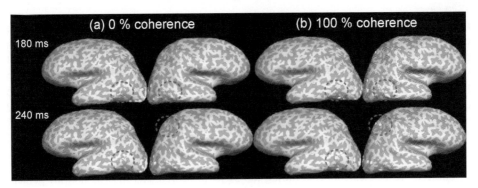

Fig. 2. Neural activity distribution estimated using MEG-fMRI combined spatio-temporal imaging for (a) the random-dot motion condition and (b) the fully coherent motion condition.

These results are in agreement with those from the previous studies of 3-D structure perception from motion using fMRI, and add further insight into the temporal characteristics of the neural activities in these regions.

These regions were also reported to be activated in mental rotation processing [3].

References

[1] A.L. Paradis, et al., Visual Perception of Motion and 3-D Structure from Motion: an fMRI Study, Cereb. Cortex 10 (2000) 772–783.
[2] A.M. Dale, et al., Spatiotemporal cortical activation patterns during semantic processing of novel and repeated words as revealed by combined fMRI and MEG, Neuron 26 (2000) 55–67.
[3] S. Iwaki, et al., Dynamic cortical activation in mental image processing revealed by biomagnetic measurement, NeuroReport 10 (1999) 1793–1797.

International Congress Series 1270 (2004) 213–215

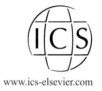

www.ics-elsevier.com

High resolution spectral analysis of visual evoked EEGs for word-recognition "Event-related spectra"

I. Shimoyama[a,*], Y. Kasagi[a,b], S. Yoshida[a,b], K. Nakazawa[a,b], A. Murata[a,c], F. Asano[a,d]

[a] Section for Human Neurophysiology, Research Center for Medical Engineering,
Chiba University,1-33, Yayoi, Inage, Chiba-City, Chiba 263-8522, Japan
[b] Department of Integrative Neurophysiology, Graduate School of Medicine, Chiba University, Japan
[c] Department of Rehabilitation, University Hospital, Chiba University, Japan
[d] Gram Corporation, Japan

Abstract. We studied precise spectra of evoked EEGs in the word recognition analyzed with multiple band-pass filters (MBFA). The filter was infinite impulse response in 2nd order. Firstly, a signal swept from 5 to 100 Hz sine wave was tested with MBFA, fast Fourier transform and Wavelet transform. Ten evoked EEGs with word visual stimuli were recorded from three volunteers. The EEGs were sampled at 1 kHz in 14 bits for 1 s, and were analyzed with MBFA to make spectra from 5 to 100 Hz, and the spectra were averaged 10 times for observation. Evoked powers were noted at alpha band over the occipital area and suppressed powers were noted at beta and alpha bands afterward. Gamma bands were noted to be evoked over the posterior central area in the normalized Event-related spectra. © 2004 Elsevier B.V. All rights reserved.

Keywords: Spectra; Filter; EEGs; ERPs; Words

1. Introduction

To study precise spectral dynamics for evoked EEGs, we studied a new technique of a multiple band-pass filter (MBFA) [1–3]. Event-related potentials are good in temporal resolution in measuring their peak-latency and amplitude; but, it takes many times to get good evoked potentials in averaging proper times with the evoked EEGs, and the background EEGs are canceled out in the process. However, alpha attenuation is another important phenomenon to estimate neural activation. To study both the background EEGs and the evoked potentials, we used MBFA for word recognition as "Event-related spectra".

---

* Corresponding author. Tel.: +81-43-290-3118; fax: +81-43-290-3118.
E-mail address: ichiro@faculty.chiba-u.jp (I. Shimoyama).

0531-5131/ © 2004 Elsevier B.V. All rights reserved.
doi:10.1016/j.ics.2004.05.093

2. Methods and subjects

Three male volunteers were participated in this study; they were all right-handed native Japanese (37/40/55 years). A Quick-cap (64 electrodes, Neuroscan, USA) was used with a reference to the midline at the frontal pole. Chinese characters were displayed on a TV monitor 1 m apart (Cambridge Research Systems, UK). The EEGs for 1 s, pre-stimulus 200 ms and post-stimulus 800 ms were recorded with a band-pass filter between 0.5 and 100 Hz (6R12, Biotop, San-ei, Japan), and the signals were digitalized in 14 bits at 1 kHz. The EEGs were analyzed with SSE-V100 (Gram, Japan), and the spectra were averaged for observation. The time window of MBFA was 20 ms, and MBFA showed spectra between 5 and 100 Hz. The algorithm of MBFA is in brief multiple band-pass filters (2nd ordered infinite impulse response)[1–3]. Before analyzing the evoked EEGs, as a control, a 1 s signal swept from 5 to 100 Hz sine wave was tested with MBFA, fast Fourier transform (FFT, 128 points with Hanning window), and Wavelet transform (Gabor8, 32/octave).

3. Results

Fig. 1 showed spectra of the test signal (A), analyzed with MBFA (B), FFT (C), and Wavelet analyses (D). The spectra with MBFA showed linear increase to time, and the resolution was 1 Hz in frequency ($df=1$ Hz); those with FFT showed rough resolution ($df=7.8$ Hz). The spectra with Wavelet showed nonlinear to time; the power showed lower and wider as time swept. Fig. 2 showed normalized spectra of examples of one channel for three subjects. Left posterior temporal spectra showed evoked power at alpha, gamma and alpha bands, suppressed power at gamma bands in subject 1. Left posterior temporal

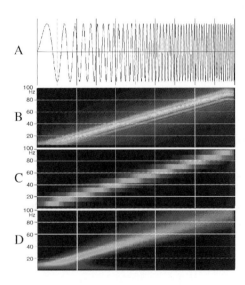

Fig. 1. Test signal (A), dynamic spectra analyzed with multiple band-pass filters (B), fast Fourier transform (C), and Wavelet transform (D). The ordinate meant frequency, and the abscissa meant time course.

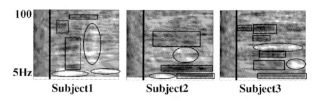

Fig. 2. Event-related spectra; examples of one channel for three subjects. The ovals showed evoked spectra and the squares showed suppressed spectra. The ordinate meant frequency, and the abscissa meant time (1 s) around the stimuli (vertical lines).

spectra showed evoked power at theta and gamma bands, suppressed power at gamma, beta, alpha and theta bands in subject 2. Right posterior temporal spectra showed suppressed power at theta, alpha, beta and gamma bands, and evoked power at gamma and beta bands in subject 3.

4. Discussion

MBFA showed us evoked and suppressed spectra in detail and MBFA is better than FFT and Wavelet in frequency domain and linearity. Evoked spectra at alpha and theta bands were the same as the reports of ERPs for word [4,5] over the occipital and posterior temporal areas. However, suppressed spectra, showed at gamma, beta, alpha, and theta bands over the posterior half of the head have never been observed in the reports. Problems about phase delay and inter-stimuli variation are left for further study.

References

[1] I. Shimoyama, et al., New algorithm for high resolution spectral analysis, J. Brain Sci. 25 (3 and 4) (1999) 147–151.
[2] I. Shimoyama, et al., Flash-related synchronization and desynchronization revealed by a multiple band frequency analysis, Jpn. J. Physiol. 50 (2000) 553–559.
[3] F. Asano, et al., Precise spectral analysis using a multiple band-pass filter for flash-visual evoked potentials, Proceeding of the 2002 Spring Conference of KOSES and The 3rd Korea–Japan International Symposium, 2002, pp. 44–50.
[4] I. Shimoyama, et al., Verbal versus non-verbal visual evoked potentials: kanji versus line drawings, Brain Topogr. 5 (1) (1992) 35–39.
[5] I. Shimoyama, et al., Visual evoked potentials relating to imagery: words for concrete objects versus absolute concepts, Brain Topogr. 9 (4) (1997) 271–274.

International Congress Series 1270 (2004) 216–219

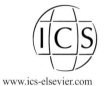

www.ics-elsevier.com

Human cortical magnetic responses to visual moving objects

K. Tsubota[a], K. Yoshino[a], M. Shintani[b,*], Y. Kato[c], M. Kato[c]

[a] Department of Ophthalmology, Ichikawa General Hospital, Tokyo Dental College, Ichikawa, Japan
[b] Laboratory of Brain Research, Oral Health Science Center, Tokyo Dental College, 1-2-2 Masago,
Mihama-ku, Chiba 261-8502, Japan
[c] Department of Neuropsychiatry, Keio University School of Medicine, Japan

Abstract. In order to clarify the brain mechanisms of visual cognition for moving objects, evoked cortical magnetic responses for horizontally moving object were measured. A major response at the latency around 140 ms appeared in the location from the right parietal region. Another distinctive response around 240 ms was observed in the right temporal region. The neural activity of the dorsal system in the right hemisphere was suggested to be necessary to visually catch the moving object and recognize it distinctively. © 2004 Elsevier B.V. All rights reserved.

Keywords: Magnetoencephalography; Visual cortex; Visual pattern recognition; Motion perception; Visual evoked fields

1. Introduction

There have been several studies which investigated the neurophysiologic mechanism and neural correlates for motion perception [1,2]. Experiments using random dot kinematogram demonstrated that the perception of coherent motion begins with the local detection of individual dot motions and subsequently proceeds to the spatial integration of these motions. Moreover, these studies showed that this integration process was supported by the neural activities of middle temporal area (MT) or V5 in the occipito-temporal lobes [3]. On the other hand, there have been few reports on the neural bases of the recognition and identification of the moving individual objects such as tools, vehicles, letters and numerals, although these dynamic activities are more essential to the human visual cognition than the recognition of resting objects in everyday life. Therefore, this study aimed to directly investigate the brain mechanisms of visual cognition for moving objects.

2. Materials and methods

Evoked cortical magnetic responses of seven healthy adults (three females) were measured with 306 ch MEG (VectorView®, Elekta-Neuromag, Finland.) All subjects were

---

* Corresponding author. Tel./fax: +81-43-270-3842.
E-mail address: shintani@tdc.ac.jp (M. Shintani).

0531-5131/ © 2004 Elsevier B.V. All rights reserved.
doi:10.1016/j.ics.2004.04.058

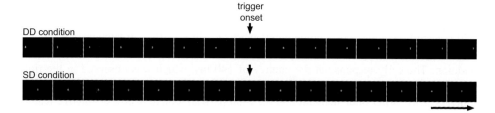

Fig. 1. Visual stimuli of DD and SD conditions. In DD condition, the target object of changing blurred figures appears from left and across the screen to the right end. In SD condition, the same object stays at the center of the screen. Of the total 45 frames (30 frames/s), 15 are shown in this figure. The trigger onset was synchronized to the midst frame of visual stimulus where the numeric figure was clearly readable in each condition at the center of screen.

right-handed and with normal or corrected-to-normal vision. The experiment was carried out in two conditions, in which the subjects were requested to read one of the changing visual numerals generated as a movie of sequential computer graphics. The movie was back-projected onto a screen, which was set 1.5 m in front of the subject.

First, in the Dynamic–Dynamic (DD) condition, subjects were instructed to read a target numeric figure, which suddenly emerged and could be clearly recognized during 70 ms at the center of the screen, among the other numerals that were quickly moving from left to right (see Fig. 1). These numerals changed at random and were dimly visible to read except at the center of screen.

Second, in the Static–Dynamic (SD) condition, the subjects were given the same task as in the DD condition, except that the changing numerals were not moving from left to right and staying at the center of screen. MEG signals obtained in 100 successful trials were averaged.

3. Results

Both spatial and temporal gradients of the subtracted waveform of DD and SD conditions were examined. A major response at the latency around 140 ms appeared mainly in the location of the right parietal region. Another distinctive response around 240 ms was observed in right temporal region (see Table 1; Figs. 2 and 3).

Since these responses were caught with gradiometers, they reflected the components derived from the cortex of the right hemisphere. In RMS analysis, the evident responses were observed in right parietal lobe.

Table 1
Peak latencies and amplitudes for M140 and M240 in seven subjects obtained from 24 channels RMS of right parietal–temporal region

Subject	M140		M240	
	Latency (ms)	Peak Amplitude (fT/cm)	Latency (ms)	Peak amplitude (fT/cm)
1	145	679	220	414
2	137	684	256	338
3	148	501	238	356
4	144	332	242	268
5	148	391	235	262
6	138	621	237	347
7	152	517	241	306
Mean	144.6	532.1	238.4	327.3
S.D.	5.5	137.7	10.7	53.4

4. Discussion

In this study, the two MEG components were clearly identified at latencies of 140 and 240 ms by comparing the DD (Dynamic–Dynamic) with the SD (Static–Dynamic) condition. The early response at the latency of 140 ms, which was observed in the right parietal lobes, is suggested to be correspondent to the process for detecting the moving numerals. This earlier brain activation in the right parietal lobe may be a distinctive feature in the recognition of the dynamically moving object. The late response, which was observed in the right temporal regions at the latency of 240 ms, corresponds to the identification process of the numerals, consisting with the previously reported findings to elucidate the object or letter recognition system. In consequence, the brain activation from the 145 ms component in the parietal lobe to the 240-ms component in the temporal lobe was integrated in the right hemisphere, resulting in the recognition and identification of moving numerals.

As for the localization of brain function, the ability to recognize the moving object should be explained in the context of the "two cortical visual systems" approach, that postulates the separation of the processes of object recognition from those involved in certain types of spatial coding: One route (the dorsal system) is dedicated to the control of action and codes a viewer-centered spatial representation. The other route (the ventral system) is concerned with object recognition and codes an object-centered representation [4,5], which is rather more static than the dorsal system. On this account, the early response at the latency of 145 ms would be seen as the operation of the dorsal system. On

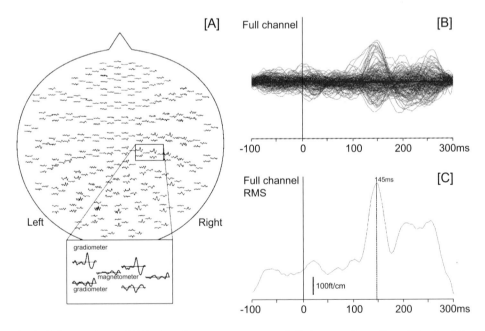

Fig. 2. VEF waveforms of 306 channels neuromagnetometer. Full-view waveforms from 102 sets of two gradiometers and a magnetometer indicate that in the corresponding channels, each gradiometer detects remarkable peaks whereas a magnetometer shows insignificant wave (A). Full-channel waveform (B) and RMS wave (C) of subject 1 show a peak at the latency of 145 ms.

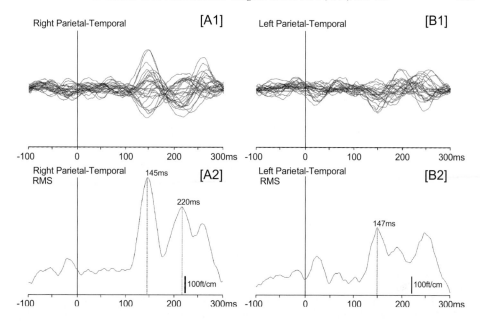

Fig. 3. Averaged MEG waveforms in subject 1 from right parietal–temporal region (A1), and from corresponding region in the left hemisphere (B1). Two significant peaks at the latencies of 145 and 220 ms were detected by RMS in the right region (A2). The highest peak in RMS waveform from left area appears at almost the same latency, but is not significant (B2).

the other hand, the late response at the latency of 240 ms could represent the contribution of the ventral system.

In summary, we suggested that the horizontal movement of the visual stimuli gave rise to the responses in right parietal lobe at the latency of 140 ms. This result indicated that the neural activity of the dorsal system in the right hemisphere was necessary to catch the moving object visually and recognize it distinctively.

Acknowledgements

Supported by HRC3B03 for High-Tech Research Center Projects from the Ministry of Education, Culture, Sports, Science and Technology of Japan granted to K.T.

References

[1] C.L. Baker Jr, R.F. Hess, J. Zihl, Residual motion perception in a "motion-blind" patient, assessed with limited-lifetime random dot stimuli, J. Neurosci. 11 (1991) 454–461.
[2] W.T. Newsome, E.B. Pare, A selective impairment of motion perception following lesions of the middle temporal visual area (MT), J. Neurosci. 8 (1988) 2201–2211.
[3] W.T. Newsome, K.H. Britten, J.A. Movshon, Neuronal correlates of a perceptual decision, Nature 341 (1989) 52–54.
[4] M. Mishkin, L.G. Ungerleider, K.A. Macko, Object vision and spatial vision: two cortical pathways, Trends Neurosci. 6 (1983) 414–417.
[5] M.A. Goodale, A.D. Milner, Separated visual pathways for perception and action, Trends Neurosci. 15 (1992) 20–25.

International Congress Series 1270 (2004) 220–224

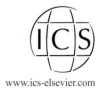

www.ics-elsevier.com

Fast responses in human extrastriate cortex using a face affect recognition task

Lichan C. Liu*, Andreas A. Ioannides

Laboratory for Human Brain Dynamics, RIKEN Brain Science Institute, 2-1 Hirosawa, Wakoshi, Saitama, Japan

Abstract. We studied magnetoencephalographic (MEG) responses to faces presented centrally and peripherally. At the center, the left and right fusiform areas showed similar activation pattern (peaked at 80 and 130 ms), but with stronger activation in the right than left fusiform. In the periphery, relative to the image presentation side, the contralateral fusiform activated much earlier and stronger than the ipsilateral fusiform. When the images were presented in the upper visual field, contralateral fusiform and V1/V2 had their first peak activation at similar latency (65 ms). © 2004 Elsevier B.V. All rights reserved.

Keywords: Magnetoencephalography (MEG); Extrastiate cortex; Fusiform gyrus; Face perception; Laterality

1. Introduction

Recent PET and fMRI studies identified face sensitive areas in the human posterior fusiform [1], lateral occipital complex [2] and middle temporal [3] areas, while EEG and magnetoencephalographic (MEG) studies found face-specific neural activity at 170 ms [4,5]. In these studies, facial images were presented centrally with a relatively large visual field. In this MEG study, we aimed to investigate spatial and temporal differences between images presented centrally and peripherally. We address how fast the human extrastriate cortex is activated and the effect of image presentation position on its activation.

2. Materials and methods

Eight healthy right-handed males participated in a face affect recognition task to name verbally the emotions shown in the images presented centrally or peripherally (Fig. 1). We recorded MEG signals using a whole-head system for 15 task runs (3 for each position) and 2 control runs (only gray background). The subjects fixated the center screen during recording. We used magnetic field tomography (MFT) [6] to track the evolution of activity over the entire brain every 1.6 ms from the cleaned and averaged data. Post-MFT statistical *t*-test [5] was further applied to identify brain areas and latencies significantly different

---

* Corresponding author. Tel.: +81-48-467-7218; fax: +81-48-467-9731.
E-mail address: lichan@brain.riken.jp (L.C. Liu).

0531-5131/ © 2004 Elsevier B.V. All rights reserved.
doi:10.1016/j.ics.2004.05.054

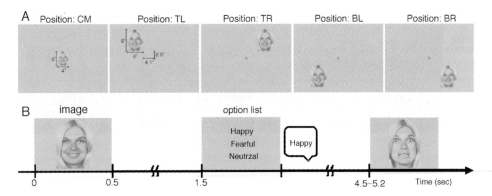

Fig. 1. Experimental setup. (A) The five image presentation positions. (B) A trial sequence.

between the task and controls runs. We then defined regions of interest (ROIs) functionally and calculated activation curves for these ROIs.

3. Results

All eight subjects performed the task without difficulty, with the best performance at the center (95.6%), followed by top-right (83.6%), top-left (81.5%), bottom-left (80.4%) and bottom-right (75.3%). The performance at the center was significantly better than the other four quadrants by ANOVA and Sheffe post hoc analyses.

Fig. 2 shows typical MEG signal waveforms as a function of the image position. The signal was averaged on image onset and from about 30 images in the first run of the three runs at one of the five positions. The peak amplitude of the MEG signal was similar in each of the five positions, but the number of peaks and peak latencies varied. Within 250 ms after the image onset, the MEG signal peaked at 40–75, 100–135 and 170–210 ms.

For each image presentation position (3 runs), we first identified strong and consistent activated areas by calculating the averaged current density smoothed with a moving window of 6.4 ms in steps of 1.6 ms. Within the first 100 ms, we observed wide spread

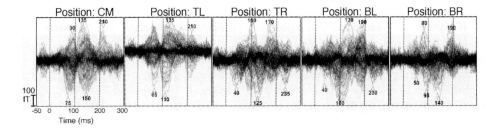

Fig. 2. Averaged MEG signal from subject 1's first run at each of the five image positions (CM, TL, TR, BL, BR) shown in the same scale. The arrows and numbers highlight the peak latencies in the signal curves.

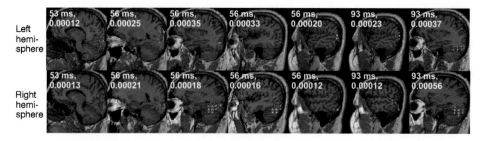

Fig. 3. The instantaneous brain activity from MFT for subject 1 when the images were presented at the center. The current density is shown using pink contours and yellow arrows (direction) and normalized separately for each image. The activation latency (ms) and strength (a.u.) are also printed on the top-left of each image.

activation in occipital and temporal areas including around the calcarine sulus, inferior, mid and superior occipital gyri, mid and superior temporal gyri, as shown in Fig. 3.

The post-MFT statistical analysis was further applied to determine whether the above activations were significant or not. Fig. 4 shows the first significant activation around the calcarine sulcus for subject 1 when the images were presented at the five positions. The significant activation in V1/V2 agrees with the well-studied retinotopical organisation in V1/2. Specifically, when the images were presented in the upper and lower visual field, the ventral and dorsal parts of V1/V2 were activated, respectively. The central presentation activated more posterior part of V1/V2 than the peripheral presentation.

We normalized the individual statistical maps into a common Talairach space to identify common significant activations from all seven or eight subjects (Table 1). We then projected these areas back to each subject and defined ROIs based on individual MFT solutions. We calculated the ROI activation curves as a function of time and compared them across runs and conditions. For two specific ROIs, V1/V2 and fusiform areas, which showed the most robust difference in activity between faces and objects [1], we found (1) V1/V2 activated earlier when the images were presented peripherally (65 ms) than centrally (70 ms) and stronger in the lower than upper visual field presentation. (2) Stronger activation in the fusiform gyri was observed when the images were presented centrally than peripherally. (3) For the central stimuli, the left and right fusiform areas showed similar activation pattern (peaked at 80 and 130 ms) but with stronger activation in the right than left fusiform. (4) When the images were presented at one of the quadrants, relative to the image presentation side, the contralateral fusiform activated much earlier

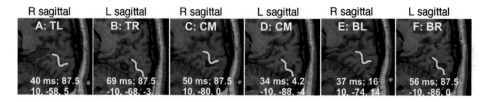

Fig. 4. The first significant activation (red contours) around the calcarine sulcus (yellow lines) for subject 1 when the images were presented at the five positions. At the bottom of each figurine, the latency, t-value and the Talairach coordinates for the centroids of the significant activation are also printed.

Table 1
Regions showing the first common significant activation ($p < 0.05$) across all seven or eight subjects

Region	Talaraich coordinates (x, y, z)	Time (ms) CM	Time (ms) TL	Time (ms) TR	Time (ms) BL	Time (ms) BR	Previous studies [1,3,7] Talaraich coordinates (x,y,z)
V1/2	−10, −88, 7 (L)	53	{85}	74	74	61	
	10, −82, 3 (R)						
Ventral occipital							
Inferior occipital gyri (LOC)	−41, −73, −7 (L)	90	146	139	144	93	−40, −72, −13
	−41, −69, −5 (R)	90	141	144	154	176	41, −69, −10 [7]
Mid-occipital gyri	−31, −78, −4 (L)	91	124	96	139	118	−37, −81, −8
	31, −81, 0 (R)	125	160		179	149	42, −79, −7 [3]
Mid-superior occipital gyri	−42, −61, 22 (L)	136		130		104	
	41, −62, 13 (R)	90	130	144	154	115	
Ventral temporal							
Posterior fusiform gyri (FEFA)	−32, −57, −9 (L)	86	118	120	128	93	−35, −63, −10
	32, −57, −11 (R)	72	{90}	{152}	149	{170}	40, −55, −10 [1]
Anterior fusiform gyri	−31, −36, −11 (L)	134	146	131	176	130	−25, −42, −10
	31, −38, −8 (R)	134	{104}	{88}	152	{186}	25, −39, −12 [7]
Mid temporal gyri	−52, −62, 3 (L)	83	122		134		
	52, −51, −3 (R)	112	125				
Superior temporal gyri	−52, −45, 16 (L)	118	147	115	128	150	−52, −61, 4
	51, −58, 16 (R)						43, −57, 12 [3]

The coordinates are the centroids of the regions. The latency under each position means, e.g., 53: all eight subjects had significant activation within a radius of 1.0 cm of the region and a time window of 19.2 ms centered at 53 ms in the Talaraich space. 85: seven out of eight subjects showed the common significant activation at 85 ms. {85}: the normalization across eight subjects is done within a radius of 1.5 cm of the region and stronger than the ipsilateral fusiform. (5) When the images were presented in the upper visual field, contralateral V1/V2 and contralateral fusiform had their first peak activation at similar latency (60–65 ms), with comparable strength (TL presentation) or weaker (TR) activation in the fusiform area.

4. Discussion

In this MEG work, we identified fast responses in human striate and extrastriate cortices well within 100 ms after the facial image onset. The reasons for our finding may be twofold: first we used a smaller image size than most of previous studies and second we did not use a narrow band filter (e.g., 1–30 Hz) which may effectively eliminate fast responses in the recorded raw data. Whether these fast responses are face selective or not still needs to be clarified with future experiments using other object categories. In divided visual field studies, it is clear which hemisphere receives the stimulus first. Our results suggest that stimuli were processed predominantly in the directly stimulated hemisphere, and visual field differences were likely due to relative differences in processing efficiency between the hemispheres.

References

[1] N. Kanwisher, et al., The fusiform face area: a module in human extrastriate cortex specialized for face perception, J. Neurosci. 17 (1997) 4302–4311.
[2] I. Gauthier, et al., The fusiform "face area" is part of a network that processes faces at the individual level, J. Cogn. Neurosci. 12 (2000) 495–504.
[3] E. Halgren, et al., Location of human face-selective cortex with respect to retinotopic areas, Hum. Brain Mapp. 7 (1999) 29–37.
[4] D.A. Jeffreys, Evoked potential studies of face and object processing, Vis. Cogn. 3 (1996) 1–38.
[5] L.C. Liu, et al., Single trial analysis of neurophysiological correlates of the recognition of complex objects and facial expressions of emotion, Brain Topogr. 11 (1999) 291–303.
[6] A.A. Ioannides, et al., Continuous probabilistic solutions to the biomagnetic inverse problem, Inverse Problems 6 (1990) 523–542.
[7] I. Levy, et al., Center-periphery organization of human object areas, Nat. Neurosci. 4 (2001) 533–539.

International Congress Series 1270 (2004) 225–228

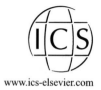

www.ics-elsevier.com

ELSEVIER

Induced gamma-band activity in a similarity grouping task

Jiuk Jung, Tetsuo Kobayashi*

Electrical Engineering, Graduate School of Engineering, Kyoto University, Kyotodaigaku-katsura, Nishikyo-ku, Kyoto 615-8510, Japan

Abstract. Perceptual grouping is a process involved in chunking of visual information and image segmentation, constituting an important aspect of visual processing. In this study, we analysed EEG gamma-band activities in a similarity grouping task to study brain mechanisms of perceptual grouping. It was found that an increase in induced gamma-band activity depended on the displayed position of the target quadrant. Induced gamma-band activity was mainly observed in the frontal and occipital areas for latencies of 370–630 ms. In addition, it was found that the duration of induced gamma-band activity reflected the level of difficulty of the task. Thus, we have shown that the neural activities involved in a similarity grouping task are characterized by the appearance of induced gamma-band activity and its continuation. © 2004 Elsevier B.V. All rights reserved.

Keywords: Perceptual grouping; EEG; Gamma rhythm

1. Introduction

Similarity is one of the most important of Gestalt's principles of perceptual grouping. According to Gestalt's theory of grouping, simple rules such as similarity of elements (shape), proximity, good continuation, common fate and connectedness dominate perceptual grouping by segmenting a visual scene into regions having some internal consistency [1]. In our previous study [2], we had measured reaction times and event-related potentials (ERPs) in a similarity grouping task in order to try to understand mechanisms underlying similarity grouping. Here, we analysed EEG gamma-band activities in the same experiments to investigate further about neural processes involved in the similarity grouping task.

2. Materials and methods

Seven healthy volunteer subjects (18–28 years old) participated in the experiments. All subjects had normal visual functions, including corrected visual acuity and visual object recognition. Each subject practiced 150 times per day during a 3- or 4-day period so that their reaction time would be fixed before the actual experiment was performed.

---

* Corresponding author. Tel.: +81-75-383-2228; fax: +81-75-383-2228.
E-mail address: tetsuo@kuee.kyoto-u.ac.jp (T. Kobayashi).

0531-5131/ © 2004 Elsevier B.V. All rights reserved.
doi:10.1016/j.ics.2004.04.056

Stimuli were generated by a computer and were presented on a Trinitron monitor at a luminance of 30 cd/m² and at a viewing distance of 60 cm. At this distance, the visual angle was 3.34°. No other contours were visible except for a small fixation point, located in the center of the display monitor.

The stimulus consisted of 80 micropattern elements, where micropattern [∨] was used in the target quadrant and micropattern [>] was used in the ground quadrant (Fig. 1). The location of the target quadrant was changed randomly at the top (quadrant 1), left (quadrant 2), bottom (quadrant 3) and right (quadrant 4). In addition, the position of each micropattern was randomly permuted, providing an approximately uniform density.

Subjects were instructed to fixate on a point before each trial and to press a button when they were ready. Stimuli were presented 2 s after the button had been pressed. Subjects were asked to press the button again as soon as they could identify with certainty the location of the disparate quadrant. A circular pattern, for which subjects selected the location of the quadrant using a computer mouse, was presented 2 s after the button had been pressed again. Each subject repeated these procedures in about 300 trials a day for 2 days. The duration from stimulus appearance until button press was measured as reaction time (RT).

EEGs at 63 scalp positions, together with electrooculrograms (EOGs), were continuously digitized (256 Hz) using a digital EEG system (Bio-logic) covering the whole scalp (according to the extended international 10–20 system) and referenced to the left earlobe. Electrode impedance was kept below 10 kΩ.

Epochs containing artifacts (eye blinks, eye movements and response errors), from 300 ms before to reaction time after stimulus onset, were rejected off-line.

The time–frequency representation based on a wavelet transform decomposition of the signals between 1 and 50 Hz was adapted. The signal convolved with complex Morlet's wavelets, $w(t, f_0)$, having a Gaussian shape both in time domain (σ_t) and frequency domain (σ_f) around its central frequency f_0 was given as

$$w(t, f_0) = A\exp(-t^2/2\sigma_t^2) \times \exp(2i\pi f_0 t), \quad \text{with } \sigma_f = 1/2\pi\sigma_t.$$

A is equal to $(\sigma_t/\pi)^{-1/2}$, which is the normalization factor, so that the wavelets' total energy was 1. A wavelet family is characterized by a constant ratio (f_0/σ_f), which should be chosen in practice greater than 5.

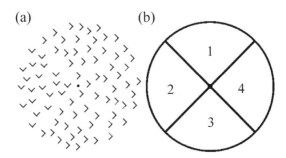

Fig. 1. An example of presented stimuli (a). A target micropattern [∨] was presented at one of the four quadrants (b).

3. Results and discussion

3.1. Reaction time

The mean percent correct for all subjects was 99.6%. There was a significant difference (ANOVA, $F(3, 2796) = 113.07$, $p < 0.01$) in the reaction times, according to the stimulus presentation position, with the reaction times for quadrants 1 and 2 significantly shorter than those for quadrants 3 and 4 (Scheffe, $p < 0.01$). On the other hand, no significant difference was seen between quadrants 1 and 2 or between quadrants 3 and 4. Therefore, we decided to handle the results for quadrants 1 and 2 together and refer to them hereafter as quadrant 1/2. We also decided to handle the results for quadrants 3 and 4 together and refer to them as quadrant 3/4 so that the original set of results was divided into two groups. The difference of reaction times between quadrants 1/2 and 3/4 was 127 ms.

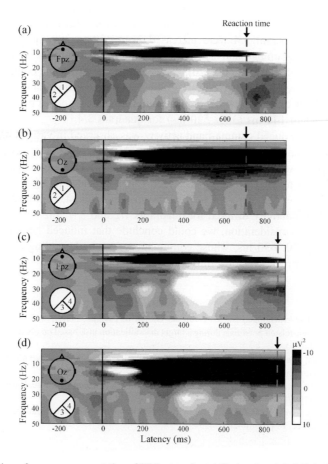

Fig. 2. Average time–frequency representation of EEGs at prefrontal (F_{PZ}) and occipital (O_Z) electrode positions for quadrants 1/2 and 3/4. (a) At F_{PZ} for quadrant 1/2, (b) at O_Z for quadrant 1/2, (c) at F_{PZ} for quadrant 3/4 and (d) at O_Z for quadrant 3/4.

We believe that it is reasonable to interpret that the degree of difficulty of the task is reflected in the difference in reaction times. Since the time required from when the subject determines the target position until he presses the button is considered fixed regardless of the degree of difficulty of the task, if a continuing brain activity that corresponds to the difference in reaction time is seen, it can be surmised that it reflects an activity concerning discrimination (correlated with the degree of difficulty).

3.2. Induced gamma response

Fig. 2 shows the time–frequency representation averaged across single trials over all subjects for quadrants 1/2 and 3/4 at electrodes F_{PZ} and O_Z from 300 ms before stimulus presentation until 900 ms after presentation. At an electrode position of F_{PZ}, the gamma-band activity was significantly increased (larger than $3 \times$ S.D. of pre-stimulus period: $P < 0.01$) from 380 ms for both quadrants 1/2 and 3/4. The increased (induced) gamma-band activities were maintained until 580 and 630 ms for quadrants 1/2 (Fig. 2a) and 3/4 (Fig. 2c), respectively. The gamma-band activities at an electrode position of O_Z for quadrant 1/2 and quadrant 3/4 were increased from 370 to 380 ms, respectively. The increased (induced) gamma-band activities were maintained until 430 and 520 ms for quadrants 1/2 (Fig. 2b) and 3/4 (Fig. 2d), respectively. Therefore, the continuation time of gamma-band activity at F_{PZ} is 200 ms (380–580 ms) for quadrant 1/2 and 250 ms (380 ~ 630 ms) for quadrant 3/4. The continuation time at O_Z is 60 ms (370 ~ 430 ms) for quadrant 1/2 and 140 ms (380–520 ms) for quadrant 3/4.

It is known that induced gamma-band activity was observed in various cognitive tasks, such as a discrimination task with the Kanizsa triangle task [3], a visual search task [4] and a memory task [5]. As shown here, it was found that the induced gamma-band activity was also observed in a similarity grouping task. Our results indicated that gamma-band activity increased from almost the same latency of 380 ms. In contrast, continuation time of the increased (induced) activity differed for quadrants 1/2 and 3/4. Taking the differences in reaction times into consideration, we could conclude that induced gamma-band activity with latencies of 370–630 ms, whose continuation time is depending on task difficulty, may reflect neural processes concerning similarity grouping.

References

[1] M. Wertheimer, Untersuchungen zur lehre von der Gestalt II, Psychol. Forsch. 4 (1923) 301–350.
[2] J. Jung, et al., Event-related potentials during a target discrimination task based on texture cue, Syst. Comput. Jpn. 34 (2003) 34–43.
[3] C. Tallon-Baudry, et al., Stimulus specificity of phase-locked and non-phase-locked 40 Hz visual responses in human, J. Neurosci. 16 (1996) 4240–4249.
[4] C. Tallon-Baudry, et al., Oscillatory γ-band (30–70 Hz) activity induced by a visual search task in human, J. Neurosci. 17 (1997) 722–734.
[5] C. Tallon-Baudry, et al., Induced γ-band activity during the delay of a visual short-term memory task in humans, J. Neurosci. 18 (1998) 4244–4254.

International Congress Series 1270 (2004) 229–232

ELSEVIER

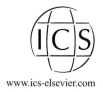

www.ics-elsevier.com

Neuromagnetic oscillatory responses related to the mirror neuron system

Eiko Honaga[a,*], Satoshi Ukai[a], Ryouhei Ishii[a],
Shunsuke Kawaguchi[a], Masakiyo Yamamoto[a], Asao Ogawa[a],
Hideto Hirotsune[a], Norihiko Fujita[b], Toshiki Yoshimine[c],
Kazuhiro Shinosaki[d], Masatoshi Takeda[a]

[a] Department of Psychiatry and Behavioral Science, Osaka University Graduate School of Medicine,
D-3, 2-2, Suita City, Osaka, Japan
[b] Department of Radiology, Osaka University Graduate School of Medicine, Osaka, Japan
[c] Department of Neurosurgery, Osaka University Graduate School of Medicine, Osaka, Japan
[d] Department of Neuropsychiatry, Wakayama Medical University, Wakayama, Japan

Abstract. Mu rhythm is the alpha (8–15 Hz) band oscillatory activity recorded over the sensorimotor cortex accompanied by a higher frequency band activity like beta (15–30 Hz) band. The contralateral sensorimotor area shows event-related desynchronization (ERD) of mu rhythm during limb movement and event-related synchronization (ERS) after the termination of the movement. Previous studies reported that ERD/ERS of mu and beta rhythm were detected during movement observation in the absence of physical movement, as well as during movement execution, suggesting that further investigations into the ERD/ERS of mu and beta rhythm in movement observation may elucidate the mechanisms of the mirror neuron system. We examined the post-movement ERS in beta band after movement observation by using MEG and Synthetic Aperture Magnetometry (SAM) analysis. The post-movement beta ERS was estimated over the bilateral, primary, sensorimotor area after the movement execution in all subjects, and estimated over the contralateral, primary, sensorimotor area after movement observation in four out of six subjects. Our results suggest that MEG SAM analysis is useful for the investigation of the mirror neuron system, which can be applied to clinical research for neurological and psychiatric diseases. © 2004 Elsevier B.V. All rights reserved.

Keywords: Mirror neuron system; Magnetoencephalography; Event-related desynchronization (ERD); Event-related synchronization (ERS); Synthetic aperture magnetometry (SAM); Beta; Mu rhythm

1. Introduction

The mirror neuron system is defined as an observation–execution matching system [1], which is considered to be responsible over the wide spectrum of emotion and cognition,

* Corresponding author. Tel.: +81-6-6879-3051; fax: +81-6-6879-3059.
E-mail address: honaga@psy.med.osaka-u.ac.jp (E. Honaga).

such as imitation, abstraction, affective contact, and understanding the meanings of actions by others. Investigation of the mirror neuron system brings significant benefits to reveal self-cognition of normal human developmental processes and pathological characteristics of several neurological and psychiatric diseases.

Mu rhythm is the alpha (8–15 Hz) band oscillatory activity recorded over the sensorimotor cortex accompanied by a higher frequency band activity like beta (15–30 Hz) band. It has been reported that motor tasks, such as self-generated movement and precision grip, result in increasing or decreasing amplitude of rhythmic activity in alpha and beta band. Pfurtscheller and Araniber [2] defined the former as event-related synchronization (ERS), and the latter as event-related desynchronization (ERD). Since previous studies have reported that ERD/ERS of mu and beta rhythm were observed during movement preparation [3], observation [4–6] and imagination [7,8], as well as during movement execution, further investigations into the ERD/ERS of mu and beta rhythm in movement observation may elucidate the mechanisms of the mirror neuron system.

Synthetic Aperture Magnetometry (SAM) [9] is a novel, spatial, filtering technique based on a nonlinear, constrained, minimum beam former. SAM can estimate spatial and temporal neuromagnetic oscillatory responses in a prescribed frequency band [10–12]. The aim of this study was to examine the post-movement beta ERS after movement observation by using MEG SAM analysis.

2. Subjects and methods

Six normal, healthy volunteers (four males, 28–39 years of age, right-handed) participated in this study. Written informed consent was given by all subjects.

Eight trials were performed. Each trial consisted of "rest-observation-rest" and "rest-execution-rest" periods. Subjects were required to observe the action of the experimenter who was manipulating small objects (observation condition), and to manipulate objects in the same way as the experimenter did in the preceding observation condition (execution condition) for 5 s, respectively. The objects consisted of daily necessities, such as chopsticks, a knife, a ball. All subjects were required to use their right hands.

MEG signals were recorded in a magnetically shielded room using a 64-channel whole-head biomagnetometer system (CTF Systems Inc.). MEG signals were digitized at 250 Hz, filtered using a combined 60 Hz notch filter and 100 Hz low-pass filter. They were recorded on a disk and analyzed off-line.

MEG signals of eight trials were digitally filtered through a band-pass of 15–30 Hz and submitted to SAM analysis. SAM can estimate tomographic distributions of the current source density (CSD) from band-limited MEG signals, and produce a statistical parametric map using voxel-to-voxel comparison by the Student's t-test of the CSD mappings taken in active and control states. In this study, we regarded the observation/execution periods as an active state and the following rest periods as control, and examined increase (corresponding to ERS) or decrease (corresponding to ERD) of CSD.

3. Results

The SAM tomographic images of the post-movement beta ERS in a subject are shown in the Fig. 1. The post-movement beta ERS was estimated over the bilateral primary

Execution   Observation

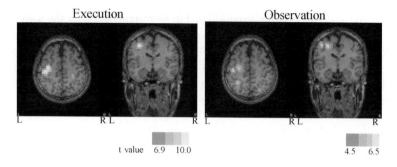

t value   6.9   10.0   4.5   6.5

Fig. 1. The SAM tomographic images of the post-movement beta ERS in Subject 1.

sensorimotor area after movement execution in all subjects, and estimated over the contralateral, primary, sensorimotor area after movement observation in four subjects (Table 1). In addition, during movement observation, the post-movement beta ERS was estimated over the superior and middle temporal gyrus (three out of six subjects), supramarginal/angular gyrus (3/6), parietal area (4/6) and occipital area (6/6).

4. Discussion

In this study, the post-movement beta ERS was estimated over the contralateral sensorimotor area during the movement observation, as well as during the movement execution using MEG SAM analysis. Our results have confirmed the previous studies claiming that ERD/ERS of beta rhythms over the sensorimotor area during movement observation might be related to the mirror neuron system [1].

Previous fMRI and SPECT studies reported that during the observation of goal-directed hand movements, rCBF increased in various brain areas, including premotor cortex, middle temporal gyrus, inferior and middle frontal gyri, and parietal cortex in the contralateral hemisphere [13]. Previous EEG studies showed interindividual variability in the localization and frequency of the post-movement ERD/ERS [5,14,15]. In the current study, the post-movement beta ERS was estimated over some other brain areas than the sensorimotor area during movement observation. In order to investigate the neural basis in various brain areas related to the mirror neuron system, MEG SAM analysis of ERD/ERS in other frequency bands is needed in future study.

Table 1
Number of post-movement beta ERS (over the sensorimotor area)

Subjects	Execution		Observation	
	Left	Right	Left	Right
1	O	O	O	
2	O		O	
3	O	O	O	
4	O	O	O	
5	O	O		
6	O			
Total	6/6	4/6	4/6	0/6

Since the mirror neuron system is considered to be responsible over the wide spectrum of emotion and cognition, it might be related to pathophysiology of several diseases, such as neurological degenerative diseases, including Parkinson's disease, cerebrovascular diseases, schizophrenia and developmental disorders. Our results suggest that MEG SAM analysis is useful for clinical research to investigate the mirror neuron system of various neurological and psychiatric diseases.

References

[1] G. Rizzolatti, L. Fogassi, V. Gallese, Neurophysiological mechanisims underlying the understanding and imitation of action, Neuroscience 12 (2001) 661–670.

[2] G. Pfurtscheller, Graphical display and statistical evaluation of event-related desynchronization, Electro-encephalogr. Clin. Neurophysiol. 43 (1977) 757–760.

[3] G. Pfurtscheller, A. Berghold, Patterns of cortical activation during planning of voluntary movement, Electroencephalogr. Clin. Neurophysiol. 72 (3) (1989) 250–258.

[4] R. Hari, et al., Activation of human primary motor cortex during action observation: a neuromagnetic study, Proc. Natl. Acad. Sci. U. S. A. 95 (25) (1998) 15061–15065.

[5] C. Babiloni, F. Babiloni, F. Carducci, Human cortical electroencephalography (EEG) rhythms during the observation of simple aimless movemets: a high-resolution EEG study, NeuroImage 17 (2002) 559–572.

[6] S.D. Muthukumaraswamy, B.W. Johnson, N.A. McNair, Mu rhythm modulation during observation of an object-directed grasp, Brain Res. Cogn. Brain Res. 19 (2) (2004) 195–201.

[7] G. Pfurtscheller, C. Neuper, Motor Imagery activates primary sensorimotir area in humans, Neurosci. Lett. 239 (1997) 65–68.

[8] J. Decety, The neurophysiological basis of motor imagery, Behav. Brain Res. 77 (1996) 45–52.

[9] S.E. Robinson, J. Vrba, Functional neuroimaging by synthetic aperature magnetometry (SAM), in: T. Yoshitomo, M. Kotani, S. Kuriki, et al. (Eds.), Recent Advances in Biomagnetism, Tohoku Univ. Press, Sendai, 1999, pp. 232–235.

[10] R. Ishii, et al., Medial prefrontal cortex generates frontal midline theta rhythm, NeuroReport 10 (4) (1999) 675–679.

[11] M. Taniguchi, et al., Movement-related desynchronization of the cerebral cortex studied with spatially filtered magnetoencephalography, NeuroImage 12 (2000) 298–306.

[12] D. Cheyne, et al., Neuromagnetic imaging of cortical oscillations accompanying tactile stimulation, Brain Res. Cogn. Brain Res. 17 (3) (2003) 599–611.

[13] J. Grezes, J. Decety, Functional anatomy of execution, mental simulation, observation, and verb generation of actions: a metaanalysis, Hum. Brain Mapp. 12 (2001) 1–19.

[14] G. Pfurtscheller, et al., Foot and hand area mu rhythms, Int. J. Psychophysiol. 26 (1–3) (1997) 121–123.

[15] G. Pfurtscheller, Functional brain imaging based on ERD/ERS, Vis. Res. 41 (10–11) (2001) 1257–1260.

ELSEVIER

International Congress Series 1270 (2004) 233–236

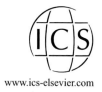

www.ics-elsevier.com

Remote effect of repetitive transcranial magnetic stimulation on the cerebellum of spinocerebellar degeneration patients

Yasushi Hada[a,*], Tatsuro Kaminaga[b], Masahiro Mikami[a]

[a] Department of Rehabilitation Medicine, Teikyo University School of Medicine, 2-11-1 Kaga, Itabashi 173-8605, Tokyo, Japan
[b] Department of Radiology, Teikyo University School of Medicine, Itabashi 173-8605, Tokyo, Japan

Abstract. In order to investigate the effect of repetitive transcranial magnetic stimulation (rTMS) on the cerebellum of spinocerebellar degeneration (SCD) patients, the hemodynamic changes of the brain during rTMS was measured using noninvasive dynamic multi-channel near-infrared optical topography (OT). Two SCD patients diagnosed as OPCA participated in this study. Both had been having rTMS administered to their cerebellum once a week for more than 2 years for therapeutic purposes under the permission of the local ethical committee. Three sessions of 15 times application of 1 Hz rTMS were applied at 3-min intervals. OT probes were set on the scalp and the hemodynamic changes of the fronto-paretal lobe were measured during each session. Changes in hemoglobin were recorded at 15-s prestimulus intervals and consecutively 195 s during and after stimulus. Increased blood flow around the premotor area was observed during rTMS, and the effects were prolonged for more than at least a couple of minutes after rTMS. These results suggest that rTMS administered to the cerebellum of SCD patients may have a remote effect on the frontal lobe and that the blood flow of the frontal lobe may change during and after rTMS. © 2004 Elsevier B.V. All rights reserved.

Keywords: Repetitive transcranial magnetic stimulation (rTMS); Spinocerebellar degeneration (SCD); Near-infrared optical topography (OT); Remote effect

1. Introduction

Transcranial magnetic stimulation (TMS) is used for treatment of such ailments as depression, Parkinson's disease and dystonia as well as for research and diagnosis. TMS is also used as a treatment for spinocerebellar degeneration (SCD). Shimizu et al. [1] applied repetitive TMS (rTMS) to SCD patients and reported improvements in walking speed and body balance after 21 days.

---

* Corresponding author. Tel.: +81-3-3964-2597; fax: +81-3-3962-4087.
E-mail address: y-hada@umin.ac.jp (Y. Hada).

0531-5131/ © 2004 Elsevier B.V. All rights reserved.
doi:10.1016/j.ics.2004.04.030

We have two SCD patients who have undergone once-weekly rTMS over their cerebellum for more than 2 years, and no remarkable aggravation has been observed during this period. The efficacy and exact mechanisms of rTMS over the cerebellum of SCD patients still remain unclear, however. In addition to the direct effect on the cerebellum, remote effects like diaschisis to regions of the cerebral cortex, such as the primary motor cortex, premotor cortex and primary sensory cortex, may be involved.

In order to investigate the effect of rTMS over the cerebellum of SCD patients, we measured the hemodynamic changes of the brain during and after rTMS using noninvasive dynamic multi-channel near-infrared optical topography (OT).

2. Material and methods/patients

Two SCD patients formerly diagnosed as OPCA participated in this study. Both had been undergoing once-weekly rTMS to their cerebellum for more than 2 years under the permission of the local ethical committee.

We used a magnetic stimulator SMN1200 (Nihon Kohden, Tokyo, Japan) with a 14-cm circular coil for rTMS. Maximum magnetic power of this stimulator was 0.51 T. Magnetic stimulations consisted of three sessions of 15 stimuli, with 3-min intervals. The center of the coil was held 5 cm left of the inion during the first session, 5 cm right of the inion during the second session, and at the inion during the third session. After every three stimuli, the coil at each position was turned over to change the direction of the current from clockwise to counter-clockwise or vice-versa. We think that this method enabled us to give magnetic stimulations widely over the cerebellum. Because the purpose of this study was to investigate what occurs on the cerebral cortex during the rTMS that had been performed once weekly to SCD patients, we did not perform sham stimulations. In this experiment, we had 3-min intervals between sessions to observe the prolonged effect after stimulations. Stimulus intensity was as strong as possible without subjecting patients to discomfort.

Near-infrared OT was performed using ETG-4000 (Hitachi Medical, Tokyo, Japan). A pair of 15 probes enabled us to monitor 22 channels (44 channels totally). Those two sets of probes were mounted on the scalp front parietally. The coronal center-line of those probes was adjusted to the C3-Cz-C4 line based on the EEG 10–20 system, with 6-cm separation. Changes in hemoglobin were recorded at 15-s pre-stimulus intervals, 15 s during stimulation and for 180 consecutive seconds after stimulus.

3. Results

Stimulus intensity was 80% of maximum power in subject 1 and 90% in subject 2. We obtained three sessions of OT images from each subject. Optical topography images of the first session of each subject are displayed in Figs. 1 and 2.

These effects appeared during rTMS and were maintained after rTMS for a while, at least until the end of our observation. There were no side effects or complaints from the subjects during this experiment.

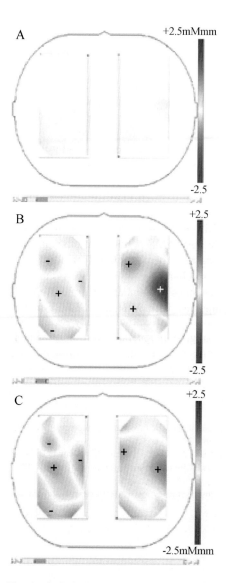

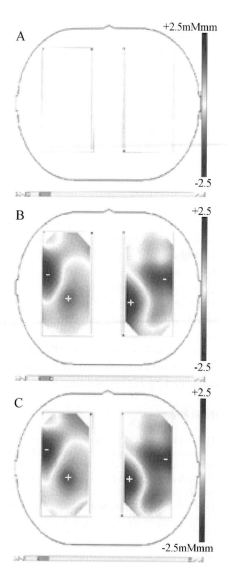

Fig. 1. Optical topography of subject 1, first session. (A) Before rTMS, (B) during rTMS, (C) 3 min after rTMS. +, increment of total Hb; −, decrement of total Hb (mM mm). An increase in total Hb was prominent at mid-lateral, front-central part of the right-hemisphere OT and at the center part of the left-hemisphere OT, during and after the first session of rTMS.

Fig. 2. Optical topography of subject 2, first session. (A) Before rTMS, (B) during rTMS, (C) 3 min after rTMS. +, increment of total Hb; −, decrement of total Hb (mM mm). The increase of total Hb in the first session was prominent at the mid-medial part of the right-hemisphere OT, and at the central to medial part of the left-hemisphere OT. A decrease was prominent at the mid-lateral part of both hemispheres.

4. Discussion

In the present study, positive and negative hemodynamic change was observed during and after rTMS over cerebellum. In the first session of subject 2, there seemed to exist a positive effect in the primary motor area and a negative effect in the premotor area; in that of subject 1, a positive effect existed in both the primary motor and premotor areas. However, we cannot argue about the cortical location in detail in the present study, because of a lack of information about the cortical map, TMS mapping and MRI linkages.

Gerschlager et al. [2] reported that much of the persisting effects of rTMS over cerebellum on cortico-spinal excitability appear to be mediated through the stimulation of peripheral rather than central structures. We used a large diameter ring coil for stimulation in the present study, so that the stimulated area would be wide and vague. Hence, our stimulations might have affected not only the cerebellum but also peripheral structures and the occipital lobe.

Enhancement and depression of cerebral blood flow through rTMS over cerebellum was prolonged for some time after rTMS, at least until the end of our observation in the present study. Chen et al. [3] found that 0.9 Hz rTMS on motor cortex decreased cortical excitability, and lasted for at least 15 min during the post-rTMS period. They thought that the depression they observed was mediated by long-term depression (LTD). Repetitive TMS over the cerebellum may create the same mechanisms as LTD and long-term potentiation, so we will need to observe the OT changes in a much longer post-rTMS period, using another experimental design accompanied with MRI and SPECT in the future.

In conclusion, rTMS administered to the cerebellum of SCD patients may have a remote effect on the frontal lobe. The blood flow of the frontal and parietal cortex may be modulated by rTMS, and this effect may linger after rTMS.

References

[1] H. Shimizu, et al., Therapeutic efficacy of trans magnetic stimulation for hereditary spinocerebellar degeneration, Tohoku Journal of Experimental Medicine 189 (1999) 203–211.

[2] W. Gerschlager, et al., rTMS over the cerebellum can increase corticospinal excitability through a spinal mechanism involving activation of peripheral nerve fibres, Clinical Neurophysiology 113 (9) (2002) 1435–1440.

[3] R. Chen, et al., Depression of motor cortex excitability by low-frequency transcranial magnetic stimulation, Neurology 48 (5) (1997) 1398–1403.

International Congress Series 1270 (2004) 237–240

ELSEVIER

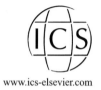

www.ics-elsevier.com

Estimation of the number of brain sources using two system identification methods

X. Bai[a,*], Q. Zhang[a], Z. Li[a], M. Akutagawa[b], Y. Kinouchi[a]

[a]Department of Electrical and Electronic Engineering, University of Tokushima, 2-1 Minamijosanjima-cho, Tokushima 770-8506, Japan
[b]School of Medicine, University of Tokushima, Japan

Abstract. The goal of source localization in the brain is to estimate a set of parameters that can represent the characteristics of the source. One of the parameters is the source number. In order to determine the dipole number with an EEG topography, we use two system identification methods, e.g., the information criterion and F-test methods. Some investigations are presented here to show that the information criterion method is an advanced approach for determining the dipole number with an EEG topography. © 2004 Elsevier B.V. All rights reserved.

Keywords: EEG topography; Powell algorithm; Information criterion; F-test

1. Introduction

The electric activity in the human brain can be recorded with surface EEG electrodes applied to the scalp. The source of recorded EEG signals can be approximated to one or more equivalent current dipoles within the brain. Much work of dipole source localization has been reported such as the moving dipole, the dipole tracing method and the neural network methods [1]. But researchers must assume to know the dipole number in the brain in these methods. A multiple signal classification (MUSIC) method has been proposed to solve this problem. However, MUSIC cannot be used to determine the dipole number with only an EEG topography [2].

In order to solve this problem, we propose a method that combines the Powell algorithm with two system identification methods, e.g., the information criterion (IC) and F-test (FT) methods [3]. And the different penalty functions in IC method are used in our study.

2. Method

System Identification deals with the problem of building mathematical models of systems based on observed data from the system. It involves at least two steps: (1) to

* Corresponding author. Tel./fax: +81-88-656-7475.
E-mail address: bai@ee.tokushima-u.ac.jp (X. Bai).

0531-5131/ © 2004 Elsevier B.V. All rights reserved.
doi:10.1016/j.ics.2004.05.034

choose the type of model, (2) to choose the order of model. In our study, the type of forward model has been determined, e.g., the current dipole model and the concentric 4-sphere head model (see Fig. 1B). The parameter number of the forward model (the dipole number) will be identified by the IC or FT method.

The combined method involves two steps: (1) the measured data are fed to source localization section, the different potential errors E_n can be calculated with the forward model set μ_n by the Powell algorithm, where n is the dipole number ($n = 1\ldots5$); (2) the IC or FT method is to use these potential errors to determine the dipole number (see Fig. 1A).

2.1. Source localization

Let V_{meas} and V_{cal} express the measured potentials from m electrodes and theoretical potentials calculated by the forward model. The potential error for n dipoles can be obtained from

$$E_n = \sqrt{(V_{meas} - V_{cal})^T (V_{meas} - V_{cal})/m}, \tag{1}$$

where m is the number of electrodes ($m = 32$). In this study, the Powell algorithm is selected to minimize Eq. (1). The Powell algorithm is particularly suited to the small-residual case. It does not require explicit expressions for the derivative matrix, but instead it uses the successive value to build up a numerical approximation to the matrix.

2.2. Information criterion and F-test methods

(A) For a model set $\{\mu_n\}$, the model with the minimum information criterion is selected as the optimal forward model (the optimal dipole number). The information criterion IC is denoted as

$$IC_n = m\log(E_n^2) + c(m)n6, \tag{2}$$

where $c(m)$ is penalty function. In 1969, AKAIKE was the first to propose the AIC, the different penalty functions based on AIC have also been reported. In this study,

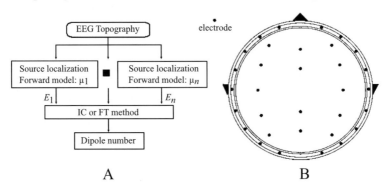

A   B

Fig. 1. (A) The flowchart of our method. (B) The head model with the concentric 4-sphere and their respective radii and conductivities, the conductivities of brain (0.33 s/m, 7.9 cm), cerebrospinal fluid (1.0 s/m, 8.1 cm), skull (0.0042 s/m, 8.5 cm), and scalp (0.33 s/m, 8.8 cm).

$c(m)$ can take one of following forms: (1) $c_1 = 2$, (2) $c_2 = 2\log(\log(m))$, (3) $c_3 = \log(m)$, (4) $c_4 = 2\log(m)$, (5) $c_5 = 3\log(m)$.

(B) Another important alternative to the IC method is the FT method. From small number m of EEG data, the test-quantity T_n can be defined as

$$T_n = \frac{E_n^2 - E_{n+1}^2}{E_{n+1}^2} \frac{m - 6(n+1)}{6} \tag{3}$$

The rule of the FT method can be expressed as

If $T_1 > F_1, \ldots, T_{n-1} > F_{n-1}, T_n < F_n, T_{n+1} < F_{n+1}, \ldots$

the optimal dipole number is n. $\tag{4}$

According to the risk of F-distribution α (in general α is 5%), F_n can be obtained from the F-distribution table as 3.87, 3.94, 4.15 and 5.14.

3. Results and discussion

In this study, several restrictions are imposed in EEG data generation. The dipoles are put randomly in the brain, and the distance between every two dipoles is set to be larger than 2 cm. The moments are generated randomly with the constant strength of 0.8. According to these conditions, five groups of EEG data are generated with different number's dipoles, e.g., one, two, three, four and five dipole cases, where each group of EEG data has 200 samples (N is the real dipole number in EEG data). In each group of EEG data, 3%, 10% and 20% white noise are inserted, respectively. Here, 3%, 10% and 20% white noise means 3%, 10% and 20% of the root mean square value of EEG data.

The optimal dipole number may be identified by comparing individual IC_n or T_n while the potential errors E_n are employed in the IC or the FT method. Table 1 shows the identification results by the IC (c_4) and FT methods for two dipoles case. In the samples, the identified dipole number using the FT method is expressed as zero. It means that the dipole number cannot be determined with the rule (Eq. (4)) of the FT method. The IC method is therefore better than FT method.

Table 2 shows the accuracy of different dipole cases by the IC method with different penalty functions. It shows the IC method with the fourth penalty function (c_4) can determine the dipole number more precisely.

The accuracy of identification in the IC method can be influenced by the different penalty functions. It may be supposed that higher accuracy can be obtained with an unknown penalty function. The different penalty functions can be obtained based on AIC theory, if this process for changing penalty function can be imitated, the better penalty

Table 1

Results for two dipole case (200 samples) using the IC ($c_4 = 2\log(m)$) and FT method

Identified dipole number	1%	2%	3%	4	5	0
FT	1	95	3.5	0	0	2
IC	2	96.5	1	0	1%	

Table 2
Accuracy using the IC method with different penalty functions ($c_{n1} = 1.8\log(m)$ and $c_{n2} = 2.2\log(m)$)

N	One			Two			Three			Four			Five		
Noise	3%	10%	20%	3%	10%	20%	3%	10%	20%	3%	10%	20%	3%	10%	20%
c_3	86	81	78	71	65	59	65.5	47	36.5	62.5	52	47.5	92.5	69	34.5
c_{n1}	100	100	100	96.5	97.5	86.5	89	72.5	43	69	45	35.5	76.5	46	29
c_4	100	100	100	97	96	86	90	67	36.5	69.5	41.5	17	69	38	5.5
c_{n2}	100	100	100	97.5	96.5	83	90.5	67	36	69.5	38	21.5	65.5	30	11
c_5	100	100	100	98.5	91.5	72.5	87.5	49	12.5	59	12.5	0.5	58.5	20	0

function may be obtained. However, it is a complex process for this unknown penalty function from the IC theory. Due to simulation results, higher accuracy is obtained by c_4. It is therefore supposed that this unknown penalty function may be close to c_4. Table 2 shows also the accuracy of two new penalty functions. But the higher accuracy of identification cannot be obtained by them. c_4 is still the optimal penalty function.

4. Conclusions

The simulation results indicate that the IC method is better than the FT method. The different penalty functions in the IC method could make impact on the accuracy of identification. c_4 can obtain the highest accuracy of identification in five penalty functions. In the simulation, we change the penalty function value, but the higher accuracy of identification cannot be obtained by them. c_4 is still the optimal penalty function.

References

[1] Y. Kinouchi, et al., Dipole source localization of MEG by BP neural network, Brain Topogr. 8 (1996) 317–321.
[2] J.C. Mosher, et al., Multiple dipole modeling and localization from spatio-temporal MEG data, IEEE Trans. Biomed. Eng. 39 (1992) 541–557.
[3] X. Bai, et al., "Multi-dipole sources identification from an EEG topography using the system identification method," IEICE Trans. Inf. and Syst., in print.

International Congress Series 1270 (2004) 241–244

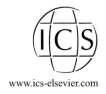

www.ics-elsevier.com

Current sources of the brain potentials before rapid eye movements in human REM sleep

Takashi Abe, Hiroshi Nittono, Tadao Hori*

Department of Behavioral Sciences, Faculty of Integrated Arts and Sciences, Hiroshima University, 1-7-1 Kagamiyama, Higashi-Hiroshima 739-8521, Japan

Abstract. In a previous study, we reported that rapid eye movements (REMs) in REM sleep were not preceded by the presaccadic positivity commonly observed before saccades in wakefulness but by a slow negative potential we called pre-REM negativity. In the present study, we examined current sources of the presaccadic positivity and pre-REM negativity using low resolution brain electromagnetic tomography (LORETA). Fourteen young healthy volunteers participated in the study. Brain potentials were recorded from 26 scalp sites and time-locked to the onsets of saccades and REMs during a visually triggered saccade task and natural nocturnal sleep. Current sources of the presaccadic positivity were estimated to be in the bilateral medial frontal gyrus, whereas those of the pre-REM negativity were estimated to be in the right amygdala, right parahippocampal gyrus, and left orbital gyrus. Different sources of these potentials give further support to the idea that different neural processes are responsible for saccades and REMs. Moreover, the findings that current sources of the pre-REM negativity were estimated to be in the limbic part of the brain suggests that this negativity might be associated with memory and emotional processing in REM sleep. © 2004 Elsevier B.V. All rights reserved.

Keywords: Presaccadic positivity; Pre-REM negativity; Electroencephalography; Event-related potentials; LORETA

1. Introduction

Rapid eye movements (REMs) are one of the prominent features of REM sleep. The similarities and differences between saccades in wakefulness and REMs in REM sleep have been under debate [1]. In wakefulness, scalp-recorded electroencephalogram (EEG) studies have revealed that the presaccadic positivity, which reflects the oculomotor planning process, appears 100–250 ms before the onset of saccades with a centro-parietal scalp distribution [2,3]. In a previous study, we found no presaccadic positivity but a slow negative potential (pre-REM negativity) before REMs in REM sleep [4]. The latter negativity had a prefrontal distribution and was larger in the right hemisphere. These

---

* Corresponding author. Tel.: +81-82-424-6580; fax: +81-82-424-0759.
E-mail address: tdhori@hiroshima-u.ac.jp (T. Hori).

0531-5131/ © 2004 Elsevier B.V. All rights reserved.
doi:10.1016/j.ics.2004.04.092

findings suggest that the generation of REMs does not involve the cortical process reflected in the presaccadic positivity but is associated with a different neural process probably reflected in the pre-REM negativity. In the present study, we examined current sources of the presaccadic positivity and pre-REM negativity using low resolution brain electromagnetic tomography (LORETA) [5].

2. Methods

We reanalyzed the data of our previous study; Abe et al. [4] described the procedure in details. Fourteen young healthy volunteers (7 women and 7 men, mean 22.8 years old) gave informed consent and participated in the study. Brain potentials associated with horizontal saccades and REMs were recorded during a visually triggered saccade task and natural nocturnal sleep after an adaptation night.

EEG was recorded from 26 scalp sites (Fp1, Fp2, F3, F4, C3, C4, P3, P4, O1, O2, F7, F8, T7, T8, P7, P8, F9, F10, P9, P10, Fpz, Fz, Cz, Pz, POz, and Oz according to the extended 10–20 system). Electrooculogram (EOG) and submental electromyogram (EMG) were recorded simultaneously. The sampling rate was 1000 Hz. Time constants were 5.0 s for EEG and EOG and 0.03 s for EMG. High cut filter was set at 300 Hz.

In the sleep session, only the periods scored as stage REM according to Rechtschaffen and Kales criteria [6] with Hori et al. supplements and amendments [7] were analyzed. EEG in the period 200 ms before and 50 ms after the onset of each eye movement were averaged. The first 50 ms of the average period was taken as a baseline.

LORETA was used to estimate current source densities of the presaccadic positivity and pre-REM negativity using the mean amplitude of the period between 150 and 20 ms before eye movements. These values were compared with zero using voxel-wise paired t tests. The resultant t values were projected into LORETA images. Correction for multiple comparisons was performed via randomization using statistical non-parametric mapping (SnPM). Corrected p values are reported.

3. Results

Fig. 1 shows the current sources of the presaccadic positivity and pre-REM negativity estimated by LORETA. In wakefulness, current sources of the presaccadic positivity were estimated in the bilateral medial frontal gyrus (BA 6), ts (13) = 9.3 and 9.3, $p < 0.05$, for the left and right hemispheres, respectively. In REM sleep, current sources of the pre-REM negativity were estimated in the right amygdala, right parahippocampal gyrus (BA 37), and left orbital gyrus (BA 11). The largest t value was found in the right amygdala and right parahippocampal gyrus, ts (13) = 11.9 and 11.9, $p < 0.05$, respectively, and the second largest t value was found in the left orbital gyrus, t (13) = 11.4, $p < 0.05$.

4. Discussion

The presaccadic positivity and pre-REM negativity showed different current sources. This result gives further support to the idea that different neural processes are responsible for saccades in wakefulness and REMs in REM sleep [4,8].

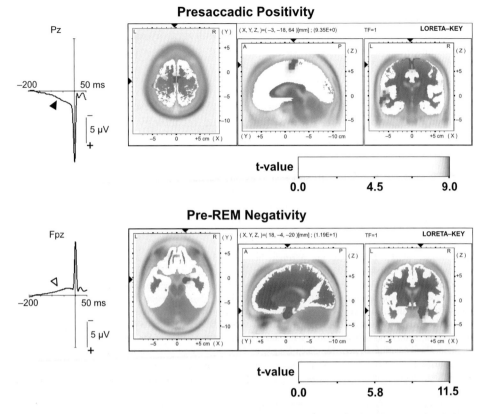

Fig. 1. Current sources of the presaccadic positivity and pre-REM negativity calculated using LORETA. Upper and lower panels show current sources of the presaccadic positivity and pre-REM negativity, respectively. Left panels show grand mean waveforms time-locked to the onsets of saccades and REMs. Recording sites were the parietal midline (Pz) and prefrontal midline (Fpz) sites, respectively, referenced to digitally linked earlobes. Vertical axes indicate the onset of eye movements. Solid and open triangles indicate the presaccadic positivity and pre-REM negativity, respectively.

The presaccadic positivity had its origin in the bilateral medial frontal gyrus. The current sources of the presaccadic positivity calculated in this study were located in somewhat upper regions above the supplementary eye fields (SEF) observed in fMRI studies [9,10]. However, considering the relatively small number of electrodes used in this study (26 sites), the current sources of the presaccadic positivity estimated in the present study might be bilateral SEFs.

In REM sleep, current sources of the pre-REM negativity were identified in the right amygdala, right parahippocampal gyrus, and left orbital gyrus. Functional imaging studies using positron emission tomography have revealed that the activations of the amygdala associated with REM sleep [11] and the right parahippocampal gyrus correlated positively with the number of REMs [12,13]. Magnetoencephalographic study showed activation in the right amygdala, right parahippocampal gyrus, and left orbitofrontal cortex in the last 100 ms before REMs [14]. Our estimation using LORETA is consistent with these findings and suggests that the pre-REM negativity reflects the activity that occurred in the limbic part of the brain and is possibly associated with memory and emotional processing in REM sleep.

Acknowledgements

This study was supported by a Grant-in-Aid for Scientific Research from the Japanese Ministry of Education, Culture, Sports, Science, and Technology (No. 14201011).

References

[1] J.A. Hobson, E.F. Pace-Schott, R. Stickgold, Dreaming and the brain: toward a cognitive neuroscience of conscious states, Behav. Brain Sci. 23 (6) (2000) 793–842.

[2] S. Everling, P. Krappmann, H. Flohr, Cortical potentials preceding pro- and antisaccades in man, Electro-encephalogr. Clin. Neurophysiol. 102 (4) (1997) 356–362.

[3] J.E. Richards, Cortical sources of event-related potentials in the prosaccade and antisaccade task, Psychophysiology 40 (6) (2003) 878–894.

[4] T. Abe, et al., Lack of presaccadic positivity before rapid eye movements in human REM sleep, Neuro-Report 15 (4) (2004) 735–738.

[5] R.D. Pascual-Marqui, C.M. Michel, D. Lehmann, Low resolution electromagnetic tomography: a new method for localizing electrical activity in the brain, Int. J. Psychophysiol. 18 (1) (1994) 49–65.

[6] A. Rechtschaffen, A. Kales, A manual of standardized terminology, techniques and scoring system for sleep stage of human subjects, UCLA, Brain Information Service/Brain Research Institute, Los Angeles, 1968.

[7] T. Hori, et al., Proposed supplements and amendments to 'A Manual of Standardized Terminology, Techniques and Scoring System for Sleep Stages of Human Subjects' the Rechtschaffen and Kales (1968) standard, Psychiatry Clin. Neurosci. 55 (3) (2001) 305–310.

[8] G. Vanni-Mercier, et al., Eye saccade dynamics during paradoxical sleep in the cat, Eur. J. Neurosci. 6 (8) (1994) 1298–1306.

[9] B. Luna, et al., Dorsal cortical regions subserving visually guided saccades in humans: an fMRI study, Cereb. Cortex 8 (1) (1998) 40–47.

[10] M.H. Grosbras, et al., An anatomical landmark for the supplementary eye fields in human revealed with functional magnetic resonance imaging, Cereb. Cortex 9 (7) (1999) 705–711.

[11] P. Maquet, et al., Functional neuroanatomy of human rapid-eye-movement sleep and dreaming, Nature 383 (6596) (1996) 163–166.

[12] A.R. Braun, et al., Dissociated pattern of activity in visual cortices and their projections during human rapid eye movement sleep, Science 279 (5347) (1998) 91–95.

[13] P. Peigneux, et al., Generation of rapid eye movements during paradoxical sleep in humans, NeuroImage 14 (3) (2001) 701–708.

[14] A.A. Ioannides, et al., MEG tomography of human cortex and brainstem activity in waking and REM sleep saccades, Cereb. Cortex 14 (1) (2004) 56–72.

International Congress Series 1270 (2004) 245–248

ELSEVIER

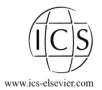

www.ics-elsevier.com

Estimation of cortical activity from noninvasive high-resolution EEG recordings

Donatella Mattia[a], Marco Mattiocco[a], Alessandro Timperi[a],
Serenella Salinari[b], Maria Grazia Marciani[a,c],
Fabio Babiloni[d,*], Cincotti Febo[a]

[a] Fondazione Santa Lucia IRCCS, Rome, Italy
[b] Department of Computer and Systems Science, University of Rome "La Sapienza", Rome, Italy
[c] Department of Neuroscience, University of Rome "Tor Vergata", Rome, Italy
[d] Department of Human Physiology and Pharmacology, University of Rome "La Sapienza", P.le A. Moro 5,
00185 Rome, Italy

Abstract. The aim of this paper is to analyze whether the use of the cortical activity estimated from noninvasive EEG recordings could be useful to detect mental states related to the imagination of limb movements. Estimation of cortical activity was performed on high-resolution EEG data related to the imagination of limb movements gathered in five normal, healthy subjects by using realistic head models. Cortical activity was estimated in region of interest (ROI) associated with the subject's Brodmann areas (BAs) by using depth-weighted minimum norm solutions. Comparisons between surface recorded EEG and the estimated cortical activity were performed. The estimated cortical activity related to the mental imagery of limbs in the five subjects is located mainly over the contralateral primary motor area. The unbalance between brain activity estimated in contralateral and ipsilateral motor cortical areas relative to the finger movement imagination is greater than those obtained in the scalp EEG recordings. Results suggest that the use of the estimated cortical activity for the motor imagery of upper limbs could be potentially superior with respect to the use of surface EEG recordings. This is due to a greater statistically significant unbalance between the activity estimated in the contralateral and ipsilateral hemisphere with respect to those observed with surface EEG. These results are useful in the context of the development of a noninvasive Brain Computer Interface. © 2004 Elsevier B.V. All rights reserved.

Keywords: Brain Computer Interface; High-resolution EEG; Imagination of movements

1. Introduction

Recently, it has been suggested that, with the use of modern high – resolution EEG technologies [1], it could be possible to estimate the cortical activity associated with the mental imagery of upper limb movements in humans [2]. However, a verification of such

* Corresponding author. Tel.: +39-649910317; fax: +39-6499103917.
E-mail address: Fabio.Babiloni@uniroma1.it (F. Babiloni).

statement on a group of normal subjects has not been yet performed. The scientific question at the base of the present work is whether the estimated cortical activity related to the mental imagery of the upper limbs returns more useful features with respect to those obtained by using scalp EEG recordings. To address this issue, we performed high-resolution EEG recordings during the imagination of upper limb movements in a group of five healthy subjects. Comparisons between the waveforms from scalp electrodes and those from the estimated cortical activity in particular regions of interest (ROIs) were then performed. These comparisons returned information about the usefulness of the use of cortical activity for the recognition of mental states with respect to the use of the scalp recorded data.

2. Methods

Five healthy subjects participated voluntarily in experiments, in which they were asked to perform the imagination of right finger movements when they perform the protrusion of their lips. EEG was recorded by using a high – resolution EEG cap with 64 electrodes disposed accordingly to an extension of the 10–20 international system. Subjects were asked to imagine the movement of their right middle finger during the simultaneous protrusion of their lips. This provided the necessary EMG trigger to synchronize the average of the recorded movements. Eighty single EEG trials were recorded for each subject. Each single EEG trial was acquired from 2 s before the arrival of the visual trigger to 1 s after. For all subjects analyzed in this study, sequential MR images were acquired and realistic head models were generated. A cortical surface reconstruction was accomplished for each subject's head with a tessellation of about 10,000 triangles on average. The estimation of cortical activity during the mental imagery task was performed in each subject by using the depth-weighted minimum norm algorithm [3]. Such estimation returns a current density estimate for each of the 5000 dipoles constituting the modeled cortical source space. Each dipole returns a time-varying amplitude representing the brain activity of a restricted patch of cerebral cortex during the entire task time-course. This rather large amount of data can be synthesized by computing the ensemble average of all the dipoles' magnitudes belonging to the same cortical region of interest (ROI). Each ROI was defined on each subject's cortical model adopted in accordance with its Brodmann areas (BAs). In the present study, the activity in the primary left and right motor area, related to the BA4 for the lips as well as hand regions have been taken into account. Artifacts correction by visual and automatic inspection was performed on each single EEG trial recorded. Threshold criteria were used to discard EEG trials contaminated by electrooculogram (EOG) or EMG activity at the resting arms. Visual inspection has been used to discard trials with unusual subthreshold artifacts. On average, about 10% of the acquired EEG trials were discarded in the recorded population. Each artifacts-free single trial was then subjected to the linear inverse procedure, and the time varying cortical distributions associated was estimated. The collapsing procedure explained above was then applied to retrieve the cortical waveforms related to each particular ROI analyzed.

3. Results

Table 1 shows the values of the measured current density in the different BAs examined at the peak of the motor potential for all the subjects employed in this study. Table 1 also

Table 1
The amplitude values at the peak of the motor potentials in all the subjects analyzed

Subject	BA4fingerL	BA4fingerR	BA4lipsL	BA4lipsR	C3	C4
#1	− 8.2	− 5.4	− 0.88	0.01	0.34	0.06
#2	− 8.6	− 7.2	− 0.57	− 0.35	− 0.48	− 0.04
#3	− 12.5	− 10.2	− 1.42	− 0.96	− 0.81	− 0.51
#4	− 5.8	− 6.9	− 0.68	− 0.34	− 0.37	0.38
#5	− 8.3	− 5.4	− 0.23	− 0.02	− 0.19	− 0.13

BA4finger label stands for Brodmann area 4 (BA; primary motor area relative to the fingers area); BA4lips label stands for BA area 4 for the lips movements while C3 and C4 labels refer to the values measured at the electrode position of the international 10–20 system. The L and R letters refer to the left and right hemispheres, respectively. Values for the C3 and C4 measurements are in μV, values for the current density measurements are in arbitrary units.

shows the potential values obtained for the scalp potentials measured at the C3 and C4 leads that are roughly placed on the central scalp areas overlying the primary motor areas. It is worth noting as the potential's amplitudes at MP peak (gathered from C3 and C4 leads) are less unbalanced between left and right scalp areas when compared with the estimated current density activity in the primary motor areas related to the finger movements (BA4Rfinger, BA4Lfinger). Furthermore, the estimated cortical current density values in the primary motor areas related to the lips' movements are rather symmetrical; that is, the values are similar for the left and right ROI considered (BA4Llips and BA4Rlips, respectively). A statistical analysis of this unbalancing for the gathered scalp potentials as well as for the estimated cortical activity was then performed by using the paired Student's t-test. Results obtained indicated: (1) a greater cortical activity estimated over the left primary motor cortical areas for finger movements (BA4Lfinger) with respect to the right one (BA4Rfinger), with a significance equal to $p < 0.0011$; (2) a statistical similar estimated cortical activity for the left (BA4Llips) and right (BA4Rlips) ROIs for the lips movement ($p < 0.36$); and (3) a statistically significant difference between the MP peak for the scalp potentials gathered from the left scalp areas (C3) with respect to the right (C4) one, with a statistical significance of $p < 0.04$.

4. Discussion

The data reported here suggest that it is possible to retrieve the cortical activity related to the mental imagery by using sophisticated high − resolution EEG techniques, obtained by solving the linear inverse problem with the use of realistic head models. Of course, the analysis of the distribution of the potential fields associated with the motor imagery in humans already has been described [4]. However, in the context of the Brain Computer Interface, it assumes importance if the activity related to the imagination of arm movement could be unbalanced between the two hemispheres. In fact, the greater this unbalance between the scalp activity gathered in scalp electrodes C3 and C4 the easier is the task of recognizing it by a classifier [5]. The relevant finding here is that the group analysis of the cortical waveforms associated with the mental imagery suggested the presence of a more pronounced unbalance between the cortical activity estimated in the primary motor areas of the right and left hemispheres with respect to those gathered from scalp electrodes. It is also worthy of note that this unbalancing of the estimated cortical activity between left and right primary motor areas related to the finger movement imagination was not found in the primary motor areas related to the actual performed lips' movements. The rather bilateral cortical activity for the lips' cortices is consistent with the bilateral activations seen in fMRI activations in a previous study [6]. On the other hand, it is worth noting that the cortical estimation methodology illustrated above is suitable for the on-line applications needed for the BCI device. In fact, despite the use of sophisticated realistic head models for scalp, skull, dura mater and cortical surface, the estimation of the instantaneous cortical distribution from the acquired potential measures required a limited amount of time necessary for a matrix multiplication. Such multiplication occurs between the data vector gathered and the pseudoinverse matrix that is stored off-line before the start of the EEG acquisition process. Enclosed in the pseudoinverse matrix is the complexity of the geometrical head modeling with the Boundary Element or with the Finite Element Modeling techniques, as well as the a priori constraints used for the minimum norm solutions.

There is a large trend in the modern neuroscience field to move toward invasive electrode implants for the recording of cortical activity in both animals and humans for the realization of an efficient BCI device [7]. In this paper, we have presented evidence that suggests an alternative methodology for the estimation of such cortical activity in a noninvasive way, by using the possibilities offered by an accurate modeling of the principal head structures involved in the transmission of the cortical potential from the brain surface to the scalp electrodes.

References

[1] A. Gevins, et al., Beyond topographic mapping: towards functional–anatomical imaging with 124-channel EEG and 3-D MRIs, Brain Topogr. 1 (1990) 53–64.
[2] F. Cincotti, et al., Classification of EEG mental patterns by using two scalp electrodes and Mahalanobis distance-based classifiers, Methods Inf. Med. 41 (4) (2002) 337–341.
[3] F. Babiloni, et al., High resolution EEG: source estimates of Laplacian-transformed somatosensory-evoked potentials using a realistic subject head model constructed from magnetic resonance images, Med. Biol. Eng. Comput. 38 (2000) 512–519.
[4] G. Pfurtscheller, C. Neuper, Motor imagery activates primary sensorimotor area in man, Neurosci. Lett. 239 (1997) 65–68.
[5] C. Neuper, A. Schlögl, G. Pfurtscheller, Enhancement of left–right sensorimotor EEG differences during motor imagery, J. Clin. Neurophysiol. 16 (1999) 373–382.
[6] M. Lotze, H. Flor, W. Grodd, Larbig and Birbaumer phantom movements and pain: an fMRI study in upper limb amputees, Brain 124 (2001) 2268–2272.
[7] J.P. Donoghue, Connecting cortex to machines: recent advances in brain interfaces, Nat. Neurosci. 5 (Suppl. 1) (2002) 1085–1088.

International Congress Series 1270 (2004) 249–253

ELSEVIER

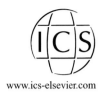

www.ics-elsevier.com

Application of multivariate autoregressive modeling for analyzing the interaction between EEG and EMG in humans

Tomohiro Shibata[a,b,c,*], Yuichi Suhara[a], Tatsuhide Oga[d],
Yoshino Ueki[e], Tatsuya Mima[e], Shin Ishii[a,c]

[a] Graduate School of Information Science, Nara Institute of Science and Technology, Nara 630-0192, Japan
[b] ATR Computational Neuroscience Laboratories, Japan
[c] CREST, Japan Science and Technology Agency, Japan
[d] Department of Neurology, Graduate School of Medicine, Kyoto University, Japan
[e] Human Brain Research Center, Graduate School of Medicine, Kyoto University, Japan

Abstract. Understanding the network of the human motor control system in noninvasive ways is beneficial not only for designing human interfaces, but also to clinical applications. This article presents applications of multivariate autoregression (MVAR) modeling for analyzing the interaction between EEG and EMG, which is challenging because of their different modalities. In contrast to previous research employing the MVAR modeling by means of frequency-domain analysis, our approach emphasizes time-domain analysis. We examined one normal subject and one mirror-movement (MM) patient. The task was a weak isotonic contraction of the right abductor pollicis brevis muscle in the normal subject, and the left extensor carpi radialis brevis in the MM patient. For each subject, three channels consisting of two EEG signals and one EMG signal were analyzed. The EMG signals were from the bilateral primary sensorimotor cortices. By using the Bayesian Information Criterion (BIC), and by choosing the appropriate data length, the model order was determined in a stable fashion. Our results provided plausible information on EEG–EMG networks: (1) Information-transmission-delay time that seems physiologically appropriate, and (2) relative contribution from the ipsi- and contralateral corticospinal pathway, which is opposite in the normal subject in comparison to MM patients. © 2004 Elsevier B.V. All rights reserved.

Keywords: Multivariate autoregression; Time-domain analysis; EEG; EMG; BIC

1. Introduction

To understand the mechanism of the brain and other systems in humans, we need to understand not only localized functions, but also effective connectivities in their networks. It has been reported that multivariate autoregressive (MVAR) modeling holds some

* Corresponding author. Graduate School of Information Science, Nara Institute of Science and Technology, 8916-5 Takayama-cho, Nara 630-0192, Japan. Tel.: +81-743-72-5981; fax: +81-743-72-5989.
E-mail address: tom@is.naist.jp (T. Shibata).

potential for such a purpose [1–3]. We have been investigating applications of the modeling to analyze the interaction between EEG and EMG, since understanding the network of the human motor control system in noninvasive ways is beneficial not only for designing human interfaces, but also to clinical applications. Moreover, it is challenging from the viewpoint of engineering because of their different modalities. Mima et al. [3] detected the information flow from the left primary sensorimotor cortices (C3) to the right abductor pollicis brevis muscle in normal humans by means of frequency-domain analysis with MVAR modeling. In this article, we also employ the MVAR modelling while emphasizing time-domain analysis. We used data from not only normal subjects, but also a mirror-movement (MM) patient [4]. The comparison of these two cases is expected to validate our approach, because it is known that the contralateral cortex controls limbs in normal humans, while it is opposite in MM patients.

2. Methods

We studied one normal subject and one MM patient, both of whom were right-handed. The protocol was approved by the Institutional Review Board and subjects gave written informed consent for the experiment. The task was a weak isotonic contraction of the right abductor pollicis brevis muscle in the normal subject, and the left extensor carpi radialis brevis in the MM patient. Subjects were instructed not to touch their thumb to the other fingers to avoid unnecessary tactile afferent feedback. Their target hand was kept covered. EEG and EMG signals were recorded during the tonic contraction for 2 min. EEG signals were recorded with a linked-ear reference, and surface EMG was recorded using pairs of electrodes and rectified. EEG and EMG signals were amplified in a bandpass of 1–200 Hz and digitized at 1000 Hz in the normal subject, and at 2000 Hz in the MM patient. Preliminary analysis using a Fast Fourier Transform (FFT) algorithm revealed that the EEG signal was significantly coherent with the EMG and was localized over the contralateral primary sensorimotor area: C3 and C4 in both subjects. Therefore, C3 and C4 were used for analysis with the MVAR model throughout this article. The EEG signals were Hjorth-transformed to increase the spatial resolution [5]. More detailed information on the data acquisition method is described elsewhere [3].

To determine the order of the MVAR model, we employed the Bayesian Information Criterion (BIC) [6] instead of the Akaike Information Criterion (AIC) [7], since we found that AIC did not work as described in the next section. The BIC is an efficient asymptotic approximation to a Bayesian model selection criterion, taking parameters of uncertainty into account. For the time-domain analysis, we employed a method for analyzing feedback systems [1], and investigated impulse responses of identified systems. The determination of the model order was significantly affected by data length, presumably due to the trade-off between asymptoticity in estimation and stationarity in data. To cope with this trade-off, we sought an appropriate block length which enabled a model order to be determined consistently over all blocks segmented from the data.

3. Results

Fig. 1 presents typical AIC (left) and BIC (right) values as a function of the model order determined with the same data. As shown in this figure, the AIC was unable to find the

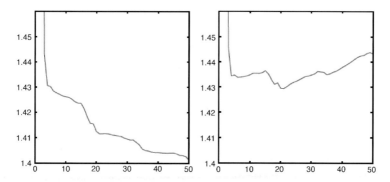

Fig. 1. Typical samples of AIC (left) and BIC (right) as functions of the model order.

minimum value within the order range that we sought, whereas the BIC robustly found it. Therefore, the BIC was employed to acquire the following results.

Table 1 shows the means and the standard deviations of the determined model order, in which the block length was varied. In the case of the normal subject, the model order was consistently determined over blocks when the block lengths were 2 and 5 s. Regarding the data for the MM subject, the model order was consistently determined over blocks when the block lengths were 40 and 50 s.

Fig. 2 illustrates that, for both subjects, the peak of the impulse response from the left EEG was significantly higher than that from the right EEG (Mann–Whitney U-test; $p < 0.01$). The impulse responses consisted of a leading noisy part followed by a certain response which was seemingly generated by a lower order linear system. The leading noisy part revealed white (Ljung–Box; $p < 0.01$), and its time length was almost the same with its corresponding model order. The model order, such as 20.3 (15.5) in the normal (MM) subject, consistently determined over blocks, can be interpreted as the information-transmission-delay time from the brain to the target muscle, since it is physiologically plausible. Thus, we chose a block length of 2 s for the normal subject, and of 40 s for the MM patient.

Fig. 3 shows the mean coherence spectra between the EEGs and the EMG of both the normal (A) and the MM patient (B). Thin lines were computed by the FFT method and thick lines by the 3-channel MVAR model; each thin line and the corresponding thick line

Table 1
Mean and standard deviation (S.D.) of the determined model order (in ms)

Normal		MM	
Block length [s]	Model order [ms]	Block length [s]	Model order [ms]
1	18.7 ± 4.44	10	5.27 ± 1.50
2	20.3 ± 0.468	20	8.09 ± 0.465
3	30.0 ± 7.60	30	14.6 ± 1.99
4	34.9 ± 4.00	40	15.5 ± 0.00
5	36.0 ± 0.175	50	15.5 ± 0.00

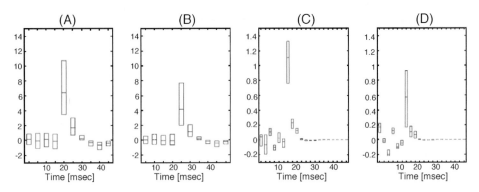

Fig. 2. The lower quartile, median and upper quartile values of the impulse responses; from the left EEG (A) and the right EEG (B) to the right EMG in the normal subject; from the left EEG (C) and the right EEG (D) to the left EMG in the MM patient.

were very similar. In the case of the normal subject, the left EEG had larger coherence than the right EEG, while this phenomenon was reversed in the MM patient.

4. Discussion

By emphasizing the time-domain analysis, we have demonstrated that the MVAR modeling approach provided plausible information about EEG–EMG networks: (1) Information-transmission-delay time, and (2) relative contribution from the ipsi- and contralateral corticospinal pathways. It is noteworthy that the known ipsilateral cortico-spinal contribution in the MM patient could not be detected by the coherence spectra (Fig. 3C,D), but could be found using the impulse responses (Fig. 2C,D).

The fact that the AIC did not work very well for our data indicates that the EEG–EMG network in our data cannot be completely modeled by the true MVAR process. Nevertheless, the following results support our approach: (1) the model order consistently determined by BIC over blocks with a specific block length seems physiologically appropriate, and (2) coherence spectra computed by the 3-channel MVAR model were

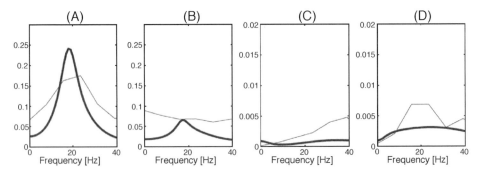

Fig. 3. Mean coherence spectra computed by the FFT method (thin line) and by the 3-channel MVAR model (thick line) between the EEGs and the EMG; from the left EEG (A) and the right EEG (B) to the right EMG in the normal subject; from the left EEG (C) and the right EEG (D) to the left EMG in the MM patient.

very similar to the one by the FFT method. The 10-fold difference in the appropriate block lengths for the normal and the MM subjects (Table 1) seems to be improved in the data acquisition step, since very low coherence spectra were observed between the EEGs and the EMG in the MM patient (Fig. 3C,D).

References

[1] H. Akaike, On the use of a linear model for the identification of feedback systems, Ann. Inst. Stat. Math. 20 (1968) 425–439.
[2] M.J. Kaminski, K.J. Blinowska, A new method of the description of the information flow in the structures, Biol. Cybern. 65 (1991) 203–210.
[3] T. Mima, T. Matsuoka, M. Hallet, Information flow from the sensorimotor cortex to muscle in humans, Clin. Neurophysiol. 112 (2001) 122–126.
[4] S.F. Farmer, et al., Abnormal cortex–muscle interactions in subjects with X-linked Kallman's syndrome and mirror movement, Brain 127 (2004) 385–397.
[5] B. Hjorth, Source derivation simplifies topographical EEG interpretation, Am. J. E.E.G. Technol. 20 (1980) 121–132.
[6] G. Schwartz, Estimating the dimension of a model, Ann. Stat. 8 (1978) 147–164.
[7] H. Akaike, A new look at the statistical model identification, IEEE Transaction on Automatic Control AC 19 (6) (1974) 716–723.

International Congress Series 1270 (2004) 254–257

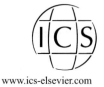

www.ics-elsevier.com

Longitudinal change of ERP during cued continuous performance test in child with attention-deficit/hyperactivity disorder

Shinji Okazaki[a,*], Hisaki Ozaki[b], Hisao Maekawa[a],
Satoshi Futakami[c]

[a] *Institute of Disability Sciences, University of Tsukuba, 1-1-1 Tennodai, Tsukuba, Ibaraki 305-8572, Japan*
[b] *Laboratory of Physiology, Ibaraki University, Ibaraki, Japan*
[c] *Department of Child Rehabilitation, Nippon Telegraph and Telephone East Corporation, Izu Medical Center, Kannami, 919-0107, Japan*

Abstract. In this study, we focused our interests on longitudinal development of motor control in attention-deficit/hyperactivity disorder (ADHD). Performance and EEG recordings during continuous performance test (CPT-AX) were obtained from a male child suffering from ADHD when he was 9.6 years old with and without psychostimulant (methylphenidate). Follow-up examinations were done when he was 10.6 and 11.6 years old. Hit rate of CPT-AX under non-medicated condition remained low, while hit rate under medication improved significantly. However, hit rate under non-medicated condition in third recording reached the behavioral level as that of the control. Longitudinal improvement in CPT-AX was also observed in ERP data. That is, P2/N2 and P3 in the first recording maintained a lower intensity with short duration. However, intensity levels in the third recording improved in comparison with control data, and the longitudinal change of ERP corresponded with intra-individual change of behavioral performance. Therefore, longitudinal examination of ERP might complement and extend the findings obtained from cross-sectional data, but also reveal a developmental course of an individual with ADHD. © 2004 Elsevier B.V. All rights reserved.

Keywords: Attention-deficit/hyperactivity disorder; Motor control; Development; Psychostimulant

1. Introduction

Many studies have reported that children with attention-deficit/hyperactivity disorder (ADHD) exhibit deficit in response to control of motor action [6]. To disclose their behavioural nature, cued continuous performance test (CPT-AX) has been used in many studies [2,3,4,6]. Recent electrophysiological approaches on ADHD have revealed their insufficient cerebral motor regulation during CPT-AX [1,5,7,8]. Although poor response with extended reaction time in CPT-AX has been reported in ADHD, cross-sectional data

* Corresponding author. Tel./fax: +81-29-853-6804
E-mail address: sokazaki@human.tsukuba.ac.jp (S. Okazaki).

0531-5131/ © 2004 Elsevier B.V. All rights reserved.
doi:10.1016/j.ics.2004.04.032

revealed the developmental change along the course of maturation with wide variation among individuals with ADHD. Therefore, we considered that follow-up study in the same individual would not only complement and extend the findings obtained from cross-sectional data, but also reveal a developmental course of an individual with ADHD.

In this study, ERP during CPT-AX were obtained longitudinally from a single case of ADHD with and without psychostimulant dosage, and developmental change of the cerebral motor control was investigated.

2. Method

2.1. Subject

One male child participated in this study. He was diagnosed as ADHD combined type in DSM-IV. He was 9.6 years old at the time of the first examination. Behavioral and electrophysiological data were obtained under medication-free conditions (non-medicated; at least 24 h prior to testing) and of 10 mg/kg methylphenidate dosage (medicated). Follow-up recordings were also carried at when he was 10.6 and 11.6 years old. Informed consent was obtained from the subject and his parent.

2.2. CPT task

A series of single digits were presented on CRT by STIM software (NeuroScan). Subject was asked to press a button when "9" was presented immediately after "1" (warning stimulus). To maintain uncertainty in the stimulus series, we implemented three different inter-stimulus intervals (ISIs) between the warning stimulus and the subsequent target (short ISI; 800 ms, medium ISI; 1500 ms, long ISI; 3000 ms). The probabilities of the target ("9" after "1") and the nontarget (a single digit except "9" after "1") was 5% in each ISI condition. Therefore, the probability of cues ("1") was 10%. A series of 400 digits were presented per block and two blocks were done. Percentage of correct response to the target (hit rate) and reaction time (RT) under medium ISI were examined. The data obtained were compared with that of normal control subjects ($N=46$, 26 boys and 20 girls; age range: 8.6–12.10 years).

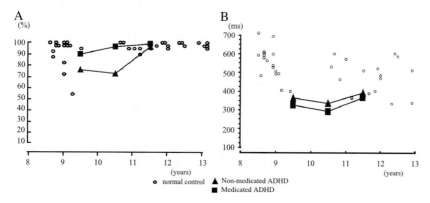

Fig. 1. Hit rate (A) and hit RT (B) in a child with ADHD (non-medicated and medicated) and in normal control.

2.3. EEG recording and ERP

EEGs were recorded from 17 locations on the scalp (10–20 system without Fp1 and Fp2) against the linked earlobes as a common reference. EEG was digitized at a sampling rate of 500 Hz. After 0.05–30 Hz band-pass filtering, artifact-free EEGs were averaged for target after warnings in medium ISI condition. Trials with response failure and with false alarms were also excluded. ERP data at 9.6 years were compared with data from a 9-year-old group (male = 4, female = 4, mean age 9.0 years, age range: 8.7–9.5) and ERP data at 11.6 years, with data from an 11-year-old group (male = 7, female = 2, mean age 11.3 years, age range: 10.10–11.10), respectively.

3. Results

3.1. Longitudinal change of performance in CPT-AX

In normal control, hit rate at medium ISI increased with age (Fig. 1A). Hit rate in non-medicated ADHD subject remained lower than that in age-matched normal control under first and second examination. However, in the third examination, hit rate of ADHD under non-medicated condition improved compared with that of normal control. Due to medication, performance in CPT-AX under first and second examinations improved as well as the level of normal controls.

Hit RT in normal control tended to shorten with age (Fig. 1B). A child with ADHD tended to perform with shorter hit RT compared with those in age-matched normal control. And developmental change of hit RT was not observed under the conditions with and without medication.

3.2. Longitudinal change of ERP in CPT-AX

Two distinct ERP components were observed during the time period 200–500 ms regardless of CA or condition, i.e. posterior-positivity/anterior-negativity around 300 ms (P2/N2), and vertex positivity around 450 ms (P3). We focused our interest on the spatio-temporal feature of those two components in this study.

ERP map series were characterized by posterior positivity (Fig. 2). In the first examination (CA 9.6), amplitudes of P2/N2 and P3 under non-medicated condition were smaller with shorter duration than those in normal controls. Due to the medication,

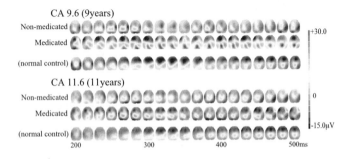

Fig. 2. ERP map series from 200 to 500 ms (per 16 ms) to targets after warning in first and third examinations.

amplitude of P2/N2 increased and its duration lengthened. Medication effects were also observed both in terms of amplitude and duration of P3. In the third examination at 11.6 years, spatio-temporal characteristics of ERP under non-medication became similar to those under Medication, except the amplitude of P2/N2.

4. Discussion

Many prior studies have reported poor performance in children with ADHD in the inhibitory control task [2,4,6]. Neurophysiological characteristics of children with ADHD were also revealed by decreased amplitudes of N200 (comparable with P2/N2 in this study) and of P300 response [1,5,7,8]. These findings were derived from cross-sectional data across different age groups. As each child with ADHD has a unique developmental process, a longitudinal study as to how an individual ADHD acquires his/her ability to control motor action will supplement and extend the findings of the developmental course of motor control. In this study, we examined the performance and neurophysiological follow-up data of CPT-AX. It turned out that the subject with ADHD at the age of 11 improved his cerebral control as well as his performance comparable with the level of normal control. And not only performance, but also neurophysiological data revealed how medication of psychostimulant drug affected the child with ADHD.

Because of the diversity of individual developmental course, both cross-sectional and longitudinal follow-up data will be needed to disclose the developmental feature of response control in children with ADHD. And the findings obtained through this strategy might offer important information to evaluate intervention and therapy provided to children with ADHD.

References

[1] A.J. Fallgatter, et al., Altered response control and anterior cingulated function in attention-deficit/hyperactivity disorder boys, Clin. Neurophysiol. 115 (2004) 973–981.
[2] B.J. Losier, P.J. McGrath, R.M. Klein, Error patterns on the continuous performance test in non-medicated and medicated samples of children with and without ADHD: a meta-analytic review, J. Chil. Psychol. Psychiatry 37 (1996) 971–987.
[3] S. Okazaki, et al., Developmental change of neurocognitive motor behavior in a continuous performance test with different interstimulus intervals, Clin. Neurophysiol. 115 (2004) 1104–1113.
[4] S. Okazaki, H. Maekawa, S. Futakami, Control of response inhibition in children with ADHD on the CPT under various intervals, Jpn. J. Spec. Educ. 38 (2001) 97–103.
[5] S. Okazaki, et al., Topographic changes of ERP during a CPT-AX task at pre- and post-medication of methylphenidate in children with ADHD, in: H. Hirata, Y. Koga, K. Nagata, H. Yamazaki (Eds.), Recent advances in human brain mapping, International Congress Series, vol. 1232, Elsevier, Amsterdam, 2002, pp. 705–710.
[6] B.F. Pennington, S. Ozonoff, Executive functions and developmental psychopathology, J. Chil. Psychol. Psychiatry 37 (1996) 51–87.
[7] T.H. van Leeuwen, et al., The continuous performance test revisited with neuroelectric mapping: impaired orienting in children with attention deficits, Behav. Brain Res. 94 (1998) 97–110.
[8] M.N. Verbaten, et al., Methylphenidate influences on both early and late ERP waves of ADHD children in a continuous performance test, J. Abnorm. Child Psychol. 22 (1994) 561–578.

ELSEVIER

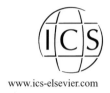

www.ics-elsevier.com

The role of memory consolidation in motor learning: a positron emission tomography study

D. Wright[a,b], G. Box[a], K. Nagata[a,*], I. Kanno[b], D. Rottenberg[c]

[a] Department of Neurology, Research Institute for Brain and Blood Vessels, 6-10 Senshu Kubota Machi, Akita 010-0874, Japan
[b] Department of Radiology, Research Institute for Brain and Blood Vessels, Japan
[c] Department of Neurology, School of Medicine, University of Minnesota, USA

Abstract. While it has been well documented that the process of motor learning is accompanied by a shift in cortical processing regions, there has been little investigation into the effects of memory consolidation. The present study builds on earlier work and aims to investigate changes in the functional anatomy of motor learning that occur when the process of motor memory consolidation is disrupted. Ten healthy, right-handed males took part in the new experimental protocol. A star shape was presented to the subject on a computer monitor positioned above the PET gantry. During each trial, the subject used a 'Felix' computer-pointing device to guide a small red dot around the star shape in an anticlockwise direction. Subjects were instructed to perform the trace as quickly and accurately as possible using their left hand. After the 10th trial, the Felix was reconfigured so that hand movements were 'mirrored' on the computer screen. In the original study, subjects performed the mirror task 15 times while in the second study a distracter task was inserted between each mirror trial in order to disrupt memory consolidation. PET images were recorded during the seventh trial and then every other trial, culminating in 10 images. The resulting images were analysed using the Minoshima analysis package and the two groups were compared to determine the effects of disrupting memory consolidation. The results showed that there was less transfer from frontal and parietal areas to the occipital and primary motor cortices in the second study. This suggests that interference with motor memory consolidation disrupts the shifts in cortical activation normally seen in motor learning. © 2004 Elsevier B.V. All rights reserved.

Keywords: Motor learning; Memory consolidation; PET

1. Introduction

While it has been well documented that the process of motor learning is accompanied by a shift in cortical processing regions, there has been little investigation into the effects

* Corresponding author. Tel.: +81-18-833-0115; fax: +81-18-836-0635.
E-mail address: nagata@akita-noken.go.jp (K. Nagata).

of memory consolidation. The present study builds on earlier work and aims to investigate changes in the functional anatomy of motor learning that occur when the process of motor memory consolidation is disrupted.

2. Methods

An original study into the functional anatomy of motor learning (study 1) was extended to investigate the effects of disrupting memory consolidation. Study 1 consisted of 30 subjects and to date, 10 subjects have taken part in the second study. All subjects were university educated, healthy, right-handed males.

A star shape was presented to the subject on a computer monitor positioned above the PET gantry. During each trial, the subject used a 'Felix' computer-pointing device to guide a small red dot around the star shape in an anticlockwise direction. Subjects were instructed to perform the trace as quickly and accurately as possible using their left hand. After the 10th trial, the Felix was reconfigured so that hand movements were 'mirrored' on the computer screen. In the original study (study 1) subjects performed the mirror task fifteen times while in the new study (study 2) a distracter task, in the form of a regular trial, was inserted between mirror trials. As such, study 2 subjects only performed the mirror trial eight times.

In both studies 1 and 2, CBF measurements were conducted in the seventh regular trial and then every other trial, culminating in 10 images. In study 1, this meant that each odd mirror trial was scanned. In study 2, as there was a distracter task in the form of a regular trial between each mirror trial, all mirror trials were scanned.

3. Results

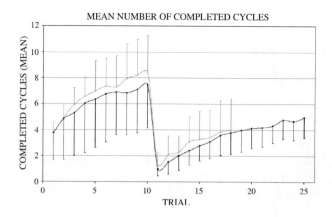

Fig. 1. Mean number of cycles per trial for both studies 1 (black) and 2 (grey). NB: Distracter trials removed from study 2.

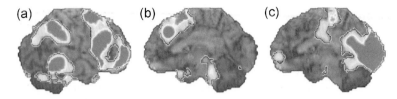

Fig. 2. (a) Right lateral view for naïve tracing performance. Activation is visible in the posterior parietal, temporal, prefrontal and premotor cortices. (b) Right medial view for naïve tracing performance. Significant activation in supplementary and presupplementary motor cortices. (c) Right medial view for practiced tracing performance. Shift in activation to occipital and primary motor cortical areas.

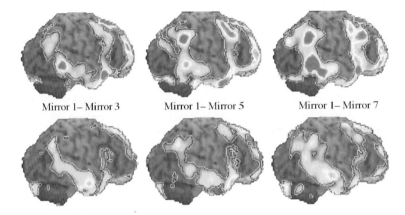

Fig. 3. Right lateral images for both studies 1 (top) and 2 (bottom).

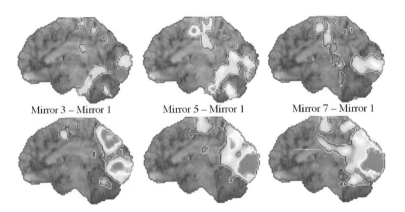

Fig. 4. Right medial images for both studies 1 (top) and 2 (bottom).

4. Discussion

Fig. 1 shows the mean number of completed cycles for both the normal and distracter groups. Although each subject was instructed to trace as quickly and accurately as possible, individuals will tend to place more emphasis on either speed or accuracy. Hence, intersubject comparisons show large variations in recorded behavioral data.

For both studies 1 and 2, a general logarithmic increase is observed throughout the regular trials as subject motor skills improve with practice. As expected, the number of cycles decreased significantly after implementation of the mirror parameters. Movements became hesitant as subjects spent more time correcting erroneous movements and planning subsequent actions. As the mirror trials progressed and subjects became accustomed to the reconfigured Felix device, tracing performance improved and the mean number of cycles increased.

While the performance of the second group who had to contend with the distracter task appears to be better, there was no significant difference between the two groups. This was surprising as we expected the subjects from study 2 to perform worse, given that they had to perform a regular trial between mirror trials.

Fig. 2a and b shows activation associated with the performance of a naïve task. Significant activation was visible in both the left and right posterior parietal cortices, extending bilaterally to the temporal cortices, suggesting visuo-spatial cognition. Right side dominant activation was observed in the prefrontal association cortex, as subjects utilised working memory to plan Felix movements, and the premotor cortex, suggested to be involved in the initiation of movement in contralateral limbs. Right side dominant activation was also visible in the supplementary motor area, associated with motor planning and the presupplementary motor area, thought to be involved in motor learning.

As the task becomes more practiced, activation shifts away from the aforementioned areas to the occipital and primary motor cortices suggesting more fundamental motor control (Fig. 2c).

Figs. 3 and 4 show the changes in activation with motor learning for both the original study and study 2 (distraction task). As subjects become more familiar with the mirror paradigm, there is a reduction in the use of prefrontal, premotor, posterior parietal and temporal cortical areas. However, after insertion of the distraction task, this reduction is not as significant, suggesting that subjects are still placing large demands on frontal, parietal and temporal areas to perform at the same level as subjects in the first study in later mirror trials. This was emphasized in Fig. 4, which shows less shift to occipital and primary motor cortical regions for the second study.

5. Conclusion

Implementation of the distracter task resulted in less reduction in frontal and parietal cortical activity and less transfer to the occipital and primary motor cortices in later mirror trials. This suggests that interference with motor memory consolidation disrupts the transfer of motor processing regions.

International Congress Series 1270 (2004) 262–265

ELSEVIER

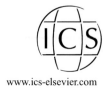

www.ics-elsevier.com

Event-related potential P2 derived from visual attention to the hemi-space. Source localization with LORETA

Takashi Maeno[a,b,*], Klevest Gjini[a], Keiji Iramina[a], Fumio Eto[b], Shoogo Ueno[a]

[a]*Department of Biomedical Engineering, Graduate School of Medicine, University of Tokyo, Bunkyo, Tokyo, Japan*
[b]*Department of Rehabilitation, University of Tokyo Hospital, Tokyo, Japan*

Abstract. This study aimed to measure event-related potential P2 using electroencephalography (EEG), and to locate equivalent current sources related to visual attention in the hemi-space. The amplitude of P2 increases when subjects perceive the stimuli or pay attention to the stimuli. Six volunteer subjects were directed to look at a train of visual oddball stimuli. The oddball stimuli consisted of a square on one side and a circle on the other side of the visual field. Subjects were requested to push a button at the visual cue 800 ms after the target stimuli were displayed. EEG activities were recorded at 64 points over the head. Low-resolution brain electromagnetic tomography (LORETA) was used for the source estimation. Event-related potential P2 was observed at around 200 ms after the onset of the target stimuli. The activity of the parietal and frontal region at P2 changed according to the attention to the hemi-visual field. The activity of the P2 may be located on the parietal lobe, and the frontal lobe (the frontal eye field) may be also activated according to the attention. © 2004 Elsevier B.V. All rights reserved.

Keywords: Electroencephalography; Attention; Vision

1. Introduction

The event-related potential P2 is the peak waveform evoked about 200 ms after the presentation of visual stimuli. The amplitude of P2 changes as the subject pays attention to the visual stimuli [1]. However, the region of the source of P2 has not been determined yet.

This study aimed to measure event-related potential P2 using electroencephalography (EEG), and to locate the equivalent current sources related to visual attention in the hemi-

---

* Corresponding author. Department of Biomedical Engineering, Graduate School of Medicine, University of Tokyo, 7-3-1 Hongo, Bunkyo Tokyo, Japan. Tel.: +81-3-5841-3389; fax: +81-3-5689-7215.

E-mail address: tmaeno-tky@umin.ac.jp (T. Maeno).

0531-5131/ © 2004 Elsevier B.V. All rights reserved.
doi:10.1016/j.ics.2004.04.034

space. Multiple equivalent current dipoles were estimated from the P2 waveforms obtained from visual oddball paradigm tasks.

2. Method

Six right-handed volunteers (three males and three females, 24–32 years old) were studied. Subjects were requested to look at a train of visual stimuli containing 20% of target stimuli (Fig. 1). The target stimuli consisted of a square on one side and a circle on the other side of the visual field. The control stimuli consisted of two circles on both sides of the visual field. Subjects were directed to push a button with their left index finger at the visual cue 800 ms after the target stimuli were displayed.

EEG activities were recorded at 64 points over the head (Nihon Koden system). The low-resolution electromagnetic brain tomography (LORETA) [2] was used for the source estimation. We applied a voxel-wise comparison to the LORETA results using the paired t-test of the nonparametric permutation test [3].

3. Result

The event-related potential P2 was observed at around 200 ms after the onset of the target stimuli (Fig. 2). Estimated sources of P2 were located on the wide range of the cortex (frontal lobe, parietal lobe, temporal lobe, occipital lobe).

The LORETA values changed on both sides of the occipital lobe and left parietal lobe at 200 ms when the subjects paid attention to the left hemi-space; however, the difference was not significant ($p = 0.1266$) (Fig. 3). The LORETA values changed on the left frontal lobe at 210 ms when the subjects paid attention to the right hemi-space ($p = 0.0530$) (Fig. 4).

4. Discussion

One of the hypotheses about the attention paid by the volunteers is that the right hemisphere is activated by attention to both visual hemi-spaces and the left hemisphere is activated by the attention to the right visual hemi-space. When the

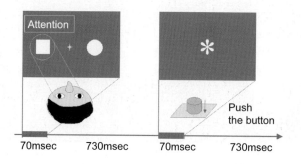

Fig. 1. Visual stimulation.

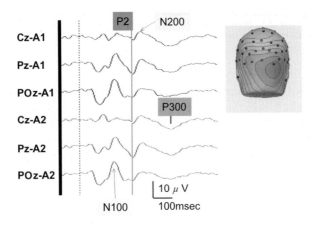

Fig. 2. The waveform and the topography of P2.

subject pays attention to the left hemi-space, the right parietal lobe is activated and the activation of the left parietal lobe relatively decreases. When the subject pays attention to the right hemi-space, both parietal lobes are activated at the same strength.

5. Conclusion

When the subjects paid attention to the left hemi-space, the activation of the left parietal lobe relatively decreased at 200 ms. When the subjects paid attention

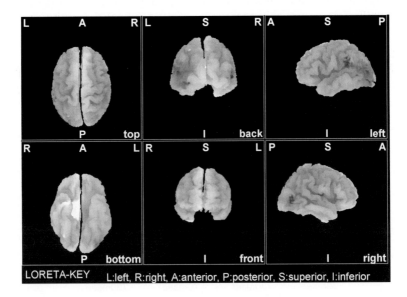

Fig. 3. The region where the LORETA values changed at 200 ms when subjects paid attention to the left hemi-space.

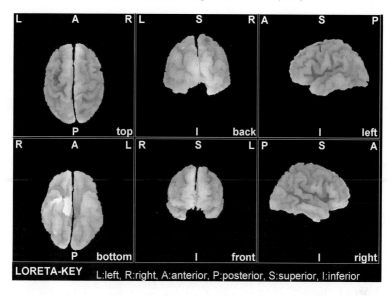

Fig. 4. The region where the LORETA values changed at 210 ms when subjects paid attention to the right hemi-space.

to the right hemi-space, the activation of the left frontal lobe relatively decreased at 210 ms.

References

[1] S. Johannes, et al., Luminance and spatial attention effects on early visual processing, Cognitive Brain Research 2 (1995) 189–205.
[2] R.D. Pascual-Marqui, et al., Low resolution electromagnetic tomography: a new method for localizing electrical activity in the brain, International Journal of Psychophysiology 18 (1994) 49–65.
[3] T. Nichols, Nonparametric permutation tests for functional neuroimaging: a primer with examples, Human Brain Mapping 15 (2001) 1–25.

International Congress Series 1270 (2004) 266–269

ELSEVIER

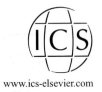

www.ics-elsevier.com

Event-related potentials in a memory scan task concerned with movement directions

Yoshimitsu Okita[a,*], Tetsuo Kobayashi[b], Noboru Ohki[c], Isao Takahashi[a], Teruhisa Kazui[d], Motohiko Kimura[e], Toshifumi Sugiura[f]

[a] Graduate School of Electronic Science and Technology, Shizuoka University, Japan
[b] Graduate School of Engineering, Kyoto University, Japan
[c] NoruPro Light Systems, Japan
[d] First Department of Surgery, Hamamatsu University School of Medicine, Japan
[e] Faculty of Engineering, Shizuoka University, Japan
[f] Research Institute of Electronics, Shizuoka University, Japan

Abstract. To study brain mechanisms of memory scan, we have measured event-related potentials (ERPs) during the execution of a Sternberg task concerned with movement directions of random dot patterns (RDPs). Five healthy male subjects participated in the experiment. Event-related potentials were recorded at 20 electrode positions over the entire head. A prominent positive ERP component peaking at 380–390 ms known as P300 was observed in the parietal region after the presentation of the probe moving random dot pattern, whereas the P300 was not observed after the presentation of a control stationary RDP. On the other hand, a positive ERP component peaking at 127 ms was commonly observed in the occipital region after the presentation of both moving and control stationary RDPs. These findings suggest that P300 may reflect cortical activities related to the memory scan of movement directions of RDP. © 2004 Elsevier B.V. All rights reserved.

Keywords: P300; Sternberg task; Working memory

1. Introduction

Although controversies still remain about the concept of memory, the process of maintenance and manipulation of information is called working memory (WM) [1]. Humans often use WM unconsciously in all scenes of everyday life. The Sternberg task [2] is known as a representative, psychological, experimental procedure to study WM which uses numbers, characters and pictures presented sequentially.

In the present study, we measured event-related potentials (ERPs) in a Sternberg task using random dot patterns (RDPs) to investigate brain activities associated with memory

---

* Corresponding author. 3-5-1, Johoku, Hamamatsu 432-8011, Japan. Tel.: +81-53-478-1353; fax: +81-53-478-1353.
E-mail address: dyokita@ipc.shizuoka.ac.jp (Y. Okita).

0531-5131/ © 2004 Elsevier B.V. All rights reserved.
doi:10.1016/j.ics.2004.05.171

scan or WM. The task was designed to require subjects to memorize directions of coherently moving RDP.

2. Material and methods

2.1. Subjects

Five healthy males (age 22–24 years) with normal or corrected to normal visual acuity participated in the experiment. All subjects except one were right-handed.

2.2. Experimental procedures

The subjects had performed a Sternberg task (Task 1) and its control task (Task 2). The time chart of stimulus presentation in the two tasks was shown in Fig. 1.

In Task 1, the coherently moving RDP was used both as target and probe. On the other hand, stationary RDP was used in Task 2. Memory set size, which is the number of target, in Task 1 was 1 and 3. Probe RDP was presented 2.0 s after the last Target RDP presentation of 0.2 s. The movement direction of the RDP was chosen from one of four vertical and horizontal directions, i.e., up, down, left and right. Subjects were instructed to press one of two buttons to distinguish whether the direction of probe was congruent with one of the targets or not. The subjects were also instructed to gaze at a " + " mark, displayed in the center of a computer screen, throughout the experiment. The size of RDP was $2.0° \times 2.0°$. The probability of the probe in RDP having the same directions as one of targets in RDP was set to about 50%.

2.3. ERP measurements and analyses

ERPs were measured at 20 electrode positions on the scalp referenced to linked ears. In order to avoid the influence of movement-related cortical potentials on the ERPs, button

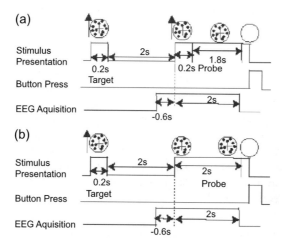

Fig. 1. The time chart of stimulus presentation in a Sternberg task (Task 1, a) and its control task (Task 2, b).

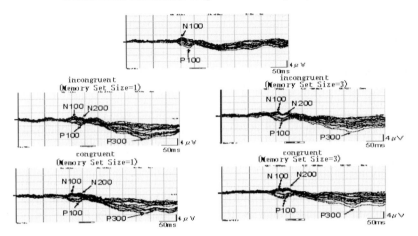

Fig. 2. Grand mean ERPs (average over five subjects) in a control task (Task 1, top) and a Sternberg task (Task 2, middle and bottom) with different memory set size of 1 and 3. The thick vertical line indicates the time of probe appearance.

press was conducted after the presentation of a white circle (Fig. 1). An epoch, which included 500 ms prestimulus and 2000 ms poststimulus period, was digitized by 1 kHz with a 0.16–100-Hz bandwidth. A total of 100 epochs, in which trials contaminated by eye blinking or eye movements (threshold potential: 50–150 μV) were excluded, were averaged to obtain ERPs. The 500 ms prestimulus period served as the baseline.

3. Results and discussion

RT for the memory set size 3 was longer than that for the memory set size 1, suggesting that RT depends on the numbers of memory set size. The percentage of correct answers was more than 92% for all subjects in all measurement.

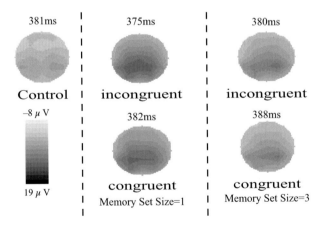

Fig. 3. Topographical maps of the potentials in the case of Task 1 and Task 2 at peak latencies of P300.

The grand mean ERPs in Tasks 1 and 2 are shown in Fig. 2.

The ERPs in all scalp potential have been superimposed in each figure. A positive component (P100) was observed peaking at 127 ms in both tasks in the occipital area (O1, O2). This component is considered to be evoked by the appearance of RDP and generated from primary or secondary visual areas. In the experiment of Task 1, a negative component (N200) was observed following P100. Taking the previous results on motion perceptions [3–5] into account, N200 may reflect cortical activities at human MT or V5. A positive ERP component (P300) can be seen at latencies of 350–390 ms in the ERPs in Task 1. However, P300 was not observed in Task 2. Fig. 3 showed topographical maps of the P300 in the cases of incongruent and congruent of probe with target at memory size of 1 and 3. P300 was mainly observed in the parietal area. As seen in this figure, we could not observe P300 component in the control task (Task 2).

These findings suggest that P300 may reflect cortical activities related to the memory scan of movement directions of RDP.

References

[1] A. Baddeley, Working memory, Science 255 (5044) (1992) 556–559.
[2] S. Sternberg, High-speed scanning in human memory, Science 153 (736) (1966) 652–654.
[3] M. Bundo, Y. Kaneoke, S. Inao, J. Yoshida, A. Nakamura, R. Kakigi, Human visual motion areas determined individually by magnetoencephalography and 3D magnetic resonance imaging, Hum. Brain Mapp. 11 (1) (2000) 33–45.
[4] O. Kawakami, Y. Kaneoke, K. Maruyama, R. Kakigi, T. Okada, N. Sadato, Y. Yonekura, Visual detection of motion speed in humans: spatiotemporal analysis by f-MRI and MEG, Hum. Brain Mapp. 16 (2) (2002) 104–118.
[5] M. Bach, D. Ullrich, Motion adaptation governs the shape of motion-evoked cortical potentials, Vis. Res. 34 (1994) 1541–1547.

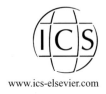
ELSEVIER

Influence of the levodopa on frontal lobe dysfunction in patients with de novo Parkinson's disease

Yuka Kobayashi, Koichi Hirata*, Akinori Hozumi, Hideaki Tanaka, Mio Arai, Yoshiaki Kaji, Taro Kadowaki, Yasuhisa Daimon

Department of Neurology, Dokkyo University School of Medicine, Kitakobayashi 880, Mibu, Tochigi 321-0293, Japan

Abstract

We investigated the efficacy of the levodopa (L-dopa) on cognitive function in patients with de novo Parkinson's disease (PD) using the event-related potential (ERP) measure and neuropsychological test batteries. We studied 20 PD patients who had never received anti-Parkinson medications. The ERP with auditory oddball P3 paradigm and neuropsychological tests such as Mini-Mental State Examination (MMSE), New Modified Wisconsin Card Sorting Test (WCST) and Trail Making Test were repeated in the patients before and after administration of levodopa plus benserazide daily 300 mg. For the ERP's components, reference-independent measures of global field power (GFP) were determined, and P3 GFP peak, peak latency and topography were assessed. After administration of levodopa, the patients revealed significant increase of the achieved categories and decrease of preservation errors in the WSCT, shortening of time in Trail Making Test although MMSE score showed no significant difference. The P3 GFP peak attenuated although there were no differences in peak latency or on scalp topography. These findings suggest that levodopa affect on the neural circuit connects frontal cortex with the striatum and normalizes its function, and it causes decrease of P3 GFP peak reflecting appropriate resource allocation. In addition, P3 GFP might be a more appropriate indicator than psychological tests. © 2004 Published by Elsevier B.V.

Keywords: De novo Parkinson's disease; Levodopa; Hoehn and Yahr; Event-related potentials; Resource allocation

1. Introduction

Parkinson's disease (PD) is characterized by the loss of dopaminergic neurons projecting from the substantia nigra to the striatum. This results in altered function of cortical–striatal–pallidal–thalamic cortical circuits that mediate normal movement, resulting in bradykinesia

* Corresponding author. Tel.: +81-282-87-2152; fax: +81-282-86-5884.
E-mail address: hirata@dokkyomed.ac.jp (K. Hirata).

0531-5131/ © 2004 Published by Elsevier B.V.
doi:10.1016/j.ics.2004.05.137

and rigidity. It has been well known that cognitive dysfunction affects patients with idiopathic PD, although they do not have clinical dementia. In 1974, Albert et al. reported that patients with subcortical disease, including PD, show cognitive disorders that differ from Alzheimer's disease [1]. There are various reports about the cognitive disorders of Parkinson's patients. PD patients are impaired on a variety of cognitive tasks that depend on frontal lobe function and/or basal ganglia. Studies using various psychological batteries demonstrated a wide variety of mental deficits in patients with PD such as impairment on tests of planning, attention set-shifting, skill leaning, habit learning [2]. P3 is affected by the dopaminergic and cholinergic systems, both of which are impaired in PD. P3 has been shown to be abnormal in PD with cognitive decline or dementia, but investigations of P3 in patients with PD without clinical dementia (nondemented PD) remain controversial [3]. A surprising result reported by Green et al. [4] was that the P3 amplitude elicited by target was increased in nonmedicated and mild PD. A similar result was reported later by Tanaka et al. [5]. The latter compared PD with differences in conditions such as duration of illness, with or without dementia, the P3 amplitude increased only in nondemented PD but not in demented patients.

Concerning the P3 latency, most studies showed consistent results in that PD did not differ from normal controls. Few studies, however, revealed the P3 with delayed latency in nondemented PD. We investigated the influence of levodopa (L-dopa) on cognitive function in de novo PD patients using the event-related potential (ERP) P3 measurement and neuropsychological test batteries. The purpose of the present study is not only to evaluate the effect of L-dopa administration changes but also the effects in difference of severity and duration of illness [6] using ERP P3 as an objective tool in mild nondemented de novo PD patients.

2. Methods

2.1. Subjects

We studied 20 patients with PD who had never received anti-Parkinson medications. We excluded subjects with clinical dementia and an MMSE score of less than 24. None of the subjects had evidence of other brain damage as confirmed by computed tomography or magnetic resonance imaging. The subjects were classified to subgroups based on duration and severity of illness. The severity of illness was determined by Hoehn and Yahr. All subjects were fully informed as to the nature and purpose of the study and gave their consent to the study. Table 1 shows the clinical background of all subjects.

2.2. Neuropsychological testing

We used neuropsychological tests such as the Mini-Mental State Examination (MMSE), New modified Wisconsin card sorting test and Trail Making Test and Stroop Test. Wisconsin Card Sorting test was used to evaluate the frontal lobe function as it is one of the few tests to detect a clear deficit specific to patients with frontal lobe dysfunction. The achieved categories classification score and the perseverance errors reported by Nelson were used to evaluate the results of this test.

Table 1
The clinical background of subjects

De novo PD patients	20
Gender (M/F)	8/12
Age (mean ± S.D.)	68.5 ± 8.92 years
Duration of illness (median)	1.475 years
<1 year	11/20
>1 year	9/20
Severity of illness (Hohen and Yahr)	
I	5/20
II	7/20
III	8/20

2.3. Stimuli and experimental conditions

Auditory oddball P3 paradigm was given for the subjects. Two tones auditory oddball paradigm was used to elicit P3. Multichannel ERPs were averaged with 21 channels using the international 10/20 system for electrode location. A topography mapping system (Brain Atlas) was used for recording and averaging. Levodopa with benserazide was administrated. Initial dose was 100 mg/day; it was then increased up to 200 mg/day per week. Finally, patient was given Levodopa with benserazide 300 mg/day. Before and after administration of the drugs we measured P3 and ran the psychological tests. For the ERP's components, reference-independent measures of global field power (GFP) were determined, and P3 GFP peak, peak latency and topography were assessed [7].

3. Results

3.1. Neuropsychological examination

MMSE score showed no significant difference before and after administration of L-dopa. On the other hand, Wisconsin Card Sorting test score showed significant increase of the achieved categories and decrease of perseverance errors after the administration, especially in patients with short duration (short group) (Fig. 1) and slight severity of

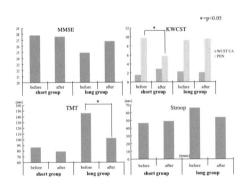
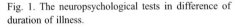
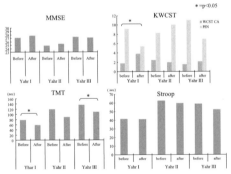

Fig. 1. The neuropsychological tests in difference of duration of illness.

Fig. 2. The neuropsychological tests in difference of severity of illness.

illness (Hoehn and Yahr I) (Fig. 2). Stroop test showed no significant difference before and after administration of L-dopa, but Trail Making test showed significant improvement especially in patients whose illness are of long duration (Fig. 1).

3.2. P3 global field power (GFP)

P3 GFP peak significantly decreased after administration of L-dopa in overall subjects. However, there is no difference of P3 latency and location in topography. P3 GFP peak decreasing is significant especially in patients with long duration (long group) (Fig. 3) and severe illness (Hoehn and Yahr III) in contrast to the results of neuropsychological examination (Fig. 4).

4. Discussion

Many studies using various psychological batteries demonstrated an attention set-shifting, skill-learning, habit-learning based on frontal lobe and basal ganglial dysfunction in patients with PD [1,2,8]. We investigated the influence of L-dopa on cognitive function in de novo PD patients using the event-related potential P3 measurement and neuropsychological test batteries. Thus, we have demonstrated that P3 GFP peak decreased significantly after administration of L-dopa, and that its ERP results may have close relationship with the results of psychological tests, especially the Wisconsin Card Sorting test. Arnsten et al. [9] administered Dopamine (DA) D1 receptor compounds in monkeys for the effects on the working memory functions of the prefrontal cortex. The partial agonist which is D1 agonist improved the aged or young reserpine-treated D1 depleted monkeys, but did not improve young control animals.

Therefore, they have concluded the importance of DA D1 mechanisms in cognitive function, and provide functional evidence of DA system degeneration. Based on their reports, our result suggests that the L-dopa improves the function of dopaminergic neural circuit between frontal lobe cortex and basal ganglia in PD.

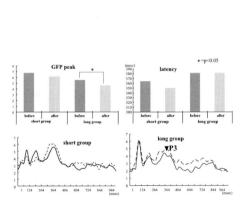
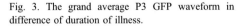

Fig. 3. The grand average P3 GFP waveform in difference of duration of illness.

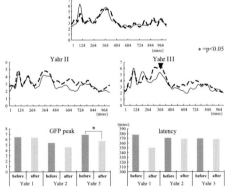

Fig. 4. The grand average P3 GFP waveform in difference of severity of illness.

P3 amplitude is related to how the stimulus delivers its task-relevant information, and that it is proportional to the amount of attention resources in terms of processing capability that is employed in a given task. P3 amplitude changes have been interpreted reflecting neural activity related to the basic aspects of cognition. P3 amplitude would be altered relative to the attention processing resources to be allocated in a task. P3 amplitude variation may provide valuable information about the intensity and the timing of energy allocation to various subprocesses of information processing. Green et al. [4] hypothesized that enlarged P3 amplitude reflects abnormality in use of attention resources to compensate for frontal dysfunction in PD. We have mentioned in the other study, P3 GFP was significantly increased in the early stage of nondemented PD patients. These results are confirmed as well as the findings of Green et al. [4] and Tanaka et al. [5]. Therefore, we think that L-dopa administration decreases P3 GFP, which reflects an improvement of attention processing resources in de novo PD patients.

The purpose of the present study is not only to evaluate the effect of L-dopa administration changes but also the effects in difference of severity and duration of illness using ERP P3 as an objective tool in mild nondemented de novo PD patients. Although the amelioration of Wisconsin Card Sorting test score was more significant in patients with short duration and slight severity of illness, P3 GFP improvement was seen only in the severe and long duration group after the administration of the drug. These results suggest that P3 GFP change linearly correlates with duration and severity of illness. The reason for discrepancy of the two measurements may be that the psychological test can be affecting learning effects. Therefore, we think that P3 GFP more objectively indicates the ameliorating effect of L-dopa than the psychological test.

References

[1] A.J. Lees, Parkinson's disease and dementia, Lancet 1 (1985) 43–44.

[2] A.J. Lees, E. Smith, Cognitive deficits in the early stage of Parkinson's disease, Brain 106 (1983) 257–270.

[3] A. Hozumi, et al., Perseveration for novel stimuli in Parkinson's disease: an evaluation based on event-related potentials topography, Mov. Disord. 15 (2000) 835–842.

[4] J. Green, et al., Event-related potential P3 change in mild Parkinson's disease, Mov. Disord. 11 (1996) 32–42.

[5] H. Tanaka, et al., Event-related potential and EEG measures in Parkinson's disease without and with dementia, Dement. Geriatr. Cogn. Disord. 11 (2000) 39–45.

[6] A. Kanazawa, Y. Mizuno, H. Narabayashi, Executive function in Parkinson's disease, Rinsho Shinkeigaku 41 (2001) 167–172 (Japanese).

[7] D. Lehmann, W. Skrandies, Reference-free identification of components of checkerboard evoked multichannel potentials field, Electroencephalogr. Clin. Neurophysiol. 48 (1980) 609–621.

[8] K.A. Flowers, C. Robertson, The effect of Parkinson's disease on the ability to maintain a mental set, J. Neurol. Neurosug. Psychiatry 48 (1985) 517–529.

[9] A.F. Arnsten, et al., Dopamin D1 receptor mechanisms in the cognitive performance of young adult and aged monkeys, Psychopharmacology (Berl.) 116 (1994) 143–151.

International Congress Series 1270 (2004) 275–278

ELSEVIER

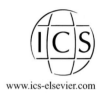

www.ics-elsevier.com

Error processing in patients with Parkinson's disease

Junko Ito*

*Central Clinical Laboratory, Division of Neurophysiology, Kyoto University Hospital,
54 Shogoin Kawaracho, Sakyo, 606-8507 Kyoto, Japan*

Abstract. To evaluate action monitoring and error detection in non-demented patients with Parkinson's disease (PD), event-related potentials (ERPs) during go and no-go reaction tasks were studied using a visually presented dual paradigm composed of Japanese phonetic characters. Error negativity (Ne) of ERPs obtained by averages time-locked to error response showed greater amplitude than the negativity for correct responses (Nc) in PDs and controls. The Ne amplitude was significantly smaller in PD, whereas there were no significant differences in Ne latency between the two subject groups. Although the Nc and error positivity (Pe) after the Ne did not show significant differences between the two subject groups, correct positivity (Pc) after the Nc showed significantly delayed latency in PD. In controls, the Ne showed frontal maximal and the Pe showed central maximal distribution, whereas the Ne and the Pe in PD tended to show diffuse scalp distribution In PD, the reaction times (RT) were significantly slower and error rates were higher. These findings suggest that the strategy for information processing and error detection, as well as action monitoring, was impaired in PD. © 2004 Elsevier B.V. All rights reserved.

Keywords: Event-related potentials; Reaction time; Error; Parkinson's disease

1. Introduction

Error negativity (Ne) or error-related negativity (ERN) of event-related potential (ERPs) is thought to be related to error detection and action monitoring [1–3]. To evaluate action monitoring and error processing in patients with Parkinson's disease (PD), ERP components time-locked to response were studied using a relatively complex oddball-type dual paradigm.

2. Patients and methods

A total of 16 non-demented, idiopathic PDs (7 males and 9 females; mean = 63.1 years) and 15 age-matched, healthy, control subjects (6 males and 9 females; mean = 63.9 years) participated in the present study. Informed consent was obtained from the PDs and controls.

Motor symptoms in the PDs ranged from Stage I to Stage III [I (2), II (8) and III (6)] on the Hoehm and Yahr scale. At the time of testing, they were treated with levodopa/dopa-decarboxylase inhibitors and dopamine agonist. None of the controls or PDs had taken any

* Tel.: +81-75-751-3658; fax: +81-75-751-3758.
E-mail address: jito@kuhp.kyoto-u.ac.jp (J. Ito).

0531-5131/ © 2004 Elsevier B.V. All rights reserved.
doi:10.1016/j.ics.2004.05.009

other drugs that might have affected the ERP components. Scores on the Mini Mental State Examination showed no significant differences between the two subject groups.

Each stimulus, composed of two Japanese phonetic characters, was displayed in the center of a computer monitor. Identical "hirakana" characters, occurring 9% of all stimuli, were designated as target stimuli (Targets). The remaining stimuli were non-target stimuli composed of different "hirakana"(73%), different "katakana" (9%) and identical "katakana" characters (9%). Each stimulus, which varied from trial-to-trial, was presented for 400 ms, and interstimulus intervals were 1800 ± 100 ms. The subjects were instructed to press a button with their preferred hand in response to targets (go) and disregard other stimuli (no-go). Speed and accuracy were equally emphasized.

EEGs recorded from the scalp were time-locked to a response in each trial and then averaged separately for correct and error trials. Negative components for error trials in the time window of 10 to 200 ms were designated as Ne. A small negative component in correct trials was designated as correct positivity (Nc). Positive components following the Ne and the Nc were designated as error positivity (Pe) and correct positivity (Pc), respectively. Peak amplitudes of individual ERP components were measured with respect to a 200-ms pre-trigger baseline, and peak latencies were defined as the points with maximal amplitudes for the respective search epochs.

ERP components were subjected to an analysis of variance (ANOVA) with the subject group (Controls, PD), condition (Correct, Error) and electrode (Fz, Cz, Pz, Oz). The criterion for significance was less than 0.05.

3. Results

The Ne amplitude was significantly reduced in the PDs ($F(1,29)=7.944$, $p=0.009$), whereas the Ne latency showed no significant differences between the two subject groups

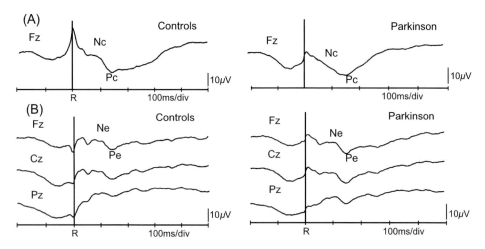

Fig. 1. Grand-averaged waveforms of ERPs time-locked to correct response (A) and error response (B). The Ne amplitude was smaller in PDs, whereas there were no significant differences in the Nc, Pc or Pe amplitude between the two subject groups. The Pc latency was delayed in PDs. (PD: Parkinson's disease, Ne: Error negativity, Pe: Error positivity, Nc: Correct negativity, Pc: Correct positivity, R: Response).

Table 1
Comparison of ERP components (mean ± S.D.)

	Controls	PD
Latency (ms)		
Ne (Fz)	72 (12)	74 (14)
Pe (Cz)	153 (10)	158 (13)
Pc (Pz)	130 (12)*	152 (15)*
Amplitude (μV)		
Ne (Fz)	− 3.6 (1.4)**	− 2.2 (0.6)**

* $p < 0.05$.
** $p < 0.01$.

(Fig. 1) (Table 1). Although the Nc and Pe components in PD did not differ significantly from those in controls, the Pc latency was significantly delayed in PDs ($F(1, 29) = 4.378$, $p = 0.045$).

The Ne amplitude showed significant differences among the electrode sites in the controls ($F(3,56) = 5.273$, $p = 0.003$), and greatest negativity at Fz. In controls, the Pe and the Pc showed significant differences among the electrode sites (Pe: $F(3,56) = 4.656$, $p = 0.006$; Pc: $F(3,56) = 2.856$, $p = 0.045$), the Pe showing central maximal and the Pc showing parietal maximal distributions. The Ne, Pe and Pc in the PDs tended to show diffuse distribution.

The PD showed significantly higher error rates (Controls: 3.5 ± 1.2, PD: 11.1 ± 3.0%) ($F(1,29) = 6.653$, $p = 0.015$). Although the reaction time (RT) in error trials (error RT) was significantly faster than in correct trials (correct RT), not only in Controls (Correct: 595 ± 52, Error: 541 ± 91 ms) ($F(1,28) = 13.310$, $p = 0.001$) but also in PDs (correct:727 ± 120, Error: 620 ± 113 ms) ($F(1,30) = 4.875$, $p = 0.035$), the error RT was significantly slower in PDs than in controls ($F(1,29) = 7.365$, $p = 0.011$). The correct RT immediately after the error RT was slower than the previous correct RT in controls (previous correct: 560 ± 69, previous error: 598 ± 76 ms) ($F(1,28) = 4.614$, $p = 0.041$), whereas PD did not show such differences (previous correct: 702 ± 161, previous error: 697 ± 196 ms).

4. Discussion

The reduced Ne amplitude was comparable with one of the previous studies on PD patients [1], while the other study did not show a reduction in Ne/ERN amplitude [2]. The Nc component was not enhanced in the PDs. These findings in PDs differed from those in patients with lateral prefrontal damage that showed enhanced Nc amplitude [3]. Personality and mood also affect the Ne amplitude [4]. As there were no significant differences in depression scores between the two subject groups, the reduced Ne amplitude in PD was not attributable to impairment of mood.

In healthy subjects, errors due to premature responding and perceived as errors were associated with large ERNs, whereas those with uncertainty were associated with smaller ERNs [5]. The RT immediately after errors was significantly slower than after correct reactions in controls. However, the PDs did not show any speed reduction in RT after errors and the error rates were significantly higher. These findings suggested that PDs had trouble detecting errors and were uncertain whether they pressed the correct button or not. Thus, the Ne amplitude was significantly reduced in PDs.

Although the error RT was faster than the correct RT, the error RT was slower in PDs. Thus, the cognitive speed of error detection and error processing might have been slowed down in PD, although Ne latency measured relative to the trigger point of slower RT was not prolonged. The Pc latency was delayed in PD. The Pc component may correspond to the P300 or P3b component. These findings suggested that information processing and stimulus evaluation were impaired in PDs.

The Pe component is thought to be a further error-specific component, which is independent of the Ne/ERN component [6]. Error awareness is thought to be associated with the Pe but not the Ne/ERN [6]. The Pe component did not differ between the two subject groups. Thus, error awareness was preserved in PD, while the smaller Ne indicated that action monitoring and information processing of errors were impaired in PDs.

References

[1] M. Falkenstein, et al., Action monitoring, error detection, and the basal ganglia: an ERP study, NeuroReport 12 (1) (2001) 157–161.
[2] C.B. Holroyd, et al., Spared error-related potentials in mild to moderate Parkinson's disease, Neuropsychologia 40 (12) (2002) 2116–2124.
[3] W.J. Gehring, R.T. Knight, Prefrontal-cingulate interactions in action monitoring, Nat. Neurosci. 3 (2000) 516–520.
[4] P. Luu, P. Collins, D.M. Tucker, Mood, personality, and self-monitoring: negative affect and emotionality in relation to frontal lobe mechanisms of error monitoring, J. Exp. Psychol. Gen. 129 (1) (2000) 43–60.
[5] M.K. Scheffers, M.G. Coles, Performance monitoring in a confusing world: error-related brain activity, judgments of response accuracy, and types of errors, J. Exp. Psychol. Hum. Percept. Perform. 26 (1) (2000) 141–151.
[6] S. Nieuwenhuis, et al., Error-related brain potentials are differentially related to awareness of response errors: evidence from an antisaccade task, Psychophysiology 38 (5) (2001) 752–760.

ELSEVIER

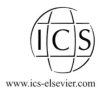

www.ics-elsevier.com

Dissociate neural correlates for incidental and intentional encoding of novel visual stimuli

Hirokazu Bokura*, Shuhei Yamaguchi, Shotai Kobayashi

Department of Neurology, Shimane University, Faculty of Medicine, 89-1 Enya-cho, 693-8501, Izumo, Shimane, Japan

Abstract. To explore neural processing of incidental and intentional encoding of novel stimuli, brain electrical activity was studied by measuring event-related brain potentials (ERPs). We used 14 healthy subjects and employed a visual novelty oddball task that included frequent triangles, rare slanted triangles, and rare novel pictures. In the incidental encoding session, subjects were instructed to press a button upon the occurrence of infrequent slanted triangles while ignoring other stimuli. In the intentional encoding session, subjects were required to memorize all novel pictures while performing the same detection task as in the incidental encoding session. Following each encoding session, a picture recognition task (memory test) was performed. ERPs were averaged separately according to whether novel pictures from each encoding session were recognized correctly or incorrectly. The rate of correct recognition of novel pictures from the intentional encoding session (86%) was better than that from the incidental encoding session (73%). There were no differences in the components of ERPs that were elicited in response to correctly and incorrectly recognized pictures from the incidental encoding session. By contrast, pictures that were successfully encoded in the intentional encoding session caused an increase in the amplitude of the N2 component relative to the magnitude of the same component for incorrectly encoded pictures. This effect was maximal over the frontal scalp. These results suggest that the frontal N2 component is involved in the intentional encoding of novel visual stimuli, but does not play a role in incidental encoding. © 2004 Elsevier B.V. All rights reserved.

Keywords: Event-related potential; Novelty; Encoding; Memory

1. Introduction

A novel stimulus provokes an orienting response and neural representation of new events is one of the most elementary forms of learning and memory [1]. Novel stimuli elicit a P3 event-related evoked potential (ERP) in the brain that is distributed fronto-centrally; this is distinct from the maximal parietal P3 component that is elicited by target stimuli [2]. Recordings of ERPs from brain-damaged patients and functional imaging

* Corresponding author. Tel.: +81-853-20-2200; fax: +81-853-20-2194.
E-mail address: bokura@med.shimane-u.ac.jp (H. Bokura).

0531-5131/ © 2004 Elsevier B.V. All rights reserved.
doi:10.1016/j.ics.2004.04.039

studies have demonstrated that the novelty detection system involves the prefrontal, temporo-parietal, and limbic regions [3,4], which are also involved in some aspects of memory processing. This suggests that the processing of novel stimuli may be linked to memory.

Although the orienting response affects encoding processes, this does not guarantee that subsequent recollection of a novel stimulus will be superior to the recollection of other events. For example, we experience novel events daily, but much of this information is forgotten. Relatively few reports have directly addressed the relationship between novelty processing and memory function [5]. In the present study, we sought to identify neural correlates that reflect subsequent effects of memory, as represented by ERPs that are elicited in response to novel stimuli. We employed two different paradigms that were based on the same visual novelty oddball task, and examined changes in ERPs that were elicited during a subsequent recognition task in response to pictures that had been memorized either incidentally or intentionally.

2. Subjects and methods

Fourteen healthy adults (six females; mean age, 24.7 ± 2.9 years) were recruited for the study. All subjects were right-handed. None of the subjects had a history of neurological disorder and none were undergoing treatment with psychotropic medication.

Frequent upright triangles (72%), infrequent slanted triangles (14%), and infrequent novel pictures (14%) were presented on a computer monitor. The novel pictures comprised 80 different images; for example, an animal, building, sport, abstract image, etc. In the first encoding session (incidental encoding session), the subjects were instructed to press a button upon presentation of a target stimulus (slanted triangle) and to ignore other stimuli. The subjects were not given any information about the novel pictures that were to be presented. In the second encoding session (intentional encoding session), the subjects were asked to memorize all novel pictures for a subsequent memory test while performing the same detection task as in the first encoding session. After each encoding session, subjects performed a task in which their memory of the novel pictures was assessed. A total of 80 pictures were presented randomly, of which 40 had been presented during the preceding encoding session and 40 were novel pictures. The reaction time (RT) for correctly and incorrectly recognized pictures was measured separately.

An electro-encephalogram (EEG) was recorded using a 128-channel Geodesic Sensor Net [6]. The band pass was set to 0.1–50 Hz, the sampling rate was 250 Hz, and all impedances were <40 kΩ. The continuous EEG was segmented into an epoch that started 200 ms before the onset of the stimulus and ended 1000 ms after the stimulus onset. Electro-oculography (EOG) was carried out using six electrodes. ERPs for novel stimuli were averaged separately, according to whether the picture that was presented during the viewing session was recognized correctly or incorrectly during the subsequent memory task. The peak latency and amplitude of components N2 (within a 220–300 ms latency window) and P3 (within 350–500 ms latency window) were measured for ERPs in response to novel pictures. Topographic distributions were also evaluated for each of the aforementioned components.

3. Results

The rates of correct recognition of novel pictures from the incidental and intentional encoding sessions were 73% and 86%, respectively. In the memory test that followed the incidental encoding session, the RTs for correct recognition of previously presented and novel pictures were 734 ± 60 and 821 ± 100 ms, respectively. The RTs for incorrect recognition (862 ± 140 and 899 ± 288 ms for previously presented and novel pictures, respectively) were significantly greater than the RTs for correct recognition. In the memory test that followed the intentional encoding session, the RTs for correct recognition of previously presented and novel pictures were 720 ± 97 and 792 ± 75 ms, respectively. The RTs for incorrect recognition (908 ± 176 and 832 ± 136 ms for previously presented and novel pictures, respectively) were significantly greater than the RTs for correct recognition.

Fig. 1 shows the grand-averaged ERPs for the novel pictures that were recognized either correctly (dark line) or incorrectly (light line) in the memory test that followed the incidental and intentional encoding sessions. There were no differences between ERPs that were elicited by correctly and incorrectly recognized pictures from the incidental encoding session. By contrast, the amplitude of N2 for pictures that were encoded successfully during the intentional encoding session was greater than that for unrecognized pictures (-3.9 ± 4.0 vs. -2.1 ± 3.9 V, $p = 0.04$). Interpolated voltage maps revealed that this effect of memory on N2 was greatest over the frontal scalp. We found no differences in the P3 component of ERPs that were elicited by correctly and incorrectly recognized pictures. The P3 component was distributed more towards the anterior scalp for pictures from the incidental encoding session as compared with the intentional encoding session, whereas N2 was maximal over the anterior site in both encoding sessions.

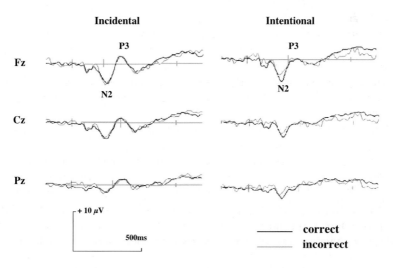

Fig. 1. Grand-averaged ERPs for the novel pictures, which were correctly (dark line) and incorrectly (light line) recognized in the subsequent memory test for the incidental and intentional sessions.

4. Discussion

The present study revealed that only the intentional condition altered the N2 component of the ERPs that were elicited by novel pictures. Because the change in N2 was independent of whether the novel pictures were recognized correctly or incorrectly in the subsequent memory test, successful incidental encoding of visual stimuli does not appear to be reflected in ERPs. The behavioral data also revealed a superior rate of recognition in the intentional condition. These results are consistent with the results of a previous auditory novelty oddball experiment [5] in which ERPs were modulated only by intentional encoding of novel auditory stimuli. However, the modulation of ERPs by memory in the aforementioned study was manifested in a latency range that was 400 ms after the end of the stimulus presentation, whereas the effect of memory on the ERPs that we observed in the present study was in the N2 latency range. The apparent discrepancy between these studies might be due to the difference in the stimulus modality or to the materials that were memorized in each study [7]. In the present study, most of the pictures that were used could easily be semantically processed, whereas auditory stimuli might be relatively more difficult to encode semantically. A subsequent effect of memory on ERPs has also been observed under incidental learning conditions [8]. In these studies, items were not memorized intentionally, but were processed semantically during a study phase. By contrast, the pictures that were used in the present study might have been processed at a shallow semantic level during the incidental encoding session. This may explain why memory did not alter ERPs for the incidental encoding condition. Alternatively, scalp-recorded ERPs might not be sufficiently sensitive to reflect the neural substrates that account for the behavioral effects of incidental memory.

In conclusion, distinct neural substrates contribute to incidental and intentional encoding of novel stimuli. The results of our study indicate that the enhanced N2 component over the anterior scalp is involved in the intentional encoding of novel visual stimuli. However, the use of scalp-recorded ERPs to elucidate the neural substrates that underlie such incidental encoding may be difficult.

References

[1] C. Ranganath, G. Rainer, Neural mechanisms for detecting and remembering novel events, Nat. Rev., Neurosci. 4 (2003) 193–202.
[2] S. Yamaguchi, R.T. Knight, P300 generation by novel somatosensory stimuli, Electroencephalogr. Clin. Neurophysiol. 78 (1991) 50–55.
[3] D. Friedman, Y.M. Cycowicz, H. Gaeta, The novelty P3: an event-related brain potential (ERP) sign of the brain's evaluation of novelty, Neurosci. Biobehav. Rev. 25 (2001) 355–373.
[4] R.T. Knight, D. Scabini, Anatomic bases of event-related potentials and their relationship to novelty detection in humans, J. Clin. Neurophysiol. 15 (1998) 3–13.
[5] Y.M. Cycowicz, D. Friedman, The effect of intention to learn novel, environmental sounds on the novelty P3 and old/new recognition memory, Biol. Psychol. 50 (1999) 35–60.
[6] D.M. Tucker, Spatial sampling of head electrical fields: the geodesic sensor net, Electroencephalogr. Clin. Neurophysiol. 87 (1993) 154–163.
[7] R. Johnson, Event-related potential insights into the neurobiology of memory systems, in: F. Boller, J. Grafman (Eds.), The Handbook of Neuropsychology, Elsevier, Amsterdam, 1995, pp. 135–164.
[8] D. Friedman, W. Ritter, J.G. Snodgrass, ERPs during study as a function of subsequent direct and indirect memory testing in young and old adults, Brain Res. Cogn. 4 (1996) 1–13.

International Congress Series 1270 (2004) 283–286

ELSEVIER

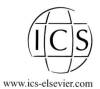

www.ics-elsevier.com

Effect of proximity and local orientation on evoked electrical brain activity in perceptual grouping

Andrey R. Nikolaev[a,b,*], Cees van Leeuwen[a,c]

[a] Laboratory for Perceptual Dynamics, RIKEN Brain Science Institute, Wako-shi, Japan
[b] Institute of Higher Nervous Activity, Moscow, Russia
[c] University of Sunderland, Sunderland, UK

Abstract. High-density, 256-channel, event-related potentials (ERP) were recorded in 12 subjects, who had to find a triangle of which only the corners were marked in an array of distracters. The orientation of the corner markers to each other and their proximity varied across trials. An early, pre-attentional, nonspatial effect of marker orientation was found at 64 and 100 ms after stimulus presentation in the right occipital areas. A spatial effect of marker proximity (triangle size) was reflected in a negative peak of 180 ms in the occipital areas and in P250 and P430 in the central areas. This result is contrary to the usual precedence of spatial over nonspatial grouping and suggests a greater flexibility in precedence based on task demands. © 2004 Elsevier B.V. All rights reserved.

Keywords: Perceptual grouping; Spatial; Nonspatial visual feature; Pre-attentive; Event-related potentials (ERP)

1. Introduction

It is traditionally accepted that spatial information is processed at a faster rate than nonspatial information in both the pre-attentive and attentive stages of visual processing. Perceptual grouping based on spatial proximity is related to an event-related potential (ERP) peak at 100 ms after stimulus presentation, and grouping by nonspatial shape similarity is reflected in a later ERP wave of about 260 ms [1]. These effects are understood as pre-attentional and bottom-up. The precedence of spatial over nonspatial processing has also been observed in top-down, attentional selection. Spatial attention is related to enhanced ERP components of about 75–150 ms after stimulus presentation, while nonspatial attention is reflected in later (120–220 ms) selection negativity [2]. Top-down influence may even affect early processing. In particular, perceptual grouping may be influenced by strategic processes in response to task demands [3]. With respect to task demands, flexibility implies that spatial, as well as nonspatial grouping mechanisms can be used in order to facilitate attentional selection [4,5]. This means that the habitual

---

* Corresponding author. Laboratory for Perceptual Dynamics, RIKEN Brain Science Institute, 2-1 Hirosawa, Wako-shi, Saitama, 351-0198 Japan. Tel.: +81-48-462-1111x7434; fax: +81-48-467-7236.
E-mail address: nikolaev@brain.riken.jp (A.R. Nikolaev).
URL: http://www.pdl.brain.riken.jp.

0531-5131/ © 2004 Elsevier B.V. All rights reserved.
doi:10.1016/j.ics.2004.04.047

precedence of spatial over nonspatial information could be found reversed in the appropriate task demands. In this study, we investigate whether certain task conditions may trigger a precedence of nonspatial over spatial processing as reflected in ERP.

2. Method

2.1. Stimuli

Gabor patches of three spatial frequencies were placed in a square array of $8°$ of visual angle (Fig. 1). Three patches of middle spatial frequency marked the corners of a rectangular triangle. There were two sizes of triangles, small and large. The orientation of target patches varied among experimental conditions: "aligned," "random," "horizontal," and "vertical." The right angle of the triangle was turned into one of four possible directions.

2.2. Procedure

Ten participants were asked to determine in which direction the right angle of the triangle was pointed. The experiment consisted of 3 series of 192 trials each. Afterwards, a control series of 70 trials was given, in which the same stimulus was always presented, and participants were asked to wait about 1–2 s and press any button.

2.3. EEG recordings and analysis

EEG was recorded using a 256-channel Geodesic Sensor Net referenced to Cz and digitized at 250 Hz. The EEG signal was bandpass filtered in 0.3–25 Hz. The data were converted to average reference and baseline-corrected. The ERP were grand-averaged in 10 subjects for each condition and voltage maps were plotted. On these maps, the areas with voltage maxima were found in time points of main ERP peaks. Maximum amplitudes in groups of adjacent channels with values within 0.1 µV from the maximum were taken

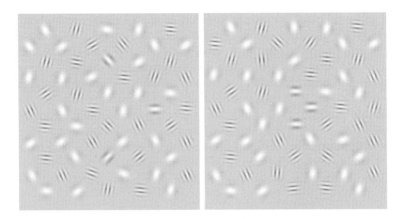

Fig. 1. Examples of displays used in the experiment. Left: large triangle with aligned orientation of component Gabor patches. Right: small triangle with horizontal orientation. Both triangles point to the right.

for statistical analysis. The amplitudes were treated with repeated measures ANOVA with two factors: triangle "size" (two levels) vs. "orientation" of their components (four levels).

3. Results

3.1. Onset of attentional processing

The difference between task and control conditions reached significance initially at N180 (Fig. 2, N180) and became more prominent for further peaks. The main difference between task and control condition was attentional demand. We may, therefore, propose that 180 ms demarcates the onset of attentional processing.

3.2. Pre-attentional effect of orientation

Gabor patch orientation resulted in significance for the peak N64 $F(3, 27) = 3.5$, $p < 0.05$, and for the peak P100 $F(3, 27) = 8.8$, $p < 0.01$ in the occipital areas. The effect at N64 was mostly contributed by the difference between random and collinear orientations in small triangles (Fig. 2, N64). It is probably related to pre-attentional grouping of close collinear elements, which may occur due to propagation of lateral interactions between flanked Gabor patches [6]. The effect at P100 was mainly based on the difference between

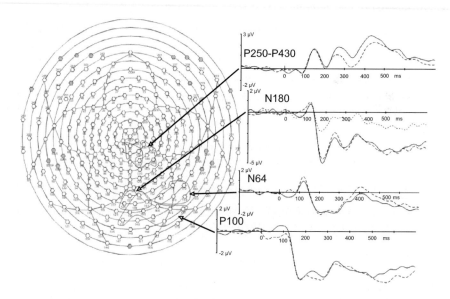

Fig. 2. Areas on the scheme of the 256-channel Geodesic Sensor Net, where significant ERP effects were found and corresponding grand averaged ERPs contributed mostly to the effects. The effect of patch orientation is indicated as follows: N64: solid line—random, dashed line—vertical orientation in small triangles; P100: solid line—aligned, dashed line—random orientation in large triangles. The effect of triangle size: N180: solid line—small, dashed line—large triangles with aligned orientation, dotted line—control condition; P250–P430: solid line—small, dashed line—large triangles with random orientation.

the random and aligned orientation ($F(1, 9) = 26.7$; $p < 0.001$) for both small and large triangles (Fig. 2, P100). Facilitation in the aligned condition is probably based on contour interpolation.

3.3. Attentional effect of size

Triangle size had its earliest effect in the negative wave N180 amplitude in the middle occipital areas $F(1, 9) = 4.8$, $p < 0.05$ (Fig. 2, N180), followed by positive waves P250 $F(1, 9) = 8.5$, $p < 0.05$ and P430 $F(1, 9) = 15.8$, $p < 0.01$ in the middle central area (Fig. 2, P250–P430). The central location of P250 and P430 may indicate processes related to response selection and preparation.

4. Discussion

We investigated the role of spatial and nonspatial features in perceptual grouping. We found early, pre-attentional effects of the nonspatial factor of component orientation, whereas the spatial feature of proximity (triangle size) has effect later.

The sequence of the effects (orientation-first, size-second) contrasts with the precedence of spatial information found in numerous studies [1,2]. This contradiction probably means that in our study, the orientational task demands reverse the established order of visual processing. Thus, any type of visual features may provide a first, coarse guidance of perceptional grouping, which facilitates target selection. This is in line with reverse hierarchy theory [4], which proposes that early, high-level perception makes a first guess at binding, and focused attention is required to confirm this guess and finally to bind features.

References

[1] S. Han, et al., Neural substrates for visual perceptual grouping in humans, Psychophysiology 38 (2001) 926–935.
[2] S.A. Hillyard, W.A. Teder-Salejarvi, T.F. Munte, Temporal dynamics of early perceptual processing, Curr. Opin. Neurobiol. 8 (1998) 202–210.
[3] J.F. Stins, C. van Leeuwen, Context influence on the perception of figures as conditional upon perceptual organization strategies, Percept. Psychophys. 53 (1993) 34–42.
[4] M. Ahissar, S. Hochstein, Task difficulty and the specificity of perceptual learning, Nature 387 (1997) 401–406.
[5] J.M. Wolfe, Moving towards solutions to some enduring controversies in visual search, Trends Cogn. Sci. 7 (2003) 70–76.
[6] U. Polat, D. Sagi, Lateral interactions between spatial channels: suppression and facilitation revealed by lateral masking experiments, Vis. Res. 33 (1993) 993–999.

International Congress Series 1270 (2004) 287–290

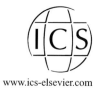

www.ics-elsevier.com

Event-related potentials to unfamiliar faces in a recognition memory task

Hisao Tachibana[a,*], Yasunobu Kida[a], Masanaka Takeda[a],
Hiroo Yoshikawa[a], Tsunetaka Okita[b]

[a] Division of Neurology and Stroke Care Unit, Department of Internal Medicine, Hyogo College of Medicine,
1-1, Mukogawa-cho, Nishinomiya 663-8501 Japan
[b] Faculty of Social Information, Sapporo Gakuin University, Japan

Abstract. The purpose of this study was to investigate electrophysiological correlates related to the recognition of repeated faces in the intact human by means of event-related potentials (ERPs). Twenty young healthy adults (mean, 24.5 years) performed a continuous face recognition task, in which unfamiliar faces were flashed upon a computer screen. Some faces were repeated immediately after initial presentation (at lag 0), while others were repeated after one intervening face (at lag 1) or at lag 3. Subjects were requested to push a button with the right thumb upon first presentation of a face and with a left thumb upon repeat presentation. Significant differences were seen in accuracy of new/old responses between at lag 0 and at lags 1 or 3. Reaction time (RT) for faces repeated at lag 0 was significantly shorter than that for first (new) presentations. RT at lag 3, however, was longer than RT for new faces. The ERPs recorded from 7 scalp sites revealed more positive going waveforms beginning at about 200 ms (old/new effect) for the correctly classified repeated faces. The ERP old/ new effects were more marked in anterior sites and were more prominent at lag 0 than at lags 1 and 3. It is thus concluded that the ERP old/new effect is demonstrated to unfamiliar faces and varies with repetition interval and scalp regions. In addition, some discrepancy was found between electrophysiological and behavioral priming effects. © 2004 Elsevier B.V. All rights resreved.

Keywords: Event-related potential (ERP); Recognition memory; ERP old/new effect

1. Introduction

Many studies have used event-related potential (ERPs) to investigate the cognitive processes involved in direct and indirect memory tests [1–3]. In both kinds of tests, the most consistent finding is that ERPs evoked by the first presentation of a stimulus (i.e., new stimulus) are relatively less positive than those elicited by the second presentation of the same item (i.e., repeated stimulus). This modulation is termed as 'ERP repetition effect' or 'ERP old/new effect' [4].

* Corresponding author. Tel.: +81-798-45-6596; fax: +81-798-45-6597.
E-mail address: htachiba@hyo-med.ac.jp (H. Tachibana).

0531-5131/ © 2004 Elsevier B.V. All rights resreved.
doi:10.1016/j.ics.2004.04.098

Table 1
Behavioral measures

	Lag 0	Lag 1	Lag 3
Reaction time (ms)			
1st presentation	623 ± 152[a]	625 ± 151	630 ± 153
2nd presentation	583 ± 128[a]	618 ± 161	658 ± 177
Accuracy (%)			
1st presentation	97.7 ± 3.9	96.6 ± 4.8	97.7 ± 2.5
2nd presentation	98.9 ± 2.0[bc]	93.8 ± 8.6[b]	88.0 ± 11.4[c]

Values are mean ± S.D.
[a] $p < 0.0001$ by Wilcoxon's signed-rank test.
[b] $p < 0.01$ by Wilcoxon's signed-rank test.
[c] $p < 0.001$ by Wilcoxon's signed-rank test.

In the present study, we investigated electrophysiological correlates related to the recognition of repeated unfamiliar faces at different intervals. Unfamiliar faces were chosen because these stimuli in the direct test foster the episodic processes by which a completely new and distinctive representation has to be formed [5].

2. Materials and methods

2.1. Subjects

Twenty young healthy adults (mean age 24.5 years, range 23–28) participated in this study. Prior to testing, informed consent was obtained from all subjects.

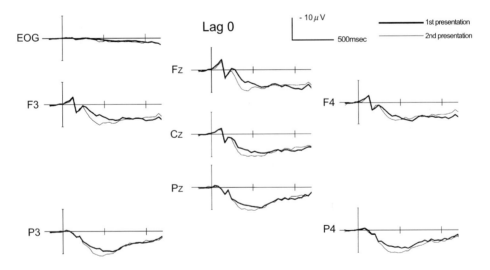

Fig. 1. Ground average ERP waveform evoked by first (new) presentation and repetition (old) faces. The ERP old/new effect was evident in all electrodes.

2.2. Stimuli and tasks

Stimuli consisted of 341 black-and-white photos representing a person's face unknown to the subjects. Thirty-one faces comprised one block. The first face was nontarget stimulus and subsequent 30 faces were targets. Ten faces were repeated immediately after the initial presentation (lag 0), while remaining each 10 faces were repeated following one intervening face (lag 1) or at lag 3. After one training block, 10 blocks of 31 faces were presented on the TV screen pseudo-randomly in a continuous repetition task sequence. The stimulus duration was 1s and the interstimulus interval was 3 s (onset to onset).

2.3. ERP recording

The subjects were seated comfortably in a dimly lit chamber and were given a thumb-switch to hold in both hands. Subjects were requested to push a button with the right thumb upon first presentation of a face on a TV screen and with the left thumb upon repeated presentation. An EEG was taken using Ag–AgCl electrodes that were placed on scalp sites Fz, Cz, Pz, F3, F4, P3 and P4 and referred to the left ear lobe. An EOG was attached below the left inferior orbital margin and the left outer canthus. The EEG and EOG activities were amplified using a 0.05–30 Hz filter.

3. Results

Significant differences were seen in the accuracy of old/new responses between lag 0 and lag 1 or 3 (Table 1). RT for faces repeated at lag 0 was significantly shorter than that of the first (new) presentations. RT at lag 3, however, was rather longer than that for new faces (Table 1). ERPs recorded from seven scalp sites revealed more positive going waveforms beginning at about 200 ms (old/new effect) for the repeated faces (Figs. 1 and

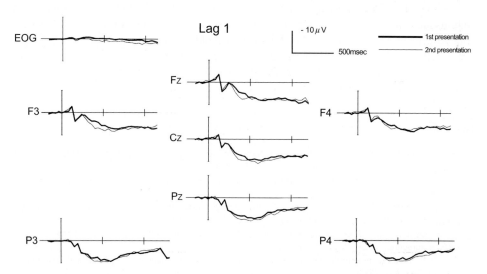

Fig. 2. Ground average ERP waveform evoked by first (new) presentation and repetition (old) faces. The ERP old/new effect is noted in the frontal and central sutes.

Table 2
ERP old/new effects between 200 and 500 ms after stimulus (μV)

	Lag 0	Lag 1	Lag 3
Fz	3.40 ± 2.2*	1.63 ± 3.0*	1.12 ± 2.5*
Cz	2.42 ± 2.3*	1.71 ± 3.0*	0.71 ± 1.9
Pz	1.71 ± 2.1*	0.95 ± 2.6	0.49 ± 2.0

$*p < 0.05$ by Wilcoxon's signed-rank test.

2). The ERP old/new effects were evaluated by subtracting the ERP for new faces from that for old faces between 200 and 500 ms after stimulus (Table 2). The old/new effects were more marked in anterior sites and were more prominent at lag 0 than at lags 1 and 3.

4. Discussion

In the present study a reliable ERP old/new effect to faces was demonstrated in a continuous recognition task. The ERP old/new effects were most prominent at the Fz site between 200 and 500 ms after stimulus. As the overall ERP repetition effect is mainly elicited within 300–500 ms over posterior sites in the direct memory test and overlaps temporally and topographically with the N400 component, it will be referred to as the 'N400 effect' [4]. Recent topographical analysis has led to the description of additional effects spanning the N400 latency range, but with frontal distribution [4]. Frontal old/new effect in the present study may correspond to the fronto-polar effect, which is reported to be elicited by unfamiliar face only in direct tasks [6].

The ERP old/new effect was more marked at lag 0 than at lags 1 and 3. This result suggests that immediate repetition facilitates stimulus identification and eliminates the need for stimulus analysis process while making categorical decisions [1], although at longer lags the episodic trace is weak.

The present study showed that the RT repetition effect at lag 0 reflects the facilitation of stimulus recognition, categorization, and decision process. On the other hand, no RT facilitation effect was noted at lag 3 although some ERP old/new effect was found. This discrepancy between ERP and behavioral measures suggests differing correlates of distinct psychological processes. Whereas the RTs reflect the combined contribution of all the sources of the repetition effect, ERPs are primarily modulated by episodic, decision-related factors [1].

References

[1] S. Bentin, G. McCarthy, The effects of immediate stimulus repetition on reaction time and event-related potentials in tasks of different complexity, J. Exp. Psychol. 20 (1994) 130–149.
[2] H. Tachibana, et al., Event-related potentials reveal memory deficits in Parkinson's disease, Cogn. Brain Res. 8 (1999) 165–172.
[3] H. Minamoto, et al., Recognition memory in normal aging and Parkinson's disease: behavioral and electrophysiologic measures, Cogn. Brain Res. 11 (2001) 23–32.
[4] F. Guillem, M. Bicu, J.B. Debruille, Dissociating memory process involved in direct and indirect tests with ERPs to unfamiliar faces, Cogn. Brain Res. 11 (2001) 113–125.
[5] D.L. Nelson, et al., Interpreting the influence of implicitly activated memories on recall and recognition, Psychol. Rev. 2 (1998) 299–324.
[6] T. Curran, The electrophysiology of incidental and intentional retrieval: ERP old/new effects in lexical decision and recognition memory, Neuropsychologia 37 (1999) 771–785.

International Congress Series 1270 (2004) 291–294

ELSEVIER

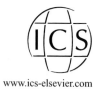

www.ics-elsevier.com

LORETA analysis of CNV in time perception

Keiichi Onoda, Jun Suzuki, Hiroshi Nittono,
Shogo Sakata, Tadao Hori*

*Graduate School of Biosphere Science, Hiroshima University, 1-7-1, Kagamiyama, Higashi-Hiroshima,
Hiroshima,739-8521, Japan*

Abstract. The aim of this study was to specify when and where "pure" temporal processing occurred in the brain. Event-related potentials were recorded from 13 young, healthy volunteers performing interval and pitch discrimination tasks. In the interval task, two 1000-Hz tones (S1 and S2) were presented with an interval of 1000 or 1500 ms. Participants were asked to judge whether the S1–S2 interval was short or long. In the pitch task, the S1 (1000 Hz) was followed by the S2 (1000 or 1050 Hz) with a fixed interval of 1000 ms. Participants were asked to judge whether the pitch of the S2 was the same as or different from that of the S1. In both tasks, contingent negative variation (CNV) was observed in the period between 500 and 1000 ms after the S1. The amplitude of the CNV was larger in the interval task than in the pitch task. The data were analyzed using low-resolution electromagnetic tomography (LORETA). The right dorsolateral prefrontal cortex (DLPFC) showed more activation in the interval task than in the pitch task. This result suggests that the right DLPFC may play an important role in time perception and processing the temporal dimension of events. © 2004 Elsevier B.V. All rights reserved.

Keywords: Time perception; Contingent negative variation (CNV); LORETA; Dorsolateral prefrontal cortex (DLPFC)

1. Introduction

Time is an important source of information influencing behavior. However, the neurophysiological basis of time perception remains a matter for debate. Recent studies using functional brain mapping have suggested some brain structures where time-related attributes of an event are processed [1]; nevertheless, these structures are also involved in the perception of other dimensions, such as the intensity, pitch, color, shape, and location of auditory and visual stimuli. In order to conclude that the perception of time is responsible for the observed pattern of activation, it should be demonstrated that this pattern is not elicited by the perception of other attributes of stimuli. In functional brain mapping studies, some patterns of activation described in the timing task are similar to

---

* Corresponding author. Tel.: +81-824-24-6580; fax: +81-824-24-0759.
  E-mail address: tdhori@hiroshima-u.ac.jp (T. Hori).

those in working memory and attention tasks. As fMRI and PET integrate an activity over a period of many seconds, temporal resolution is often insufficient to specify areas only involved when temporal processing is performed. Therefore, Pouthas et al. [2] examined contingent negative variation (CNV) observed in duration discrimination tasks using dipole analysis. They discovered that the right frontal dipole is active during the CNV, and proposed that the processing of temporal information would specifically involve the right frontal area. The CNV, however, reflects not only temporal processing but also others, such as attention and motivation. In order to argue the contribution of the right frontal lobe in time perception, it is necessary to distinguish the processing of time from other processing tasks. This study used two tasks based on the S1–S2 paradigm, a task in which the interval of the S1 and S2 was judged, and a task in which the pitch of the S1 and S2 were judged. Sources of the CNV observed in the two tasks were compared using low-resolution brain electromagnetic tomography (LORETA) [3].

2. Method

2.1. Subjects

Participants were 13 (5 females and 8 males) young volunteers between 21 and 25 years old with normal audition. The experiment was conducted with the informed consent of each subject.

2.2. Tasks

In the interval task, two 1000-Hz tones (S1 and S2, 70 dB) were presented with an interval of 1000 or 1500 ms. Participants were asked to judge whether the S1–S2 interval was short or long. The tone duration was 50 ms. The intensity of the stimulus was 70 dB. The ISI lasted between 2600 and 3400 ms (on average, 3000 ms). The probabilities were 0.5/0.5. The button press responses were made with the thumbs of each hand. They were instructed to delay their responses for about 1000 ms in both tasks. Each participant was given 100 trials in this task.

In the pitch task, the S1 (1000 Hz) was followed by the S2 (1000 or 1050 Hz) with a fixed interval of 1000 ms. Participants were required to judge whether the pitch of the S2 was the same as or different from that of the S1. Other variables were the same as that of the interval task. The response hands and the task order were counterbalanced across participants.

2.3. ERP recording and analysis

Electroencephalograms (EEGs) were recorded digitally from 24 electrode sites and re-referenced to the nose tip. Horizontal and vertical electro-oculograms (EOGs) were simultaneously recorded. The sampling rate was 500 Hz. A bandpass filter of 0.016–100 Hz was used. Event-related potentials (ERPs) were obtained for each task. The averaging period was 1200 ms with a 200 ms baseline before the onset of S1. A repeated measure analysis of variance was performed on the mean amplitudes at Cz between 500 and 1000 ms after the S1. LORETA [3,4] was used to find differences in intracerebral

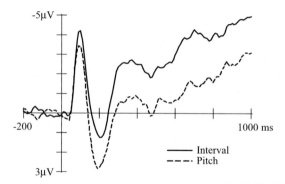

Fig. 1. Grand mean ERP waveforms recorded at Cz during the S1–S2 interval period (N = 13). The vertical line shows the onset of S1.

sources of the CNV between the two tasks. The pairwise t-test was performed on a voxel-by-voxel basis.

3. Results

3.1. Behavior

The correct response rates in the two tasks were 97.8% (S.D. 2.7) for the interval task, and 97.4% (5.0) for the pitch task. No difference in performance was found between the tasks, $t(12)$ = 0.24, n.s.

3.2. ERP

Fig. 1 shows ERP waveforms at the vertex (Cz) averaged across subjects in the interval and the pitch discrimination tasks. Following the sensory-evoked potentials, a clear CNV can be observed from 500 to 1000 ms after the S1 in both tasks. The mean amplitude between 500 and 1000 ms was larger in the interval task than in the pitch task, $F(1,12)$ = 13.28, $p < 0.01$.

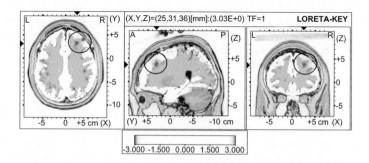

Fig. 2. Statistical maps of t value illustrating the differences in current source density between the interval and pitch tasks at the epoch between 500 and 1000 ms. Highlighted voxels ($t > 3.00$) appear in the right dorsolateral prefrontal cortex (DLPFC).

3.3. LORETA

To compare the differences in current source density between the CNVs (500–1000 ms) in the two tasks, the pairwise *t*-test was used on a voxel-by-voxel basis. The maximal t value was observed in the right dorsolateral prefrontal cortex (DLPFC) at the Talairach coordinates (25, 31, 36) (Fig. 2).

4. Discussion

In the present study, we examined the spatio-temporal organization of cerebral areas involved in temporal processing by LORETA analysis of ERP. The activation of the right DLPFC was found during the CNV in the interval task. Since sustained attention and working memory were also involved in the pitch task, the differential activation in the right DLPFC suggests an important role of this area processing the temporal dimension of the event.

Using ERPs combined with PET, Pouthas et al. [2] found the timing of activation in the right inferior prefrontal cortex during time discrimination was strongly aligned with the durations. The contribution of the right dorsolateral and inferior prefrontal cortices in time perception was supported by fMRI studies (e.g. Ref. [4]), although the differences between the roles of these regions are not clear.

Some hypotheses about the role of the right DLPFC in time perception proposed that the role of the region may act as a central "clock" mechanism, "accumulator" storing temporal information, "mediator" of time estimation process, and "maker of decisions" [5]. Although the results of this study cannot directly mention the role of the right DLPFC, a more detailed, temporal–spatial analysis using LORETA may help to understand the process of time perception.

References

[1] P.A. Lewis, R.C. Miall, Distinct systems for automatic and cognitively controlled time measurement: evidence from neuroimaging, Curr. Opin. Neurobiol. 13 (2003) 250–255.
[2] V. Pouthas, et al., ERPs and PET analysis of time perception: spatial and temporal brain mapping during visual discrimination tasks, Hum. Brain Mapp. 10 (2000) 49–60.
[3] R.D. Pascual-Marqui, C.M. Michel, D. Lehmann, Low resolution electromagnetic tomography: a new method for localizing electrical activity in the brain, Int. J. Psychophysiol. 18 (1994) 49–65.
[4] A. Smith, et al., Right hemispheric frontocerebellar network for time discrimination of several hundreds of milliseconds, NeuroImage 20 (2003) 344–350.
[5] J.A. Mangels, R.B. Ivry, N. Shimizu, Dissociable contributions of the prefrontal and neocerebellar cortex to time perception, Brain Res. Cogn. Brain Res. 7 (1998) 15–39.

International Congress Series 1270 (2004) 295–298

ELSEVIER

www.ics-elsevier.com

SERPs due to vibration presented at index fingers and selective-attention in the blind

Megumi Masuzawa[a], Hiroaki Shoji[b], Hisaki Ozaki[b],*

[a]Graduate School of Education, Ibaraki University, Mito, Japan
[b]Laboratory of Physiology, Ibaraki University, 2-1-1 Bunkyou, Mito, Ibaraki 310-8512, Japan

Abstract. Somatosensory event-related potential (SERP) was recorded in the blind and cerebral process of vibration pattern discrimination was examined. A large vibration pattern or a small one was delivered at a ratio of 8.5:1.5 to the left or the right index finger. Subjects were asked to push a foot switch when small-size pattern was presented at an attended side. EEG was recorded from 18 locations and SERPs due to large-size pattern to the left index finger were obtained. Regardless whether the left index finger was the attended side or the non-attended one, N80, N140 and P300 were observed in both subject groups. SERP within 200–230 ms under left-attended condition shifted toward negativity than those under right-attended one ($p < 0.05$) in both subject groups. As a difficult task was used in this study, this negative shift might be processing negativity (PN) with the prolonged latency at the central area. PN was also observed in the blind, but at the parietal area. PN in the blind might infer an involvement of posterior cerebral structure to execute selective attention. Under left-attended condition, sustained positivity after P300 remained until 580 ms in both subject groups. However, sustained positivity was not observed under right-attended condition in the sighted. As the subjects ignored stimulus to the left index finger under right-attended condition, sustained positivity might be concerned with slow wave (SW). However, SW was also observed under right-attended condition in the blind. Therefore, the blind might perceive not only vibration patterns delivered to the attended side but also to the non-attended side. © 2004 Elsevier B.V. All rights reserved.

Keywords: Blind; Somatosensory event-related potential (SERP); Selective attention; Vibratory stimuli

1. Introduction

As the blind are restricted in taking information through visual system, they tend to depend upon other sensory modalities, i.e., tactile and auditory systems. In braille reading, tactile system might be an absolutely necessary sensory channel. And blind people tend to be more dependent upon tactile information in shape recognition. Recent brain imaging studies have been disclosing a higher tactile sensitivity concerned with brain plasticity [1].

* Corresponding author. Tel./fax: +81-29-228-8292.
E-mail address: ozaki@mx.ibaraki.ac.jp (H. Ozaki).

0531-5131/ © 2004 Elsevier B.V. All rights reserved.
doi:10.1016/j.ics.2004.04.097

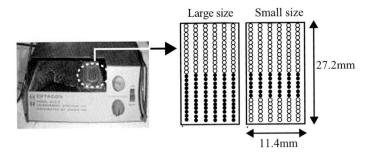

Fig. 1. Optacon and patterns of vibratory stimuli presented to the left and the right index fingers.

Dynamic process of tactile sensation has been studied using somatosensory evoked potential (SEP) [2]. Kujala et al. [3] also reported centro-posterior distribution of N250 in the blind, suggesting the cerebral plasticity might be concerned with their higher sensitivity in tactile sensation. Both findings were obtained while subjects were engaged in discrimination of tactile stimuli. Therefore, effects of attention should be taken into consideration to study somatosensory event-related potential (SERP). In this study, we recorded SERP due to vibratory stimuli in the blind as well as in the sighted, and examined cerebral information processing of vibration pattern stimuli to which selective attention was directed or not.

2. Materials and methods

Ten sighted (aged 21–24 years) and six totally blind (aged 15–55 years) participated in this experiment. Two Optacons (tactile reading device, Telesensory Systems) were used for stimulus presentation. Square pattern on CRT was detected by camera and was transformed into vibration pattern with 230 Hz. The vibration plate contains 144 solenoids (6×24) and 72 solenoids (6×12) were driven in large-size pattern and 36 solenoids in small-size pattern. Large-size and small-size patterns were delivered at a ratio of 8.5:1.5 to the left or the right index finger with various inter-stimulus intervals within 1.5–2.0 s (Fig. 1). Subjects were asked to push the foot switch when small-size pattern was presented at the attended side. EEGs were recorded from 18 locations including C3P (on equidistant location from C3 and P3) and C4P (on equidistant location from C4 and P4) with the linked earlobes as a reference. Vertical and horizontal EOGs were also recorded. After the artifact rejection, SERPs to large-size stimulus at the left index finger were obtained. After SERPs were offset by the baseline within 120–20 ms before stimulus, grand averaged SERPs were calculated. Then, two-factor analysis of variance was performed on mean amplitudes of each search window indicated in Table 1.

Table 1
Search windows used for measuring mean amplitudes of SERP components

Component	N80	N140	Processing negativity	P300	Slow wave
Search window	60–80 ms	140–160 ms	200–230 ms	280–380 ms	380–580 ms

3. Results and discussion

3.1. Selective-attention revealed by SERPs due to vibratory stimulus

In this study, subjects were asked to discriminate vibration pattern presented to the left or the right index finger. During subjects attended to either of index fingers, however, vibration patterns were also delivered to the other index finger. SERPs due to large-size stimulus at the left index finger were examined during left-attended condition and during right-attended condition as well. Therefore, difference between those two conditions might be concerned with whether the left index finger was the attentive side or the non-attentive one. Regardless whether the left index finger was the attentive side or the non-attentive one, various components were observed in SERP, i.e., N80, N140 and P300 (Figs. 2 and 3). And amplitude of these components did not differ significantly between conditions when subjects directed their attention to another side.

Therefore, those components might not be affected whether subjects attend to the left index finger or to the right one. Such finding was observed in the blind subjects as well. SERP within 200–230 ms under left-attended condition shifted toward negativity compared with those under right-attended one ($p < 0.05$) in both subject groups. Minami et al. [4] reported processing negativity (PN) in somatosensory modality, i.e., amplitude of N140 increased at the attended side compared with that at the non-attended one. However, the latency of PN might be extended when a difficult discrimination task was used in somatosensory modality [5,6]. We asked subjects to discriminate small-size pattern from large-size one. Hit rate of the target detection was rather low (40% in average) and pattern discrimination in this study might be difficult for the subjects. Therefore, negative shift within 200–230 ms might be also PN with the prolonged latency due to task difficulty. Such PN was also observed in the blind at the contra-lateral parietal, but not at the contra-lateral central area. As posterior contribution to tactile discrimination had been reported in the blind [3], PN in the blind might infer an involvement of the posterior cerebral structure to selective attention.

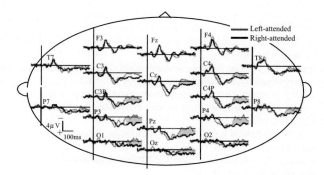

Fig. 2. Grand averaged waveforms of SERP due to vibratory stimuli at the left index finger in the sighted. SERP waveforms under left-attended condition are shown in thick lines and those under right-attended condition are shown in thin lines. Upward deflections designate a negativity. Significant difference was observed at search windows indicated by gray band.

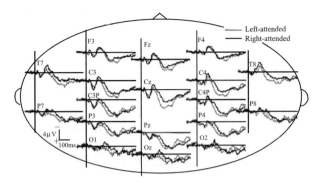

Fig. 3. Grand averaged waveforms of SERP due to vibratory stimuli at the left index finger in the blind. See explanation in Fig. 2.

3.2. Cerebral process of tactile pattern discrimination

Under left-attended condition, sustained positivity after P300 remained for a longer time, until 580ms after stimulus presentation in both subject groups. Such positivity was not observed under right-attended condition in the sighted. As the subjects had ignored stimulus to the left index finger under right-attended condition, sustained positivity under left-attended condition may be regarded as slow wave (SW), which might be concerned with discrimination [7]. However, sustained positivity in SERP in the blind was observed under both conditions. Therefore, the blind might perceive not only vibration patterns delivered to the attended side but also vibration patterns to the non-attended side. These results indicate the unconscious strategy of the tactile activation implying the semi-automatic information uptakes in the blind.

References

[1] N. Sadato, et al., Critical period for cross-modal plasticity in blind humans: a functional MRI study, Neuro-Image 16 (2002) 389–400.
[2] I. Okamoto, H. Ozaki, Somatosensory ERP in discrimination of patterned vibratory stimuli in persons with visual impairment, Clinical Electroencephalography (In Japanese) 43 (7) (2001) 448–453.
[3] T. Kujala, et al., Auditory and somatosensory event-related potentials in early blind humans, Experimental Brain Research 104 (1995) 519–526.
[4] E. Minami, K. Hosokawa, Y. Okita, Selective attention effect on the somatosensory event-related potential, Clinical Electroencephalography (In Japanese) 31 (7) (1989) 457–462.
[5] T.M. Patricia, Selective attention effects on somatosensory event-related potentials, in: R. Karrer, J. Cohen, P. Tueting (Eds.), Brain and Information. Event-Related Potentials, Annals of the New York Academy of Sciences, vol. 425, 1984, pp. 250–255.
[6] T.M. Patricia, et al., The effects of spatial selective attention on the somatosensory event-related potential, Psychophysiology 24 (1987) 449–463.
[7] D.S. Ruchkin, S. Sutton, L. Mitchell, Slow wave and P300 in signal detection, Electroencephalography and Clinical Neurophysiology 50 (1980) 35–47.

International Congress Series 1270 (2004) 299–301

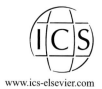

www.ics-elsevier.com

Changes in cerebral hemodynamics during a cognitive task after caffeine ingestion

T. Niioka*, M. Sasaki

Graduate School of Environmental Earth Science, Hokkaido University, Kita 10 Nishi 5, Kita-ku, Sapporo 060-0810, Japan

Abstract. The present study was carried out to clarify whether caffeine affects cerebral hemodynamics in the prefrontal cortex association area in young male subjects during a cognitive task. Relative changes in blood volume and oxygenation in the prefrontal association cortex were measured noninvasively using continuous-wave near-infrared spectroscopy. A modified Stroop color-word task we developed was employed as a cognitive task to activate the prefrontal association cortex. The results showed that caffeine ingestion affects cerebral hemodynamics during the modified Stroop task, and suggested that the decrease in oxygenated hemoglobin may be related to deterioration of performance on the cognitive task following caffeine ingestion. © 2004 Elsevier B.V. All rights reserved.

Keywords: Caffeine; Cognitive task; Task performance; Cerebral oxygenation; Cerebral activity

1. Introduction

The central nervous system stimulating action of caffeine is well known [1]. On the other hand, it is also established that caffeine acts as a vasoconstrictor of cerebral arteries and reduces cerebral blood flow [2]. However, changes in cerebral hemodynamics after caffeine ingestion during a cognitive task in which oxygen supply is required are so far unknown. Near-infrared spectroscopy (NIRS) is a new technique for noninvasive measurements of blood volume and oxygenation in the brain [3,4]. The Stroop color-word task, which is a cognitive psychological test, has been proven to be a useful tool to elucidate brain function [5,6].

The purpose of this study is to determine whether caffeine influences blood volume and oxygenation, which are measured noninvasively by NIRS, in the prefrontal association cortex during a modified Stroop color-word task, which we have recently developed [7].

---

* Corresponding author. Tel.: +81-11-706-2242; fax: +81-11-706-4864.
E-mail address: niioka@ees.hokudai.ac.jp (T. Niioka).

0531-5131/ © 2004 Elsevier B.V. All rights reserved.
doi:10.1016/j.ics.2004.04.055

2. Methods

Ten healthy, right-handed, young, male volunteers participated in this study. Subjects were instructed to refrain from drinking caffeine-containing beverages, such as coffee, tea, and cola on the day of the experiment.

The modified Stroop color-word task we developed is described elsewhere [7]. Briefly, the subject is instructed to select one of three colored disks presented simultaneously with one color word on a computer screen, according to the instruction (i.e., "color" or "meaning"). The color of the presented word on the screen is discordant with the meaning of the word. Three colors (i.e., red, blue, and green) are used. The order of appearance of the instructions and color words is randomized. Each trial is started by the tapping of subject himself immediately after finishing one trial. Subjects are encouraged to do their best to earn money prizes.

The blood volume and oxygenation in the brain were measured using a tissue oximeter (HEO-200; Omron, Tokyo, Japan). The oximeter [8] provides relative changes in concentrations of oxygenated hemoglobin (Δoxy-Hb), deoxygenated hemoglobin (Δdeoxy-Hb), and total hemoglobin (Δtotal-Hb=Δoxy-Hb+Δdeoxy-Hb) based on continuous-wave NIRS using two wavelengths (760 and 840 nm). Optodes of the NIRS device with a source-detector distance of 4 cm were positioned high on the left side of the forehead (below the hairline) of the subject.

Two successive performing sessions (pre and post) were administered as an experimental procedure. After a resting period, subjects participated in a 4-min performance session—the first task (pretreatment). After a resting period following the first task, each subject drank 100 ml of decaffeinated coffee supplemented with 200 mg of caffeine on a double-blind basis. A resting period of 18 min plus a 2-min anticipation period followed, and the subject again participated in the same performance session—the second task (posttreatment). As controls, the same subject drank 100 ml of decaffeinated coffee without supplemental caffeine, and participated in the same experiment on another day. The order of participation in these two conditions was counterbalanced across subjects.

Each session consisted of Baseline (one block, the last 2-min average of the resting period), Anticipation (two blocks, each 1-min average), and Performance (four blocks, each 1-min average) for three cerebral blood variables (Δoxy-Hb, Δdeoxy-Hb, and Δtotal-Hb). These experimental blocks were used for time course analysis. One of several indexes of performance employed to evaluate performance changes in the modified Stroop task was change in the number of correct answers in the posttreatment task compared with that in the pretreatment task. Alteration of the average value during the modified task from the baseline in each cerebral blood variable was used for further analyses.

3. Results and discussion

The task provoked increases in Δoxy-Hb and Δtotal-Hb, and a decrease in Δdeoxy-Hb during the modified Stroop task in general. The results were similar to our previous study using a mental arithmetic task as a cognitive task [4].

In contrast, the modified Stroop task after caffeine ingestion induced a significant decrease in time-averaged Δoxy-Hb or Δtotal-Hb compared with that in this task without caffeine ($p<0.05$; paired t-test). A direct vasoconstrictive action of caffeine on the cerebral blood vessels is reported [2]. Thus, the present results would be accounted for by the vasoconstrictive action of caffeine.

Change in the time-averaged Δoxy-Hb during the task was found to be positively correlated with the change in the number of correct answers in the posttreatment task compared with that in the pretreatment task under a caffeine condition ($p<0.05$).

These results obtained in the present study may imply that the decrease in oxygenated hemoglobin in the prefrontal association cortex was related to the deterioration of performance on the cognitive task following caffeine ingestion.

In conclusion, it was shown that caffeine ingestion decreased cerebral blood volume and oxygenated hemoglobin concentration during a cognitive task, and that caffeine might deteriorate cerebral activity.

Acknowledgements

Part of this work was supported by a grant from the Ministry of Education, Science, Sports and Culture, Japan.

References

[1] A. Nehlig, J.L. Daval, G. Debry, Caffeine and the central nervous system: mechanisms of action, biochemical, metabolic and psychostimulant effects, Brain Res. Rev. 17 (1992) 139–170.

[2] R.M. Julien, A primer of drug action, 7th ed., Freeman, New York, 1995, pp. 158–162, Chapter 7.

[3] C.E. Elwell, et al., Quantification of adult cerebral hemodynamics by near-infrared spectroscopy, J. Appl. Physiol. 77 (1994) 2753–2760.

[4] T. Niioka, M. Shiraiwa, K. Hasegawa, Changes in the regional cerebral blood volume and oxygenation during a mental arithmetic task and their relationships to personality and stress coping traits, Ther. Res. 22 (2001) 2004–2007.

[5] J.R. Stroop, Studies of interference in serial verbal reactions, J. Exp. Psychol. 18 (1935) 643–662.

[6] N.E. Adleman, et al., A developmental fMRI study of the Stroop Color-Word task, Neuroimage 16 (2002) 61–75.

[7] T. Niioka, M. Sasaki, Individual cerebral hemodynamic response to caffeine was related to performance on a newly developed Stroop color-word task, Opt. Rev. 10 (2003) 607–608.

[8] T. Shiga, et al., Study of an algorithm based on model experiments and diffusion theory for a portable tissue oximeter, J. Biomed. Opt. 2 (1997) 154–161.

International Congress Series 1270 (2004) 302–305

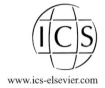

www.ics-elsevier.com

Cortical oxyhemoglobin dynamics during caloric test with near-infrared spectroscopy

I. Shimoyama[a,*], Y. Kasagi[a,b], S. Yoshida[a,b], K. Nakazawa[a,b], A. Murata[a,c], Y. Miyake[a,d]

[a] Section for Human Neurophysiology, Research center for Frontier Medical Engineering, Chiba University, 1-33, Yayoi, Inage, Chiba City, Chiba, 263-8522, Japan
[b] Department of Integrative Neurophysiology, Graduate School of Medicine, Chiba University, Chiba City, Chiba, Japan
[c] Department of Rehabilitation, University Hospital, Chiba City, Chiba, Japan
[d] Information and Image Sciences, Faculty Engineering, Chiba University, Chiba City, Chiba, Japan

Abstract. To study cerebral cortical function in equilibrium, cortical oxyhemoglobin saturation rate was measured during Caloric test for five volunteers. Near-infrared spectroscopy (NIRS) measuring backscattered reflection is a non-invasive, good method to study human cortical activation. Over both temporal areas, the oxyhemoglobin saturation rate changed during the irrigation to the auricle, the irrigation to the ear meatus, and during nystagmus. Caloric test induced various cortical activation; e.g., the sensation in irrigating iced water, vestibulo-autonomic response, vestibulo-ocular response, anticipation to the stimuli and so on. © 2004 Elsevier B.V. All rights reserved.

Keywords: Caloric test; Near infra-red spectroscopy; Oxyhemoglobin; Nystagmus

1. Introduction

Equilibrium is inevitable for humans to walk. The brain stem and cerebellum are well studied in animal experiments [1], but cerebral contribution in maintaining equilibrium remains unknown. Caloric test is good way to stimulate equilibrium as nystagmus [2]. Near-infrared spectroscopy (NIRS) is a non-invasive and good method to study human cortical activation [3,4]. We measured oxyhemoglobin saturation rate during the caloric test with iced water for five volunteers.

2. Methods and subjects

Oxyhemoglobin saturation rate was measured over the bilateral temporal areas with near-infrared backscattered reflection. The distance of the emitting and receiving probes

---

* Corresponding author. Tel:+81-43-290-3118; fax: +81-43-290-3118.
E-mail address: ichiro@faculty.chiba-u.jp (I. Shimoyama).

0531-5131/ © 2004 Elsevier B.V. All rights reserved.
doi:10.1016/j.ics.2004.04.094

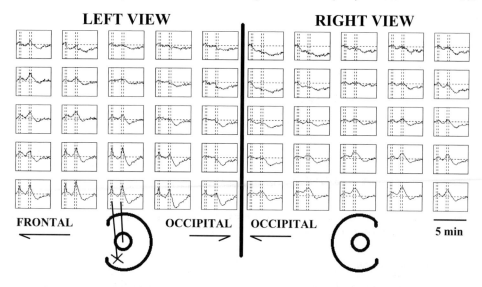

Fig. 1. One example of oxyhemoglobin saturation rate for subject-2. Saturation rate of oxyhemoglobin changed during at rest, irrigation to the left auricle, at rest, irrigation to the left ear meatus and nystagmus.

was 3 cm and the probes were arrayed 3 × 3 (ETG-100, Hitachi Medical, Japan) and 4 × 4 (OMM-2001, Shimadzu, Japan) for each hemisphere. The array was placed on the temporal area just above the auricle. Five volunteers, aged 36–55 years, lay at supine position with head up 30°. Following the visual inspection of the ear canal, 10 ml iced water was injected, and the eye movement was observed until after the end of the nystagmus by one otologist.

Two subjects were observed, the oxyhemoglobin saturation rate was measured at rest and at the caloric test with OMM-2001 [3]. Five subjects were measured while they were at rest, at the application of iced water to the auricles, and at the application to the external ear meatus with ETG-100 [4].

3. Results

Fig. 1 shows one example of subject-2 during resting, irrigation to the auricle, resting, irrigation to the ear meatus and nystagmus. A sharp upward increase was noted over the frontal temporal area in the left view by the irrigation to the left auricle. A sharp increase

Table 1
Auricle irrigation

Subjects	First irrigation (right auricle)	Second irrigation (left auricle)
1	no change	no change
2	no change	increase at left lower temporal
3	increase at right posterior temporal	no change
4	increase at right posterior temporal	increase at posterior right
5	increase at left central	increase both sides

Table 2
Ear meatus irrigation

Subjects	First Irrigation (right meatus)	Second Irrigation (left meatus)
1	decrease at both sides	decrease at both sides
2	decrease at left side	decrease at both sides
3	decrease at both sides	increase at left lower posterior temporal
4	increase at left lower temporal increase at right lower posterior temporal	decrease at both sides
5	increase at right posterior	no change
6	decrease at both sides	decrease at both central but increase at both anterior temporal
7	increase at right posterior	no change

was also noted by the irrigation to the ear meatus over the same area, and after the peak, the rate decreased on both sides diffusely.

3.1. Auricle irrigation

Table 1 summarizes the results for five subjects. The irrigation either induced an increase in the rates of the subjects or there was no change at all.

3.2. Ear meatus irrigation

Table 2 shows the summary for seven subjects. The irrigation either induced their rates to increase or decrease, or not at all.

4. Discussion

Increase of the oxyhemoglobin saturation rate has been reported in cortical activation [3,4]. Increase induced by auricle irrigation was suspected to be evoked by the sensation for water; increase by the meatus irrigation was also suspected to be evoked by the sensation for water and, moreover, by the noise of irrigation. Several seconds after meatus irrigation, nystagmus occurred gradually and lasted for a few minutes. Therefore, cortical activation in the caloric test is complex; caloric stimuli may induce not only vestibulo-ocular reflex as nystagmus, but also vestibulo-autonomic response as nausea or cardiovascular response. Some subjects had experience of the caloric test, while the others had none. Experienced subjects reported known anticipation to the whole course of the caloric stimuli, while naïve subjects reported unknown anticipation in the form of anxiety and being scared or experiencing amazing sensation, after the experiment. NIRS could be used to measure backscattered reflection for oxyhemoglobin and deoxyhemo-globin; therefore, the results showed cortical responses in the caloric stimuli. However, we cannot conclude about cortical activation specific to nystagmus from these results at present.

Acknowledgements

The authors are grateful to Shimadzu and Hitachi Medical for their courtesy in allowing us to use their instruments; OMM-2001 and ETG-100.

References

[1] M. Ito, The Cerebellum and Neural Control, Raven Press, New York, 1984.
[2] P.G. Jacobson, W.C. Newman, M.J. Kartush, Handbook of Balance Function Testing, Mosby Year Book, St. Louis, 1993.
[3] I. Miyai, et al., Mapping of gait in humans: a near-infrared spectroscopic topography study, NueroImage 14 (2001) 1186–1192.
[4] G. Taga, et al., Brain imaging in awake infants by near-infrared optical topography, PNAS 100 (19) (2003) 10722–10727.

ELSEVIER

International Congress Series 1270 (2004) 306–310

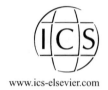

www.ics-elsevier.com

An fMRI study on autobiographical memory retrieval

Aki Horiike[a,*], Takahiro Kuroki[b], Katsumasa Sato[c],
Kazuko Terada[a], Wang Li-qun[d], Hiroshi Nakane[c], Chiaki Nishimura[a]

[a] *Department of Medical Informatics, Toho University School of Medicine, 5-12-16 Omorinshi, Ota Tokyo 143-8540, Japan*
[b] *Department of Information and Communication Engineering, Tokyo Denki University, Japan*
[c] *Faculty of Electronic Engineering, Kogakuin University, Japan*
[d] *Applied Superconductivity Research Laboratory, Tokyo Denki University, Japan*

Abstract. Autobiographical memory is a memory for events and issues related to oneself and may be differently structured from other memories. To clarify the difference, we investigated an fMRI study of activated regions in the human brain in autobiographical memory retrieval. Each subject experienced two types of tasks, TASK1 and TASK2. In TASK1, the subject was requested to read a brief sentence in which an episode in his/her own past was described, then to silently make an image of the situation in his/her mind. In TASK2, in contrast, the subject was requested to read a sentence describing the other person's episode, and to make its image. The block-designed fMRI measurement was performed in three conditions: TASK1 vs. REST where the subject laid at rest, TASK2 vs. REST, and TASK1 vs. TASK2. Both in TASK1 vs. REST and in TASK2 vs. REST, increasing relative regional cerebral blood flow (rCBF) was observed in the striate cortex, the supplementary motor area, the frontal eye field, the frontal association area, and the cerebellum. The area of activated regions in autobiographical memory retrieval was larger than that in nonautobiographical memory retrieval. In the comparison of TASK1 vs. TASK2, relative rCBF increased in the frontal association area and inferior parietal lobule. The result in the TASK1 vs. TASK2 condition shows the possibility that the neural activity in the prefrontal area is specifically related to an ecphory of autobiographical information. © 2004 Published by Elsevier B.V.

Keywords: Autobiographical memory; Functional MRI; Frontal association area

1. Introduction

Memory is commonly classified into two categories, declarative memory and procedural memory, and it is assumed that different brain regions contribute to various forms of memory processing. Declarative memory is further subdivided into episodic and semantic memory. Within episodic memory, a type of memory for events and issues strongly related

---

* Corresponding author. Tel.: +81-3-3762-4151; fax: +81-3-5493-5419.
E-mail address: akiho@med.toho-u.ac.jp (A. Horiike).

0531-5131/ © 2004 Published by Elsevier B.V.
doi:10.1016/j.ics.2004.05.011

to oneself is called autobiographical memory. It relies on complex interactions between episodic memory contents, associated emotions and a sense of self-continuity in the time course of one's life history.

Recently, PET studies [1,3] on autobiographical memory revealed the activation in the left inferior frontal gyrus, the left perihippocampal gyrus, anterior cingulate gyrus, and medial frontal cortex in the encoding process, and the activation in the basilic frontal area, right medial frontal gyrus, right posterior cingulate gyrus, right parietal cortex, and right insula in the retrieval process. In this study, we focused on the retrieval process in autobiographical memory and investigated the brain regions activated by an ecphory of autobiographical materials with event-related fMRI.

2. Materials and methods

2.1. Participants

Six healthy adults (five males and one female) were recruited. Mean age was 32.7 years old, ranging in age from 22 to 56 years. All were native Japanese speakers with normal vision and reported no history of neurological profiles. They were all right-handed.

2.2. fMRI measurement

Functional imaging was conducted on the STRATISII MRI system (Hitachi Medical). Visual stimuli were generated on a Windows computer as a brief text describing an episode and projected onto a screen beside the MRI apparatus, which was viewed by subjects using a binocular-mirror apparatus. First, anatomical images were acquired using a T_1-weighted sequence. Functional images were then acquired using an echo-planar sequence.

2.3. fMRI data analysis and modeling

Image preprocessing was performed using SPM99 software (the Wellcome Department of Cognitive Neurology, Institute of Neurology, UK). All statistical modeling was performed using a general linear model as implemented on an SPM99.

2.4. Preprocessing

For each subject, images were realigned to the original volume and resampled into a standardized atlas space defined by Talairach and Tournoux [5], using 2 mm isotropic voxels. They were then smoothed to a 14 mm full width at half of the maximum (FWHM) Gaussian spatial filter.

2.5. Statistical analysis

All measurements per condition were averaged across subjects. State dependent differences in global flow were detected using ANCOVA. Main effects and interactions were assessed by the t-statistics, subsequently transformed into the z-statistics. The resulting set of z values constituted a statistical parametric map (SPM$\{z\}$). Localization of maxima was reported within the standard space and their locations were superimposed on the group mean MRI image spatially normalized into the same anatomical space.

2.6. Experimental design

Each subject experienced two types of tasks, TASK1 and TASK2. In TASK1, the subject was requested to read a brief sentence in which an episode in his/her own past was described, then to silently make an image of the situation in his/her mind. In TASK2, the subject was requested to read a sentence describing the other person's episode and to make its image. A block-designed fMRI measurement was performed under three conditions: TASK1 vs. REST where the subject laid at rest, TASK2 vs. REST, and TASK1 vs. TASK2.

3. Results

The results in the three conditions were summarized in Table 1.

Table 1
The regions of increasing relative rCBF during TASK vs. baseline condition

Stereotaxic coordinate					
x	y	z (mm)	T	Side	Brain area
Nonautobiographical memory ecphory					
− 18	− 102	0	12.25	L	Striate cortex (BA17)
12	− 100	2	9.81	R	Striate cortex (BA17)
0	62	− 4	6.30	R	Frontal association area (BA10)
56	26	− 4	5.69	R	Frontal association area (BA10/47)
− 42	10	42	5.63	L	Supplementary motor area (BA6)
− 12	58	34	5.15	L	Frontal association area (BA9)
0	18	60	4.83	R	Supplementary motor area (BA6)
10	52	46	4.80	R	Frontal association area (BA9)
− 54	24	− 4	4.72	L	Frontal association area (BA47)
Autobiographical memory ecphory					
− 20	− 98	− 4	14.83	L	Striate cortex (BA17)
22	− 92	− 18	10.74	R	Striate cortex (BA17)
− 46	14	44	7.93	L	Frontal eye field (BA8)
− 6	8	68	7.73	L	Supplementary motor area (BA6)
− 2	62	− 2	5.85	L	Frontal association area (BA10)
42	34	− 22	5.71	R	Frontal association area (BA47)
− 14	58	30	5.64	L	Frontal association area (BA9)
66	− 50	6	5.23	R	Temporo-occipital area (BA37)
2	− 58	− 44	5.19	R	Cerebellum
2	− 30	8	4.97	R	Cingulate cortex (BA26)
− 4	34	56	4.92	L	Parietal association area (BA5)
Autobiographical vs. nonautobiographical memory ecphory					
− 26	60	4	6.03	L	Frontal association area (BA10)
− 48	− 80	26	5.00	L	Inferior parietal lobule (BA39)
10	48	44	4.78	R	Frontal eye field (BA8)
18	36	8	4.42	R	Frontal association area (BA10)
50	− 76	26	4.24	R	Inferior parietal lobule (BA39)

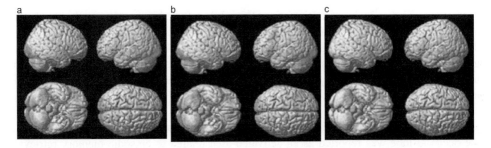

Fig. 1. Areas where increased relative rCBF was observed, in (a) TASK1 vs. REST condition, (b) TASK2 vs. REST condition, and (c) TASK1 vs. TASK2 condition.

3.1. TASK1 vs. REST condition

In this condition, increased relative regional cerebral blood flow (rCBF) was observed in the bilateral superior occipital gyrus and the inferior occipital gyrus (BA17, 18), the left frontal eye field (BA8), the bilateral supplementary motor area (BA6), the bilateral frontal association area (BA9, 10, 11), the Broca's area (BA44, 45), and the bilateral cerebellum. Fig. 1a is a pictorial demonstration of the situation.

3.2. TASK2 vs. REST condition

In this condition, increased relative rCBF was observed in the bilateral superior occipital gyrus, the inferior occipital gyrus (BA17, 18), the left frontal eye field (BA8), the bilateral supplementary motor area (BA6), the bilateral frontal association area (BA9, 10, 11), the Broca's area (BA44, 45), and the bilateral cerebellum. Fig. 1b is a pictorial demonstration of the situation.

3.3. TASK1 vs. TASK2 condition

In this condition, increased relative rCBF was observed in the left superior parietal lobule (BA7), and the bilateral frontal association area (BA9, 10, 11). Fig. 1c is a pictorial demonstration of the situation.

4. Discussion

We hypothesized that autobiographical memory is somewhat differently structured compared with other episodic memory. In this study, we compared autobiographical memory ecphory with nonautobiographical ecphory in fMRI measurement. The three experimental conditions, TASK1 vs. REST, TASK2 vs. REST, and TASK1 vs. TASK2, correspond to nonautobiographical episodic memory ecphory vs. baseline, autobiographical episodic memory ecphory vs. baseline, and nonautobiographical episodic memory ecphory vs. autobiographical episodic memory ecphory, respectively. Compared with baseline, both autobiographical and nonautobiographical memory ecphory demonstrated increased relative rCBF, commonly in the superior and inferior occipital gyri, the frontal eye field, the supplementary motor area, the frontal association area and the cerebellum. The volume of each activated region was larger in the autobiographical memory ecphory (Table 1). The difference in the volume is considered to reflect the difference in the mode of memory retrieval between autobiographical and nonautobiographical memory ecphories. In the retrieval of autobiographical episodes, more information might have been recollected and arranged along time axes of oneself than in simple imagery.

Activation in the occipital area would be partly caused by visual stimulus input (i.e. sentences), but it could be caused by the subject's visual imagery as well. In some studies, the occipital lobe was reported as an activated area related to episodic memory retrieval [2]. The activation in the frontal eye field and the Broca's area is supposed to be related to reading and interpretation of the input sentence.

Neural activation was also observed in the supplementary motor area. While the reason for this is still unclear, in some studies on episodic memory retrieval activation in this area was reported [2]. It would be speculated that the activation was related to an image in which some kind of body movement was involved.

Many studies reported activation in the prefrontal cortex during episodic memory-associated tasks, and it has been speculated that it may be related to a function of the prefrontal area, namely a center for controlling, sequencing and organizing relevant information [4]. The results of our study were in good agreement with the previous reports.

The activation in the cerebellum was observed in our study like many other studies on episodic memory retrieval [2]. Recently, the function of the cerebellum has attracted attention in relation to cognition, but it remains unanswered what the activation in the cerebellum during episodic memory retrieval means. Further investigation is necessary on this point.

5. Conclusions

We investigated the activated regions in the human brain related to autobiographical memory ecphory using fMRI. The activated areas in autobiographical memory ecphory were larger than in nonautobiographical memory ecphory, and the activation of the prefrontal area was specifically observed.

References

[1] G. Fink, et al., Cerebral representation of one's own past: Neural networks involved in autobiographical memory, The Journal of Neuroscience 16 (13) (1996) 4275–4282.
[2] R. Cabeza, L. Nyberg, Imaging cognition: an empirical review of 275 PET and fMRI studies, Journal of Cognitive Neuroscience 12 (1) (2000) 1–47.
[3] H. Fuji, Memory study with neuroimaging methods, Saishin Igaku 58 (3) (2003) 409–414.
[4] H. Niki, The role of the frontal area, Shinkeigaku No Shinpo 32 (4) (1988) 598–603.
[5] J. Talairach, P. Tournoux, Co-planar Stereotaxic Atlas of the Human Brain, Georg Thieme Verlag, Stuttgart, New York, 1988.

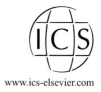
Functional MRI study on neural network dysfunction in schizophrenia and epileptic psychosis

Masato Matsuura[a,*], Mai Fukumoto[b], Eisuke Matsushima[b],
Tetsuya Matsuda[c], Tatsunobu Ohkubo[d], Hiromi Ohkubo[d],
Yasundo Nemoto[d], Noriko Kanaka[d], Takuya Kojima[d], Masato Taira[e]

[a] Section of Life Sciences and Bio-informatics, Graduate School of Tokyo Medical and Dental University, Japan
[b] Section of Liaison Psychiatry and Palliative Medicine,
Graduate School of Tokyo Medical and Dental University, Japan
[c] Brain Activity Imaging Center, Tamagawa University Research Institute, Japan
[d] Department of Neuropsychiatry, Nihon University School of Medicine, Japan
[e] Department of Physiology, Nihon University School of Medicine, Japan

Abstract. To elucidate whether there is a common or a different neural substrate deficit between schizophrenia and epileptic psychosis, we have investigated brain activation patterns during various eye movement tasks using functional magnetic resonance imaging (fMRI). Compared with normal controls, low capacity or inefficiency in frontal function during visually guided saccade task and striate–thalamic hypo-function during anti-saccade task was found both in schizophrenia and epileptic psychosis. Therefore, these findings may not be attributable to disease but to a psychotic state. On the other hand, right hemisphere hypo-function during a smooth pursuit eye movement (SPEM) task with attention-enhanced procedure was found only in schizophrenia and may be a specific finding in schizophrenia. © 2004 Elsevier B.V. All rights reserved.

Keywords: Functional MRI; Schizophrenia; Epileptic psychosis; Anti-saccade; Smooth pursuit eye movement

1. Introduction

The ability to suppress unwanted reflexive saccades and to generate voluntary eye movements is crucial for everyday life in the achievement of goal-directed behavior. The neural circuitry for eye movements has been elucidated in healthy subjects [1], and this circuitry is known to be common with the neural network for attention control. The abnormal voluntary eye movements are reported to be a genetic vulnerability marker for schizophrenia. Therefore, we have studied brain activation patterns during various eye

* Corresponding author. Section of Biofunctional Informatics, Graduate School of Allied Health Sciences, Tokyo Medical and Dental University, 1-5-45 Yushima, Bunkyo, 113-8519 Tokyo, Japan. Tel.: +81-03-5803-5372; fax: +81-03-5803-0165.
E-mail address: matsu.mtec@tmd.ac.jp (M. Matsuura).

0531-5131/ © 2004 Elsevier B.V. All rights reserved.
doi:10.1016/j.ics.2004.05.047

movement tasks to elucidate abnormal neural circuitry for schizophrenia using functional magnetic resonance imaging (fMRI). We have also investigated the patients with epileptic psychosis, whose symptoms are similar to those with schizophrenia [2], to clarify whether the same neural circuit is affected or not. If abnormal activation patterns are similar in both schizophrenia and epileptic psychosis, then findings may be attributable to psychosis. Conversely, if abnormal activation patterns are different between the two patient groups, those may be disease specific.

2. Subject and methods

2.1. Subjects

This research obtained approval from the ethical committee of the Nihon University School of Medicine. Written informed consent was obtained from all the participants after the procedure of the experiments was fully explained. The participants with brain structural abnormalities and those with gross movement of 2 mm or more while performing eye movement tasks in the MRI scanner were excluded. As a result, 21 normal controls (11 males/10 females, mean age 39.2 ± 10.2 years), 18 patients with schizophrenia (12/6, 34.8 ± 8.5 years), and five patients with epileptic psychosis (5/0, 34.8 ± 14.4 years) were invited. All subjects were right-handed according to the Edinburgh Handedness Inventory.

Because poor performance may result in bias toward reduced brain activations, the patients with schizophrenia were divided into good performance and poor performance groups. Between the two schizophrenic groups, the mean ages at the onset of psychosis (24.9 and 26.7 years), psychopathology determined using the Brief Psychiatric Rating Scale (41.6 and 42.1 scores), and total doses of antipsychotic medications converted to haloperidol equivalency (16.2 and 15.7 mg) were similar.

2.2. Methods

Using a 1.5-T clinical MRI scanner (Siemens Symphony System, Erlangen), brain imaging data were acquired with gradient-recalled echo planar imaging (EPI) to obtain blood oxygen level-dependent (BOLD) contrast encompassing the entire brain (TR 4000 ms, TE 62 ms, pixel size 3.0×3.0 mm, number of slices 40, FOV 192 mm, matrix 64×64, flip angle $90°$, slice thickness 3 mm). Each subject performed five series of tasks, alternating between 40 s of eye movement task and 40 s of baseline. Baseline is a fixation task on a central visual target ($1°$ visual angle) illuminated on a dark background.

An eye tracking instrument (Visible Eye, Avotec) was used for task display and eye movement monitoring. The eye movement tasks consisted of: (1) visually guided saccade task: generates a saccade when a visual target jumps to the periphery ($10°$ visual angle from the center, randomly allocated to the left or right on the horizontal axis) with a random interval from 500 to 1500 ms; (2) anti-saccade task: generates a saccade towards the mirror position of the target jumped; (3) smooth pursuit eye movement (SPEM) task: pursues a visual target that moves like a pendulum at a $20°$ visual angle with 0.5 Hz frequency; and (4) SPEM task with an attention enhancement procedure: counts the moving target that randomly flashes with a mean frequency of 1 Hz during pursuit.

2.3. Statistical analysis

Image analysis was performed using Statistical Parametric Mapping 99 (SPM99, Wellcome Department of Cognitive Neurology, London). Cognitive load-dependent activations can be obtained by contrasting between two tasks by random-effect analysis at a significant level of uncorrected $p < 0.001$ and cluster level corrected at $p < 0.05$. However, in the case of epileptic psychosis, the number of subjects was small and they were analyzed by fix-effect analysis.

3. Results

During the saccade task, the frontal, supplementary, and parietal eye fields (fronto-parietal eye movement circuitry) were activated in the normal control group. Among the patient groups, in addition to the fronto-parietal hyper-activations, the bilateral dorsolateral prefrontal cortex (DLPFC) was also activated during the saccade task (Fig. 1).

During the anti-saccade task, physiological enhancement of the fronto-parietal activations was found in controls and the good performance schizophrenia groups. In contrast, these cortical hyper-activations were not found in the poor performance schizophrenia, as well as the epileptic psychosis groups.

In addition to the cortical activations, the striate–thalamic activations were found during the anti-saccade task in the normal control group. However, these striate–thalamic activations during the anti-saccade task were not found in all the patient groups.

During the standard SPEM task, the fronto-parietal circuitry, especially in the left hemisphere, as well as the lateral occipito-temporal cortex (MT/MST) were activated in all

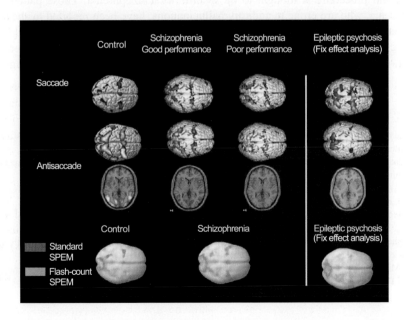

Fig. 1. Group averaged brain activation patterns during various eye movement tasks.

groups. (Because the brain activation patterns during SPEM were similar between the good/poor performance schizophrenia groups, they were averaged together).

During the flash-counting SPEM task, fronto-parietal activations in the right hemisphere were enhanced in the normal controls. While these attention-related right hemisphere hyper-activations were found in the epileptic psychosis group, these were not found in the schizophrenia group.

4. Discussion

Visually guided saccade is a reflexive saccade that requires a low demand on neural resources. In spite of this, fronto-parietal hyper-activation, including DLPFC, was found in patients with schizophrenia, as well as those with epileptic psychosis. This may stem from a low capacity or inefficiency in frontal function in these patient groups.

On the other hand, anti-saccade tasks need to suppress reflexive saccades and to generate voluntary saccades that place increased demand on higher cognitive resources. Physiological enhancement at the fronto-parietal activations was not found in the poor performance schizophrenia and epileptic psychosis groups. Therefore, this cortical activation deficit may not be disease specific, but may be performance related.

The striato-thalamic circuitry is capable of exerting both facilitatory and inhibitory saccades via two parallel pathways [3]. Although the present result was in accordance with the hypothesis that schizophrenia possesses a distributed cortico-striato-thalamic dysfunction [4], the striate–thalamic hypo-activation during the anti-saccade task may be attributable to the psychotic state.

In contrast, right hemisphere hypo-activation during the SPEM task with attention enhancement procedure is thought to be specific to schizophrenia. Those patients with schizophrenia, who are prone to auditory hallucinations, have been reported to show right hemisphere hypo-activity that is implicated in aberrant verbal self-monitoring [5]. The present results are in accordance with the evidence for abnormal hemispherical laterality in schizophrenia, which has been reported by recent fMRI studies on various language tasks [6].

References

[1] T. Matsuda, et al., Functional MRI mapping of brain activation during visually guided saccades and anti-saccades: cortical and sub-cortical networks, Psychiatry Res.: Neuroimaging (2004) (in press).

[2] M. Matsuura, et al., A polydiagnostic and dimensional comparison of epileptic psychoses and schizophrenia spectrum disorders, Schizophr. Res. (2004) (in press).

[3] G.E. Alexander, M.D. Crutcher, M.R. Delong, Basal ganglia–thalamocortical circuits: parallel substrates for motor, oculomotor, "prefrontal" and "limbic" functions, Prog. Brain Res. 85 (1990) 119–146.

[4] A. Carlsson, et al., Network interactions in schizophrenia–therapeutic implications, Brain Res. Rev. 31 (2000) 342–349.

[5] S.S. Shergill, et al., Engagement of brain areas implicated in processing inner speech in people with auditory hallucinations, Br. J. Psychiatry 182 (2003) 525–531.

[6] R.L. Mitchell, R. Elliott, P.W. Woodruff, fMRI and cognitive dysfunction in schizophrenia, Trends Cogn. Sci. 5 (2001) 71–81.

International Congress Series 1270 (2004) 315–319

www.ics-elsevier.com

The response of brain with chronic pain during spinal cord stimulation, using FDG-PET

T. Nihashi[a,b,*], S. Shiraishi[a], K. Kato[a], S. Ito[a], S. Abe[a], M. Nishino[a],
T. Ishigaki[a], M. Ikeda[c], T. Kimura[d], M. Tadokoro[e], H. Kobayashi[f],
T. Kato[g], K. Ito[g]

[a] Department of Radiology, Nagoya University School of Medicine, 466-8585,
65 Tsurumai, Shouwa, Nagoya, Japan
[b] Department of Radiology, National Hospital for Geriatric Medicine, Japan
[c] Department of Medical Information and Medical Records, Nagoya University School of Medicine, Japan
[d] Department of Anesthesia, Nagoya University School of Medicine, Japan
[e] Department of Radiology, Toyota Memorial Hospital, Japan
[f] Department of Health Sciences, Fujita Health University, Graduate School of Medicine, Japan
[g] Department of Biofunctional Research, National Institute for Longevity Sciences, Japan

Abstract. To evaluate the effect of epidural spinal cord electrical stimulation (SCS), the response of the brain with chronic pain was examined "before" and "during" stimulation, using fluorine-18 fluorodeoxyglucose (FDG) positron emission tomography (PET). The thalamus was considered to have an important role for the response. © 2004 Elsevier B.V. All rights reserved.

Keywords: Chronic pain; FDG-PET; Spinal cord stimulation; Thalamus

1. Introduction

Chronic pain is a widespread problem in the neurological and anaesthetic fields. Many studies, using brain imaging, have reported on this [1–3]. However, there has been no report to show the relation between SCS and FDG metabolism. In the present study, we analysed seven patients treated by SCS.

2. Material and methods

2.1. Patients

All patients complained of severe pain in the limb [complex regional pain syndrome (CRPS)] for at least 6 months and had no neurological disease.

---

* Corresponding author. Department of Radiology, Nagoya University School of Medicine, 466-8585, 65 Tsurumai, Shouwa, Nagoya, Japan. Tel.: +81-52-744-2327.
E-mail address: dr284@hotmail.com (T. Nihashi).

0531-5131/ © 2004 Elsevier B.V. All rights reserved.
doi:10.1016/j.ics.2004.05.010

Table 1

Individual analysis (each subject compared to normal subjects)

Subject	Condition	Side	Ant. ins.	Post. ins.	SII	ACC	PCC	Thal.	SI	DLPFC	MPFC	Pari.	Amy.	SMA	Mid.	Cerebel.	Temp.	MI
1	before	L	L↑R↓	R↓	B↑	B↑	→	L↓		R↑	B↑	B↑	R↓		R↓	B↓		
	during		R↑	R↑	B↑	B↑	→	B↓	R↑	R↑	B↑	B↑↓	B↓		R↓	B↓		
2	before	L		R↑	B↑	R↓			R↑	R↑	B↑	B↑↓	R↓			R↓	B↑	
	during				B↑	R↓			R↑			B↑↓	B↓					
3	before	L		B↑	B↓	B↓	R↓		L↓	R↑	R↑	B↑		B↑		B↓	B↓	R↓
	during		B↑	L↑	B↓	B↓	R↓		L↓	R↑	R↑	B↑→	B↑	B↑		B↑	B↓	
4	before	R	L↑	L↑	L↑R↓			L↑	L↓	B↓	L↑	L↑R↓	B↑		B↑	B↑		L↓
	during		R↑	L↑	L↑R↓	R↓		L↑	L↓	B↓	L↑	R↑	B↑	R↑	L↑	R↑	R↑	
5	before	R	R↑	R↑	B↓			L↑	B↓	R↑	B↑	R↑	B↑	B↑			B↓
	during			R↓	L↓				L↓	R↑	R↑	R↑	B↑			B↓
6	before	R							L↑	R↑	B↑	B↑	B↑	B↑		B↓
	during								R↑	B↑	B↑	B↑	L↓	R↑
7	before	R	L↑	R↑	R↑				L↑	B↑	B↑	R↑			R↓	R↑
	during			R↑	R↑	R↑			L↓	B↑	B↑		L↓		L↓

Group analysis (subjects 2–7)

			Ant. ins.	Post. ins.	SII	ACC	PCC	Thal.	SI	DLPFC	MPFC	Pari.	Amy.	Mid.	Cerebel.	Temp.	MI
			B↑	L↑	R↑	R↑	→	L↑	L↑	L↑	R↑	B↑	R↓	L↑	B↑	B↑	R↓

Left side (L), right side (R), bilateral (B), anterior insula (Ant. ins.), posterior insula (post. ins.), secondary somatosensory cortex (SII), anterior cingulate cortex (ACC), posterior cingulate cortex (PCC), thalamus (thal.), primary somatosensory cortex (SI), dorsolateral prefrontal cortex (DLPFC), medial prefrontal cortex (MPFC), parietal (pari.), amygdara (amy.), supplementary motor cortex (SMA), midbrain (mid.), cerebellum (cerebel.), temporal (temp.), primary motor cortex (MI).

Table 2

	Sex	Age	Disease and painful part	VAS		Stimulus sites
				Before	During	
1	F	54	lt. upper and rt. Lower CRPS	10	9	Th12
2	M	40	lt. upper CRPS	10	2	C7-Th1
3	M	35	lt. upper phantom pain	9	1	C5
4	M	64	rt. upper CRPS	7	1	C6
5	M	44	rt. upper CRPS	7	2	C5/6
6	M	52	rt. upper CRPS	7	3	C6/7
7	M	50	rt. lower CRPS	10	2.5	Th11/12

For subject 1, the spinal cord was stimulated at Th12 for the right lower limb pain.

2.2. Evaluation of the pain

We used a visual analogue scale (VAS) to evaluate the magnitudes of pain before and during SCS, and divided our results into two groups, i.e., an effective group and not effective group. When VAS decreased by more than 50%, SCS was effective for the patients.

2.3. PET scan and analysis

Data were obtained twice from seven patients. These patients received the initial FDG-PET scan before SCS; labelled "before". Then, FDG-PET scan was performed on the stimulus condition of SCS; "during". A Headtome-V PET camera (Shimadzu, Kyoto, Japan) was used. All conditions of the patients were compared with 13 normal subjects (11 men, two women, aged 27–58, mean 38.7). Especially, as an effective group, the "during" conditions were compared with the "before" conditions.

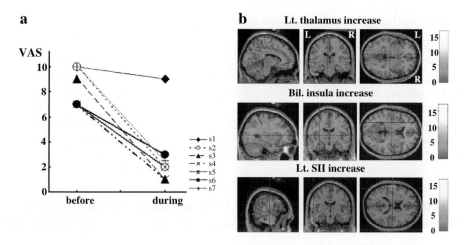

Fig. 1. (a) Showed good response of SCS for six patients. (b) Group analysis Effective patients ($P < 0.01$, uncorrected). The increase in FD6 was shown in the representative locations.

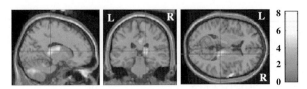

Fig. 2. The decrease of FDG was shown at the bilateral thalamus during stimulation of Th12 for left upper pain ($P<0.05$, uncorrected in subject 1).

SPM 99 (Welcome Department of Cognitive Neurology, London, UK) was used for statistical analysis.

2.4. Stimulus conditions

The electrical stimulus was delivered at a rate of 2–50 Hz, stimulus duration (0.3 ms). The stimulus intensity was 1–3 V. Each stimulus condition was decided for the patient. The patients felt the stimulation of the area innerved by stimulus sites on the spinal cord.

3. Results

Table 1 showed all results of both the individual and group analyses.

3.1. For the effective group (group and individual analysis)

Six patients showed a good response for SCS (Table 2, Fig. 1a). FDG uptake increased in the left thalamus, secondary somatosensory cortex, ACC, bilateral insula, DLPFC and bilateral superior temporal gyrus. On the other hand, FDG uptake decreased in the PCC, right temporal tip, amygdala, MI, MPFC and secondary somatosensory area. Representative responses were shown in Fig. 1b.

3.2. For the not effective patient (individual analysis)

SCS was not effective for subject 1. In the "during" condition, FDG uptake increased in the right primary somatosensory cortex, bilateral secondary somatosensory cortex, parietal, MPFC, and DLPFC. On the other hand, FDG uptake decreased in the bilateral thalamus, ACC, midbrain, and cerebellum. On the "before" condition, the pattern of FDG uptake was similar to the "during" condition.

However, the decrease of FDG in the right thalamus was observed not in the "before" condition, but in the "during" condition, following the stimulation of the right side at Th12. Representative responses were shown in Fig. 2.

4. Discussion

In the present study, during SCS, we found an increase of FDG metabolism in the thalamus for the effective group. However, for the not effective patient, FDG was decreased in the contralateral thalamus following electrical stimulation. This showed that thalamus uptake of FDG might be related to whether or not SCS was effective.

References

[1] M.J. Iadarola, et al., Unilateral decrease in thalamus activity observed with positron emission tomography in patients with chronic neuropathic pain, Pain 63 (1995) 55–64.

[2] R. Peyron, et al., Functional imaging of the brain responses to pain. A review and meta-analysis, Neurophysiol. Clin. 30 (2000) 263–288.

[3] M.S. Matharu, et al., Central neuromodulation in chronic migraine patients with suboccipital stimulators: a PET study, Brain 127 (2004) 220–230.

International Congress Series 1270 (2004) 320–323

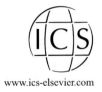

www.ics-elsevier.com

The relationship between the prognosis of motor dysfunction and pyramidal tract injuries

Keiichiro Kasai[a,*], Morikazu Ueda[b], Genn Kusaka[a], Hideaki Izukura[a], Keisuke Ito[a], Hirotsugu Samejima[b]

[a] *Tokyo Rinkai Hospital, 2-4-1 Rinkaicho Edogawa, Tokyo 134-0086, Japan*
[b] *Toho University Ohashi Hospital, Japan*

Abstract. MRI-estimated pyramidal tract injuries of 33 hypertensive cerebral hemorrhages in acute phase. The motor function prognosis of the hypertensive cerebral hemorrhage is highly related to the degrees of pyramidal tract injuries. © 2004 Elsevier B.V. All rights reserved.

Keywords: Pyramidal tract; MRI; Diffusion image; Motor function

1. Introduction

It is very important for the rehabilitation of hypertensive cerebral hemorrhage patients to estimate the degrees of the pyramidal tracts. MRI diffusion images of the coronal brain sections were used to estimate pyramidal tract injuries and motor function recovery after 6 months rehabilitation compared with the degrees of the pyramidal tract injuries.

2. Objects

Hypertensive cerebral hemorrhage 33 cases (Thalamic H., 14 cases and Putaminal H., 19 cases).

3. Methods

MRI diffusion images of the coronal brain sections were performed within 2 weeks of the hemorrhage attacks in all 33 cases (Toshiba 1.5 T, 2-mm serial scans, multi-slice scan,

* Corresponding author. Tokyo Rinkai Hospital, 2-4-1 Rinkaicho Edogawa, Tokyo 134-0086, Japan. Tel.: +81-3-5605-8811; fax: +81-3-5605-8113.
  E-mail address: kkasai-lj@infoseek.jp (K. Kasai).

0531-5131/ © 2004 Elsevier B.V. All rights reserved.
doi:10.1016/j.ics.2004.05.045

b-factor = 1000, MPG; three directions). Subtraction images were made subtracting isotropic images from anisotropic images. MIP images of pyramidal tracts were also made and evaluated three-dimensionally.

Motor function was estimated by MMT method in six degrees (0/5, 1/5, 2/5, 3/5, 4/5 and 5/5) at onset, 1 and 6 months after the onset.

The degree of the muscle power was degreed in six.

4. Results

Pyramidal tract injuries were estimated in three degrees. The degrees of pyramidal tract injuries were classified to three groups. Compression type (Fig. 1a): these pyramidal tracts were only compressed by hematoma and not injured. There were 15 compression type cases. The motor function of all 15 cases recovered completely up to 5/5 after 6 months of rehabilitation (Fig. 2a). The prognosis of the motor function of these type cases was suspected to be good and requires an early start of rehabilitation (Fig. 3a). Partial injury (Fig. 1b): these pyramidal tracts were injured partially, but not completely, by hematoma. There were 10 partial injury cases. The motor dysfunction at onset in these 10 cases was more severe than those of compression type (Fig. 2a). But in seven cases, the motor function recovered completely up to 5/5, and in the other three cases, the motor function recovered up to 4/5 after six months of rehabilitation. The prognosis of the motor function of these type cases was suspected to be moderately good and also needed an early start of rehabilitation (Fig. 3b). Complete injury (Fig. 1c): these pyramidal tracts were injured completely by hematoma. There were eight complete injury cases. In five cases, the motor function recovered up to 3/5 and in two cases recovered up to 2/5, but in the other case, there was no recovery after 6 months of rehabilitation. The prognosis of the motor function of these type cases was suspected to be very severe and require an early start of rehabilitation. The motor function, after 6 months from the onset of the hemorrhage, was highly related to the degrees of

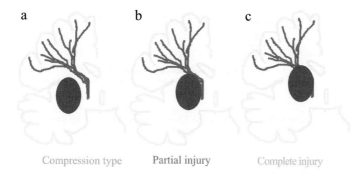

a   b   c

Compression type   Partial injury   Complete injury

Fig. 1. (a) Compression type: these pyramidal tracts were only compressed by hematoma and not injured. (b) Partial injury: these pyramidal tracts were injured partially by hematoma. (c) Complete injury: These pyramidal tracts were injured completely by hematoma.

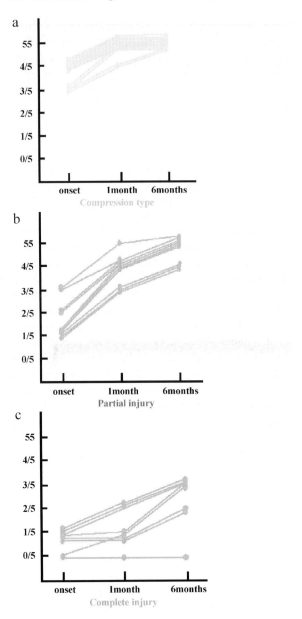

Fig. 2. (a) There were 15 compression type cases. (b) There were 10 partial injury cases. (c) There were eight complete injury cases.

pyramidal tract injuries (Fig. 3c). Compression type: the motor function after 6 months from the onset of this group is very good (Fig. 2a). Partial injury: The motor function after 6 months from the onset of this group is moderately good (Fig. 2b). Complete

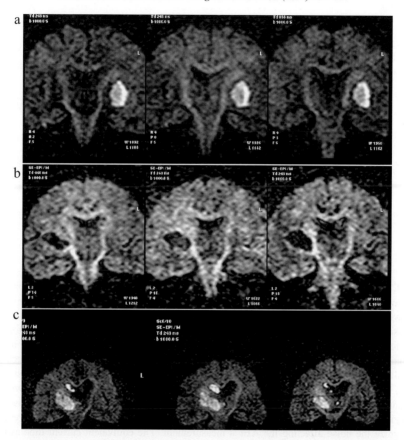

Fig. 3. (a) Case 1 (compression type): a 56-year-old man has sudden right motor weakness (MMT 2/5). The MRI coronal diffusion images (2 days after onset) show the inside shift of the left pyramidal tract, but the tracts remained continuous (a). The left motor function was recovered completely after 6 months of rehabilitation. (b) Case 2 (partial injury type): a 43-year-old man has sudden left motor weakness (MMT 2/5). The MRI coronal diffusion images (2 days after onset) show the inside shift of the left pyramidal tract and the tracts were partially injured (b). The left motor function was recovered incompletely (MMT4/5) after 6 months of rehabilitation. (c) Case 3 (complete injury type): a 63-year-old woman has sudden left motor weakness (MMT 0/5). The MRI coronal diffusion images (4 days after onset) show the discontinuation of the right pyramidal tracts (c). The left motor function was not recovered (MMT0/5) after 6 months of rehabilitation.

injury: the motor function after 6 months from the onset of this group is very severe (Fig. 2c).

5. Conclusion

The motor function prognosis of hypertensive hemorrhages are highly related to the degrees of pyramidal tract injuries, estimated by MRI coronal diffusion images in acute phase.

International Congress Series 1270 (2004) 324–328

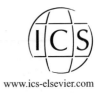

ELSEVIER

www.ics-elsevier.com

The effect of cotton roll biting on auditory evoked magnetic fields

Y. Kobayashi[a],*, T. Matsukubo[a], T. Sato[a], H. Nagasaka[a],
N. Sugihara[a], M. Yumoto[b], T. Ishikawa[a]

[a]*Laboratory of Brain Research, Oral Health Science Center, Department of Epidemiology & Public Health, Tokyo Dental College, 1-2-2 Masago, Mihama-ward, Chiba 2618502 Japan*
[b]*University of Tokyo Hospital, Japan*

Abstract. We have reported numerous clinical cases where a patient's unilateral chewing was thought to have reduced hearing ability. The purpose of this study is to determine whether occlusion and chewing function affect auditory evoked magnetic fields (AEFs). The subjects (seven males, 20–29) signed consent forms approved by the institutional ethical committee. A button sensor (FlexiForce™, Nitta) was used to monitor a subject's occlusal pressure. The subjects were instructed to maintain three ranges of their maximum occlusal pressure in each experiment. Subjects bit on cotton roll on the left or right first molar sites and were then stimulated with pure tone bursts (80 dB, 1000 Hz) from the left or right. The source localization was based on the signals recorded with the 36 planar gradiometers near both sides of the auditory area and the analysis was carried out based on the time-varying, multi-dipole model. The equipment used to monitor a subject's occlusal pressure did not recognize the noise affecting the AEF's measurement. The equivalent current dipoles (ECDs) measured at 20% or less than the maximum occlusal pressure, and between 20% and 40% of the maximum occlusal pressure confirmed existing in less than 1 mm by the MRI image as compared with control. This shows that the localization of ECDs exists in the auditory area at less than 40% of the maximum occlusal pressure. The AEF's response to a stimulus on the right shows a lower value compared with controls during cotton roll biting. Biting on cotton roll affected the AEF's response and the response was related to the strength of the occlusal force. © 2004 Elsevier B.V. All rights reserved.

Keywords: MEG; AEFs; Occlusion; Clenching; Hearing

1. Introduction

Over the past few decades, a considerable number of studies have discussed the relationship between occlusal conditions and hearing [1]. We have reported numerous clinical cases where a patient's unilateral chewing was thought to have reduced hearing

---

* Corresponding author. Tel.: +81-43-270-3747; fax: +81-43-270-3748.
E-mail address: kobayosi@tdc.ac.jp (Y. Kobayashi).

ability. We have also found that hearing ability can be improved by dental treatment and chewing instruction [2,3].

The purpose of this study is to determine whether occlusion and chewing function affect auditory evoked magnetic fields (AEFs). We wanted to find out how hearing ability changes with the improvements seen under occlusal conditions in clinical cases. We thus compared the responses in the human auditory cortex activated by auditory stimulation in healthy normal subjects biting on a cotton roll and those not biting on cotton roll by measuring their AEFs.

We used a quantitative method of measuring the AEFs of subjects biting on cotton roll on molar sites and evaluated the method of measuring AEFs under a constant occlusal pressure.

2. Subjects and methods

Seven males (right-handed, 20–29) participated in this study. The subjects signed consent forms approved by the institutional ethical committee and all procedures were undertaken according to the Declaration of Helsinki.

We monitored a subject's occlusal pressure by projecting it as a bar graph on a screen in a shield room. A button sensor (FlexiForce™, Nitta) (Fig. 1) was used for measuring the occlusal pressure. The button sensor was sandwiched between the cotton roll and fixed with double-sided tape (Fig. 1). This sensor does not generate a magnetic field when the tension is measured because the sensor film is laminated with a very thin admiration ink layer. The sensor is cylindrical and has a diameter of 9.5 mm (Fig. 1). The subjects were instructed to maintain below 20%, between 20% and 40%, or between 40 and 60% of their maximum occlusal pressure for 50 seconds in each experiment. In addition, an electromyogram (EMG) of the temporalis was recorded simultaneously with the AEFs.

A helmet-shaped, 306-channel neuromagnetometer (Vectorview™, Neuromag, Helsinki, Finland) was used for recording the magnetic field. We only analyzed signals from the 204 planar gradiometer at 102 points around the head, thus measuring the two orthogonal derivatives of the radial magnetic field.

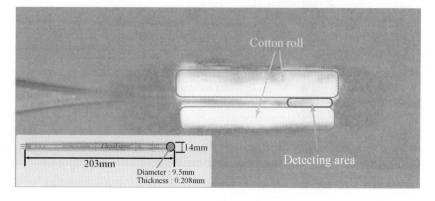

Fig. 1. Sensor sheet used for measuring.

Subjects bit on cotton roll on the left or right first molar sites and were then stimulated with pure tone bursts (80 dB, 1000 Hz) from the left or right. AEFs were then measured. The average of 50 AEF responses was taken for each condition.

All signals were digitized at 999 Hz and were band-pass-filtered (0.1–330 Hz). The EMG was measured to monitor the action potential of the masseters during biting. Each participant was monitored by electroencephalography (Fp$_1$, Fp$_2$, C$_3$, C$_4$, O$_1$, O$_2$) to check alertness. When epochs contained an MEG signal exceeding 1500 fT/cm, or when the subjects appeared to be drowsy, the measurement was excluded from analysis and an additional set of data was collected. Magnetic signals over fifty trials in a session were averaged with trigger pulses. The analysis period was set to 900 ms (100 ms before the trigger pulse and 800 ms after).

The locations of four head position indicator coils attached to the scalp and the anatomical landmarks (the bilateral preauricular points and nasion) in subjects were measured with a three-dimensional digitizer (Isotrak, Polhemus, Colchester, Vermont). At the beginning of each recording session, weak currents were fed into these coils, and the resulting magnetic fields were measured with the sensor array to find the head location with respect to the sensors. This information was used to align the MEG and MRI coordinate systems and to show the source locations with respect to the anatomical structure. The head MRIs were obtained with the 1.5-T Siemens Symphony system (Erlangen, Germany).

The source localization was based on the signals recorded with the 36-planar gradiometers near both sides of the auditory area, and the analysis was carried out based on the time-varying, multi-dipole model. We predicted the AEFs in each measurement. The localization of equivalent current dipoles (ECDs) is integrated on the MRI image. The moment of the ECDs for each experiment was compared using the graph (Neuromag) after confirming each ECD existed in the auditory area. The frequency analysis used the average of 50 AEF responses by means of Fast Fourier Transformation (FFT). The

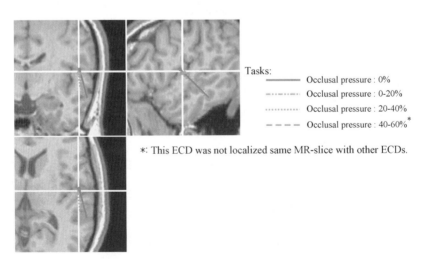

Tasks:
———— Occlusal pressure : 0%
–·–·–·– Occlusal pressure : 0-20%
·········· Occlusal pressure : 20-40%
– – – – Occlusal pressure : 40-60%[*]

[*]: This ECD was not localized same MR-slice with other ECDs.

Fig. 2. Right AEF localization in each task.

superimposed profiles of the AEFs suggest two responses related to clenching and an auditory response. Therefore, the moment of the ECD was analyzed by setting a low-pass filter at 28 Hz Fig. 2.

The averaged magnetic signals were digitally low-pass filtered at 40 Hz. The mean amplitude of the first 100 ms (from 100 to 0 ms) served as a baseline for amplitude measurements at each channel. We constructed isocontour maps of the minimum norm estimate. The sources of the dipolar magnetic field patterns were modeled as ECDs whose three-dimensional location, orientation and strength were estimated in a spherical conductor model based on the individual MRIs obtained from each subject [5]. The ECDs that best explained the measured signal at given peak latencies were first determined by a least-squares search, based on data of 36 channels over the response areas including the local signal maximum.

Only ECDs attaining more than 90% goodness-of-fit were accepted for further analysis, in which the entire time and all channels were taken into account in computing the parameters of a time-varying, multi-dipole model [4,5]. In the model, the strength of the ECDs was allowed to vary as a function of time while the ECD locations and orientations were kept fixed. The measured signals explained by the model were extracted with signal space projection [6], and a new ECD was identified on the basis of the residual field pattern.

3. Results and discussion

The equipment used to monitor a subject's occlusal pressure did not recognize the noise affecting the AEFs measurement. Using hard material, such as a splint with a button sensor to monitor occlusal pressure exerts a significant burden on subjects in such a task and can lead to problems with measurement accuracy. Therefore, we used a button sensor sandwiched between the cotton roll to monitor occlusal pressure. This made it possible to greatly reduce the burden on subjects during measurement. The method used here, then, is a useful approach to experimentally examine the effect of unilateral chewing on hearing ability. ECDs measured at up to 20% and between 20% and 40% of the maximum occlusal pressure confirmed existing in less than 1 mm by the MRI image as compared with control. This result shows that the localization of the ECDs exists in the auditory area when the occlusal pressure is less than 40% of the maximum occlusal pressure.

The FFT frequency analysis showed that the component required for sound stimulus exists in a low-frequency band, and the component required for cotton roll biting exists in a high-frequency band. Therefore, the low-frequency band was used for the analysis in the source modeling in this study. Table 1 compares the moment of the ECDs estimated with a left or right sound stimulus. The AEF's response to a stimulus on the right shows a lower value compared with controls during cotton roll biting. Moreover, although these AEF responses had an extremely low GOF (good of fitness), the low value of the moment of the ECDs was obtained during cotton roll biting.

These results indicate that biting on cotton roll affected the AEF's response and that the response was related to the strength of the occlusal force. However, we did not compare

Table 1
Localization and source strength of ECDs estimated

	Biting force change (%)	Latency (ms)	Laterality of AEFs	X (mm)	Y (mm)	Z (mm)	Q (nAm)	GOF (%)	V (mm)^2
Left-side stimulus	0%	83.2	right	42.4	6.9	54.2	62.1	91.1	75.2
		–	–	–	–	–	–	–	–
	<20%	80.5	right	51.1	8.1	58.6	32.7	88.3	66.6
		121.5	left	−40.4	13.9	52.8	37.8	74.4	4880.6
	<40%	77.8	right	52.0	4.5	55.3	25.7	82.8	107.5
		–	–	–	–	–	–	–	–
	<60%	77.8	right	47.9	−0.6	52.1	37.7	84.0	117.7
		–	–	–	–	–	–	–	–
Right-side stimulus	<0%	88.7	right	46.1	11.7	60.2	36.3	79.6	147.2
		–	–	–	–	–	–	–	–
	<20%	83.2	right	46.2	9.8	56.7	35.3	72.4	139.4
		99.6	left	−56.9	10.1	56.9	17.9	83.4	1316.0
	<40%	75.0	right	45.0	7.3	57.4	25.4	51.1	517.9
		118.8	left	−48.6	11.4	44.6	25.3	49.4	5151.0
	<60%	96.9	right	36.8	6.4	65.5	27.8	50.7	2186.5
		–	–	–	–	–	–	–	–

the AEF's response at less than 40% of the maximum occlusal pressure, so further analysis is necessary. It is difficult to consider the mechanism that biting a cotton roll has influenced AEFs directly. We need to confirm whether there is the same mechanism also in AEFs, although the gate control theory is accepted in SEF (somatosensory-evoked field).

Acknowledgements

This work was supported by a grant (HRC 3A10) and B-15390657 from the Ministry of Education, Culture, Sports, Science and Technology in Japan.

References

[1] J.B. Costen, A syndrome of ear and sinus symptoms dependent upon disturbed function of the temporo-mandibular joint, Ann. Otol. Rhinol. Laryngol. 106 (1997) 805–819.
[2] H. Nagasaka, et al., Hearing loss associated with habits. Shikwa Gakuho 100, 491–498.
[3] H. Nagasaka, et al., Changes and equalization in hearing level induced by dental treatment and instruction in bilaterally equalized chewing: a clinical report, Bull. Tokyo Dent. Coll. 43 (2002) 243–250.
[4] N. Nishitani, R. Hari, Temporal dynamics of cortical representation for action, Proc. Natl. Acad. Sci. U. S. A. 18 (2000) 913–918.
[5] M. Hamalainen, et al., Magnetoencephalography—theory, instrumentation, and applications to noninvasive studies of the working human brain, Rev. Mod. Phys. 65 (1993) 413–497.
[6] M.A. Uusitalo, R.J. Ilmoniemi, Signal-space projection method for separating MEG or EEG into components, Med. Biol. Eng. Comput. 35 (1997) 135–140.

International Congress Series 1270 (2004) 329–332

ELSEVIER

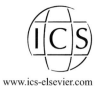

www.ics-elsevier.com

The neural basis of imaginary vocalization: an MEG study

G. Yoshimura[a,*], Y. Kato[b], M. Kato[b], M. Shintani[c], T. Uchiyama[a]

[a] Department of Oral and Maxillofacial Surgery II, Tokyo Dental College, Masago-mihama 1-2-2, Chiba City, Chiba 261-8502, Japan
[b] Department of Neuropsyhiatry, School of Medicine, Keio University, Japan
[c] Laboratory of Brain Research, Oral Health Science Center, Tokyo Dental College, Japan

Abstract. To explore the neural basis of vocalization, we measured visual evoked magnetic fields (VEFs) related to time-locked imaginary articulation using magnetoencephalography (MEG). We demonstrated a unique procedure, synchronized auditory stimulus with visually presented movies, and made comparisons before and after the auditory presentations. Since MEG measurements have high temporal resolution, we used visual stimuli with subjects to have the timing of silent articulation, and subtracted responses from each other. With this paradigm, the brain activities of the right temporal region at the latency around 160 ms were detected and supposed to relate the initial brain activity of word generation. © 2004 Elsevier B.V. All rights reserved.

Keywords: Neurosciences; Magnetoencephalography (MEG); Language; Cognition; Speech

1. Introduction

The spoken language is reported to be self-controlled by feedback mechanisms between sensory information of not only hearing but also the surface sensibilities of the oral cavity and articulation motions. The abnormality or disorder in part of the feedback mechanism may cause dysarthria, and clinically we often experienced this symptom caused by the wearing of dentures, stomatitis, or local anesthesia. But, unfortunately, there are few reports on the neural basis of vocalization and utterance [1], including these feedback mechanisms [2]. The whole function involved in speech is still unclear and controversial. The timing and location of the initial activities for vocalization in the human brain have been indeed of great interest among scientists.

Since noise deflection relating to muscle movements is a problematic confounder, specifically upon MEG measurements, experiences with actual utterance have been accompanied by great difficulties. Here we demonstrated the visual-evoked-magnetic-fields (VEFs) for imaginary articulation without actual utterance of letters through a

---

* Corresponding author. Tel.: +81-43-271-3978; fax: +81-43-270-3979.
E-mail address: yoshigen@tdc.ac.jp (G. Yoshimura).

0531-5131/ © 2004 Elsevier B.V. All rights reserved.
doi:10.1016/j.ics.2004.05.011

unique procedure in which the timing of silent articulation was controlled. We devised the new tasks that were designed to allow high temporal resolution and reduce the noise from muscle movement to a minimum.

2. Materials and methods

2.1. Subjects

Six normal subjects (two female) participated in this paradigm. They were all right-handed (according to the Edinburgh Scale) and had normal or corrected-to-normal vision. Subjects were fully informed of the MEG recording and written informed consent was obtained from each subject.

2.2. MEG recording

MEG was measured using a 306-channel, whole-scalp neuromagnetometer (Vector-view, Neuromag, Helsinki, Finland). The system was equipped with two orthogonal planar gradiometers and one magnetometer at each of the 102 measurement locations (arranged in a helmet-shaped array). The exact position of the head with respect to sensors was determined by measuring magnetic signals produced by currents leading into four indicator coils that were placed at known sites on the scalp. The location of the coils with respect to cranial landmarks was determined using a 3D digitizer (Isotrak, Polhemus, Colchester, Vermont) to allow alignment of the MEG and MRI coordinate systems. Head MRIs were obtained using a 1.5-T Siemens Symphony system (Erlangen, Germany). MEG responses were recorded using a 0.1–200 Hz bandpass filter and digitized at a sampling rate of 997 Hz. The analysis period of 400 ms included a pre-stimulus DC baseline of 100 ms. Epochs in which signals exceeding 1500 fT/cm were excluded from averaging, and an additional set of data was collected.

2.3. Stimuli and device

We prepared a unique paradigm that visual and auditory stimuli are presented parallel with synchronization in a sequential movie, which enables subjects to use timing to retrieve an auditory representation visually (Fig. 1). The task consisted of three sessions, which were performed by each subject sequentially, and event-related-magnetic-fields (ERFs) were measured separately.

1st session: Only visual stimuli were presented.
2nd session: Visual and auditory stimuli were synchronously presented.

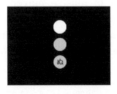

Fig. 1. An example of stimulus. In the lower circle, a Japanese letter of the pronunciation "nu" is shown.

3rd session: Subjects were required to retrieve auditory images synchronous to visual stimuli (no auditory stimuli were presented).

We presented the same movie throughout the three sessions with (2nd session) or without (1st and 3rd sessions) auditory output. In this task, a letter is fixed at the middle of the screen, and the subjects are instructed to concentrate on the letter in order to avoid the effects of extra-ocular muscle movement. A spotlight comes down toward the letter from the top of the screen in this movie, and when the spotlight hit the letter, the auditory sound of the letter is provided (only 2nd session). Thus, subtraction between the responses measured through the 3rd session from the 1st session would reflect the neural activity related to the retrieval of auditory images, which were presented again and again in the 2nd session. Ten letter words, i.e. "u", "ku", "su", "tsu", "nu", "hu", "mu", "yu", "ru", and "pu", were presented randomly in the sequential movie.

3. Results

In all subjects, three major components were identified within the time window of 0–300 ms in the waveforms measured at session 3. Peak latencies of these three components were approximately 120, 160 and 220 ms after stimulus onset. On the other hand, response measured through session 1 revealed two components, which were determined at the latencies of 120 and 220 ms in temporal processing. Subtraction waveforms between sessions 1 and 3 indicated an enhanced component at the latency around 160 ms, which was observed as the dominant at the right temporal region.

Fig. 2A denoted the grand average waveforms measured through sessions 1 and 3 and subtraction from representative subject 1. Fig. 2B also showed the spatial distribution of subtraction waveforms by means of a full view window.

Grand average waveforms from 306 channels clearly showed the temporal distribution related to imaginary vocalization, which were observed at the latency around 160ms, by means of subtraction from the response measured from session 1 to session 3. And, a full view window describing spatial distribution of the component observed at the latency of 160 ms demonstrated that this signal was dominant from the right temporal region. These

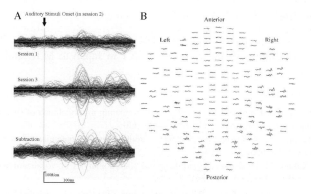

Fig. 2. (A) Grand average waveforms of 306 channels in a representative subject measured through each session. (B) Subtraction waveforms by full view window in a representative subject.

tendencies were recognized in all subjects, which suggested that the right temporal region was activated at the latency of 160 ms in this paradigm, and this component suggests imaginary vocalization.

4. Discussion

In this study, MEG responses to imaging of speech were evaluated using visual and audio stimuli. The results obtained were responses induced by imaginary vocalization, since the low-level properties evoked by visual stimulation were offset by subtraction. These results were in agreement with the report by Gunji et al. [3] in that the right insula is related to pharyngeal and laryngeal movement, and the possibility that the pharynx and larynx move during imaging of speech cannot be excluded. Another study reported by Hoshiyama et al. [4] mentioned that the brain activity for retrieval imagery of a sound occurs at the latency around 151 ms, dominant at the right insular region to the right inferior frontal sulcus. Our novel paradigm, "retrieving verbal sound," is essentially in line with sound retrieval reported by Hoshiyama et al. There was the possibility that the initial brain activity was observed from the right insular cortex, and this region may play the key role in initiating vocalization. The oral cavity, which is a peripheral organ of articulation and vocalization, cannot be separated from oral surgery, in which the prevention of diseases and treatment of postoperative dysfunction and disorders, as well as surgical treatment for diseases, are important tasks. The clarification of the mechanism of the central control of imaging of speech in healthy individuals suggests the possibility that causes of speech disorders due to sensory abnormalities of the oral cavity, such as loss of function and neuroparalysis due to congenital anomalies and surgical invasion, may be identified by central as well as peripheral approaches. Our method, which allows the determination of impaired or improved sites concerning articulation and vocalization and non-invasive examination, is considered to be effective for more precise evaluation of therapeutic methods. Our observations are considered to need verification through application of our method in patients with the above disorders.

Acknowledgements

This work was supported by Grants (HRC 3A04) for High-Tech Research Center Projects at Tokyo Dental College from the MEXT in Japan to M.K. and T.I.

References

[1] A. Gunji, R. Kakigi, M. Hoshiyama, Cortical activation relating to modulation of sound frequency: how to vocalize? Cognitive Brain Research 17 (2003) 495–506.
[2] A. Gunji, M. Hoshiyama, R. Kakigi, Identification of auditory evoked potentials of ones own voice, Clinical Neurophysiology 111 (2000) 214–219.
[3] A. Gunji, R. Kakigi, M. Hoshiyama, Spatiotemporal source analysis of vocalization-associated magnetic fields, Cognitive Brain Research 9 (1999) 157–163.
[4] M. Hoshiyama, A. Gunji, R. Kakigi, Hearing the sound of silence: a magnetoencephalographic study, NeuroReport 12 (2001) 1097–1102.

International Congress Series 1270 (2004) 333–336

ELSEVIER

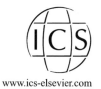

www.ics-elsevier.com

The activities of the central nervous system concerned with the recognition of periodontal tactile sensation Recording of SEFs following periodontal tactile stimulation and identification of the ECD in the postcentral gyrus in humans

Hideshi Sekine[a,b,*], Tomohiko Arataki[b], Ichiro Shimamura[b], Masataka Kishi[b], Yoshiyuki Shibukawa[a,c], Takashi Suzuki[a,c], Kiyoshi Mochizuki[a,d]

[a] Laboratory of Brain Research, Oral Health Science Center, Tokyo Dental College, 1-2-2, Masago, Mihama, Chiba 261-8502, Japan
[b] Department of Prosthodontics, Tokyo Dental College, Japan
[c] Department of Physiology, Tokyo Dental College, Japan
[d] Department of Pediatric Dentistry, Tokyo Dental College, Japan

Abstract. In this study, we confirmed the reappearance of the somatosensory-evoked field (SEF) responses following periodontal mechanical stimulation of the upper and lower teeth. And the equivalent current dipole (ECD) locations activated by the stimulation of the upper tooth were compared with those of the lower tooth. In addition, we investigated the influences of lack of periodontal pressoreceptive information under anesthetized conditions at the periodontal tissue of the upper tooth. For mechanical stimulation to the periodontal ligament, we used a nitrogen gas pressure-driven tactile stimulator. SEFs were recorded using 306-channel whole-head DC-SQUID neuromagnetmeter when the tactile stimulation was applied to the tooth. The SEFs were recorded following tactile stimulation of the tooth. Three peaks were observed in the SEF response. Although the ECDs of their peak latencies for upper and lower teeth were identified. There was no significant difference ($p < 0.05$) in the peak latencies between the upper tooth and the lower tooth. Under infiltration anesthesia conditions, disappearance of the SEFs was accepted. These results mean that the luck of periodontal ligament might lead to dysfunction of control system of mandibular movement that is related to neuro-muscular system. © 2004 Elsevier B.V. All rights reserved.

Keywords: Human; Magnetoencephalography; Periodontal tissue; Tactile sensation; Somatosensory area

* Corresponding author. Laboratory of Brain Research, Oral Health Science Center, Tokyo Dental College, 1-2-2, Masago, Mihama, Chiba 261-8502, Japan. Tel.: +81-43-270-3942; fax: +81-43-270-3943.
E-mail address: sekine@tdc.ac.jp (H. Sekine).

0531-5131/ © 2004 Elsevier B.V. All rights reserved.
doi:10.1016/j.ics.2004.05.075

1. Introduction

The purpose of this study is to record the somatosensory-evoked fields (SEFs) from the somatosensory area in the human cortices related to periodontal tactile sensation using magnetoencephalography. In the previous study, we identified the equivalent current dipole (ECD) locations in the bottom of the central sulcus near the primary somatosensory cortex (S1) and primary motor cortex (M1) areas bilaterally following periodontal tactile stimulation of the upper left central-incisor. In this study, we confirmed the reappearance of the SEF responses following periodontal mechanical stimulation of the upper and lower teeth. Then, the ECD locations activated by the stimulation of the upper tooth were compared with those of the lower tooth. In addition, we investigated the influences of lack of periodontal pressoreceptive information under anesthetized conditions at the periodontal tissue of the upper left central-incisor.

2. Materials and methods

For mechanical stimulation to the periodontal ligament, we used a nitrogen gas pressure-driven tactile stimulator which was taped to the labial surface of the tooth. The devised stimulator head with a "pin-form" was attached to the tooth surface using an individual plastic splint fixed in the mouth.

Four subjects were instructed to be seated on a reclining chair in a quiet magnetically shielded room. SEFs were recorded when the tactile stimulation was applied to the left upper central-incisor and left lower central-incisor of the subjects using 306-channel whole-head DC-SQUID neuromagnetmeter (Vectorview, Neuromag, Helsinki, Finland). In addition, three subjects were investigated regarding the influences of lack of periodontal pressoreceptive information under anesthetized conditions with infiltration anesthesia by 1.8 ml of 2% lidocaine with 1:100,000 epinephrine (Xylocaine, Fujisawa Pharmaceutical, Japan) at the periodontal tissue of the upper left central-incisor.

The stimulus was 0.15 MPa in pressure, 50 ms in duration, and 1000 ms in interval. Three hundred trials were averaged on the stimulating site. Isocontour maps were constructed from the measured data at selected points in time using the minimum-norm estimate. The sources of the magnetic fields were modeled as equivalent current dipoles (ECDs) whose three-dimensional location, orientation and strength were estimated in a spherical conductor model. ECD was first determined by a least-squares search, based on data of 20–30 channels over the response area. Only ECDs attaining more than 85% of the goodness-of-fit were accepted for further analysis in which the entire time period and all channels were taken into account in computing the parameters of a time-varying multi-dipole model. In the model, the strength of the found ECDs was allowed to change as a function of time. The ECDs were then superimposed on the subject's MR images to show the source locations with respect to anatomical structure, according to the alignment of the MEG and MR image coordinate systems.

3. Results

SEFs were recorded following tactile stimulation of the left upper central-incisor. Three peaks were observed in the SEF response (Fig. 1). At the contralateral side of the

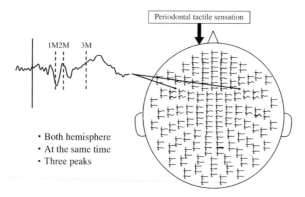

Fig. 1. Somatosensory evoked magnetic field: SEFs were recorded following tactile stimulation of the tooth.

hemisphere, the first peak was evoked at about 40 ms, the second peak at about 70 ms and the third peak at about 150 ms after stimulation, respectively. At the ipsilateral side of the hemisphere, their peak latencies were almost the same time as the peak latencies at the contralateral side.

SEFs were recorded following tactile stimulation of the left lower central-incisor. Three peaks were observed in the SEF response. At the contralateral side of the hemisphere, their peak latencies were about 40, 90 and 170 ms, respectively. At the ipsilateral side of the hemisphere, their peak latencies were almost the same time as the peak latencies at the contralatreral side.

The ECDs of the peak latencies were estimated from SEF records, in both sides of the postcentral gyrus at the same time. The ECD locations with goodness-of-fit better than 80% were transposed upon the MRI of the corresponding subject.

Under infiltration anesthesia conditions, disappearance of the SEFs was accepted in all cases.

4. Discussion

Many investigators have evaluated the SEFs in normal human subjects. SEFs after mechanical stimulation by air-pressure induced tapping which was applied to the forehead and occiput were examined by Hoshiyama et al. [1]. In this review, the ECD of the initial magnetic field was identified in the primary somatosensory cortex (SI) in the hemisphere contralateral to the stimulation. The ECD of the subsequent magnetic fields was identified in bilateral second sensory cortices (SII). Also, Kimura et al. [2] analyzed the ECD movement around primary cortical response elicited by the index finger stimulation, and SEFs were recorded over the hand area contralateral to the stimulation side. Hiraba et al. [3] mention that bilateral representation of intraoral mechanosensitive neurones in the S1 cortex might participate in recognizing the location of food in the mouth.

In our study, the SEFs were recorded following tactile stimulation of the tooth. Three peaks were observed in the SEF response. Although the ECDs of their peak latencies for upper and lower teeth were identified in both sides of the postcentral gyrus at the same time. There was no significant difference ($p < 0.05$) in the peak latencies between the upper tooth and the lower tooth. These results indicated that postcentral gyrus in the primary somatosensory cortices were responsible for processing mechanical information initially from the periodontal ligament.

The SEFs appeared in neither place of a cerebral cortex by tactile stimulation of the left upper central-incisor under infiltration anesthesia into periodontal tissue. It is considered that the disappearance of magnetoencephalo response at the somatosensory cortex following periodontal mechanical stimulation is caused with the infiltration anesthesia that influences mechanosensitive neurones from periodontal ligament and intercepts conduction of impulses from pressoreceptor around periodontal tissue. These results mean that the luck of periodontal ligament might lead to dysfunction of control system of mandibular movement that is related to neuro-muscular system.

Acknowledgements

This work was supported by Grants (HRC 3B08, 3B01) for High-Tech Research Center Projects from the Ministry of Education, Culture, Sports, Science and Technology of Japan.

References

[1] M. Hoshiyama, et al., Somatosensory evoked magnetic fields after mechanical stimulation of the scalp in humans, Neurosci. Lett. 195 (1) (1995 Jul. 28) 29–32.

[2] T. Kimura, I. Hashimoto, Source of somatosensory primary cortical evoked magnetic fields (N20 m) elicited by index finger stimulation moves toward mediolateral direction in area 3b in man, Neurosci. Lett. 299 (1–2) 2001 (Feb. 16).

[3] H. Hiraba, et al., The function of oro-facial neurons with the ispi- and bilateral receptive fields in the first somatosensory cortex of the conscious cat, Jpn. J. Oral Biol. 34 (1992) 481–493.

International Congress Series 1270 (2004) 337–340

ELSEVIER

www.ics-elsevier.com

Effect of pain alleviation by occlusal contact

K. Takahashi[a,*], Y. Muto[a], Y. Hirai[a], T. Ishikawa[a], M. Nishina[b], M. Kato[c]

[a] *The Third Department of Conservative Dentistry, Oral Health Science Center, Tokyo Dental College, 1-2-2 Masago, Mihama, Chiba, Japan*
[b] *Department of Internal Medicine, Oral Health Science Center, Tokyo Dental College, Chiba, Japan*
[c] *Department of Neuropsychiatry, School of Medicine, Keio University, Japan*

Abstract. The purpose of this study is to investigate the effect of cerebral cortex caused by clenching during stimulation of pain. Three healthy adult males were chosen. CO_2 laser stimulator was used as a stimulus of pain. Neuromagnetic activities of the cerebral cortex were recorded using a 306-channel whole-head neuromagnetometer, and the results were obtained by the averaged neuromagnetic signals in 100 times of stimulation in each rest position of mandible and intercuspal position. The peak latencies were approximately 190 ms in two out of three subjects. These amplitudes of peak latencies were reduced during intercuspal position, comparing with rest position of mandible. The ECDs were determined in temporal region. When their locations overlapped on MRI, the ECDs were located in the second sensory cortex. The ECDs were oriented towards the anterior and upper direction. These results suggested that occlusion might be a factor of pain alleviation in humans. © 2004 Elsevier B.V. All rights reserved.

Keywords: CO_2 laser; MEG; Occlusion; Stress

1. Introduction

Many authors reported that mental activity has been emphasized in orofacial function such as pronunciation and masticatory function. This is perhaps borne out by the Japanese proverb, "clench one's teeth in pain". Some studies with rats reported that biting significantly attenuates stress-induced noradrenaline release in brain and gastric ulcer formation [1–4]. The purpose of this study is to investigate the effect of cerebral cortex in human beings caused by clenching during stimulation of pain using magnetoencephalography (MEG).

* Corresponding author. Tel.: +81-43-270-3958; fax: +81-43-270-3959.
E-mail address: ketakaha@tdc.ac.jp (K. Takahashi).

2. Materials and methods

The ethical issue was considered according to the declaration of Helsinki. Three healthy adult males were chosen. CO_2 laser (OPELASER 03SIISP, Yoshida Dental Mfg., Tokyo, Japan) stimulator was used as a stimulus of pain. The laser wavelength was 10.6 m and the diameter of the irradiation beam was about 0.5 mm. The stimulus intensity was 1.5 W in output power and the stimulus duration was 50 ms. The stimulus interval of the laser beam was random, between 3 and 5 s. To avoid magnetic noises caused by the stimulator, it was placed outside of the shielded room, and the laser beam was carried through the optical fiber. The handpiece of the laser stimulator was set at 30 mm from the recipient site, central area in right carpal by using handpiece holder. The irradiated points were moved slightly for stimulus to avoid burns or habituation. Neuromagnetic activities of the cerebral cortex were recorded using a 306-channel whole-head neuromagnetometer (Vectorview, neuromag, Helsinki, Finland), and the results were obtained by the averaged neuromagnetic signals in 100 times of stimulation in each rest position of mandible and intercuspal position.

3. Results

The peak latencies of sub.1 and 2 during rest position of mandible were approximately 190 ms, while the peak latencies of sub.3 during rest position of mandible were approximately 120 ms. These amplitudes of peak latencies were reduced during intercuspal position, comparing with rest position of mandible (Fig. 1).

The position of the equivalent current dipole (ECD) of each deflection was analyzed. The ECDs were determined in temporal region during the rest position of mandible, the intensity of ECDs during intercuspal position became weaker. When their locations

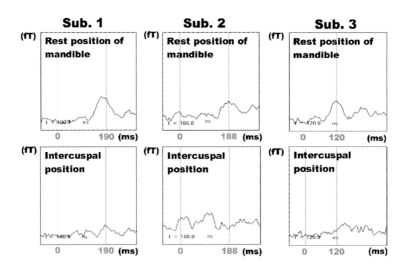

Fig. 1. Peak latencies. The amplitude of peak latencies were reduced during intercuspal position, comparing with the rest position of mandible.

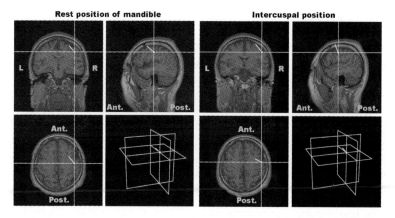

Fig. 2. ECD locations overlapped on MRI. The ECDs were determined in the temporal region. When their locations overlapped on MRI, the ECDs were located in the second sensory cortex. The ECDs were oriented towards the anterior and upper direction.

overlapped on MRI, the ECDs were located in the second sensory cortex. The ECDs were oriented towards the anterior and upper direction (Fig. 2).

The peak latency was delayed or the amplitude was reduced in some channels of temporal region during intercuspal position, compared with rest position of mandible.

4. Discussion

Kakigi et al. [5] reported that the onset and peak latencies following painful heat stimulation by CO_2 laser beam applied to upper limb varied in each subject, being about 140–170 and 180–210 ms. In our study, the peak latencies were approximately 190 ms in two out of three subjects. The same results were obtained.

Recently, some animal experimental research about stress and biting were reported.

Tanaka et al. [3] reported that when rats were exposed to a 60-min period of cold restraint stress with or without being allowed to bite a wooden stick, stress-induced noradrenaline release in the rat amygdala and ulcer formation in the biting group were significantly lower than those seen in the nonbiting group.

Gomez et al. [6] observed that stress-induced increases in central noradrenergic neurotransmission were attenuated in rats that were allowed to bite during stress caused by tail pinch, and he concluded that the expression of parafunctional masticatory activity attenuates the effect of stress on central catecholaminergic neurotransmission.

Sato et al. [7] also suggested that the masticatory activity plays a role in effecting the restraint of stress-induced psychosomatic disorders by down-regulating the limbic system.

In our study, the intensity of peak latency during intercuspal position was reduced more than that seen in the rest position of mandible. Therefore, occlusion or biting might be a factor of pain alleviation in human.

The present study reported the importance of masticatory function related to stress management. Consequently, the systemic effect of occlusal adjustment, including somatic system, will be emphasized more.

Acknowledgements

This work was supported by a Grant (HRC 3A09) for High-Tech Research Center Projects of Tokyo Dental College from the MEXT, Japanese Government.

References

[1] A. Tsuda, et al., Expression of aggression attenuates stress-induced increases in rat brain noradrenaline turnover, Brain Res. 474 (1988) 174–180.

[2] M. Tanaka, et al., Psychological stress-induced increases in noradrenaline release in rat brain regions are attenuated by diazepam, but not by morphine, Pharmacol. Biochem. Behav. 39 (1991) 191–195.

[3] T. Tanaka, et al., Expression of aggression attenuates both stress-induced gastric ulcer formation and increases in noradrenaline release in the rat amygdala assessed by intracerebral microdialysis, Pharmacol. Biochem. Behav. 59 (1998) 27–31.

[4] M. Tanaka, Emotional stress and characteristics of brain noradrenaline release in the rat, Ind. Health 37 (1999) 143–156.

[5] R. Kakigi, et al., Pain-related magnetic fields following painful CO_2 laser stimulation in man, Neurosci. Lett. 192 (1995) 45–48.

[6] F.M. Gomez, et al., A possible attenuation of stress-induced increases in striatal dopamine metabolism by the expression of non-functional masticatory activity in the rat, Eur. J. Oral Sci. 107 (1999) 461–467.

[7] S. Sato, et al., The masticatory organ, brain function, stress-release, and a proposal to add a new category to the taxonomy of the healing arts: occlusion medicine, Bull. Kanagawa Dent. Coll. 30 (2002) 117–126.

International Congress Series 1270 (2004) 341–344

www.ics-elsevier.com

Visual cognitive function of patients with unilateral spatial neglect and a new objective diagnostic method by measuring eye movement

Yu Chiba[a,b,*], Akira Yamaguchi[a], Shogo Fukushima[c], Shuji Murakami[c], Satoru Inakagata[c], Fumio Eto[b]

[a] *Department of Rehabilitation, National Center of Neurology and Psychiatry, Tokyo, Japan*
[b] *Department of Rehabilitation, Graduate School of Medicine, University of Tokyo, Tokyo, Japan*
[c] *Matsushita Electric Works, 1048 Oaza Kadoma, Kadoma, Osaka, Japan*

Abstract. Left unilateral spatial neglect is caused by brain damage in the right hemisphere. Other than a subjective method such as line bisection test in which a patient is requested to draw the mark at the center of the line, recording of eye movement has been evaluated as an objective diagnostic method. As a measurement tool, electro-oculography or an eye camera has been used for recording of eye movement. However, such conventional recording systems are interrupted by head movement. The authors have developed a new head set which has two functions simultaneously, measuring eye movement and presenting visual image for both eyes. Since the relative geometrical association with each other's coordinates system for measurement and presentation is absolutely fixed, the developed head set is robust to head movement. © 2004 Elsevier B.V. All rights reserved.

Keywords: Unilateral spatial neglect; Eye movement; Visual image presentation

1. Introduction

Unilateral neglect (UN) is a condition in which the brain-damaged patient fails to respond to stimuli on the side opposite to the lesion. Severe unilateral neglect is common after large injury to the right hemisphere. The condition is regarded as heterogeneous [1]. It is divided generally into two disorders. One is the perceptual neglect such as disorder of mental representation [2] and spatial misperception [3]. The other is motor neglect such as directional hypokinesia [4]. In addition, most of UN patients suffer from other disorders. Intelligence impairment, hypobulia and impaired consciousness are frequently observed in UN patients. Therefore, it is not easy to assess

---

* Corresponding author. Department of Rehabilitation, National Center of Neurology and Psychiatry, 4-1-1, Ogawahigashimachi, Kodaira, Tokyo 187-8511, Japan. Tel.: +81-42-341-2711; fax: +81-42-346-1705.
E-mail address: ychiba@violin.ocn.ne.jp (Y. Chiba).

0531-5131/ © 2004 Elsevier B.V. All rights reserved.
doi:10.1016/j.ics.2004.05.070

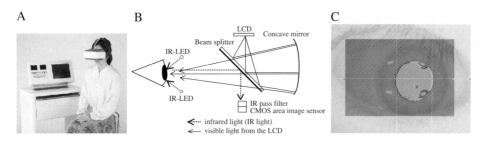

Fig. 1. (A) System appearance of the developed head set and visual image controller, (B) schematic of the optical system inside the developed head set, and (C) a sample of the processed eye image.

the severity of pure UN by conventional subjective methods such as pencil-and-paper type tests.

Many standard tests for neglect include pencil-and-paper type tests, such as line bisection [5], line cancellation [6], copying and drawing [7]. However, such conventional tests demand both sensory cognition and motor movement, which increases the difficulty of diagnosis. Furthermore, because of the intellectual demands in addition to cognitive ones in the tests, it is difficult to assess pure sensory neglect quantitatively. In order to overcome the current situation, the authors have developed a new device and designed a new method, which minimized motor bias, and then which enable us to assess pure sensory neglect.

2. Material and methods

2.1. Subjects

A 60-year-old, right-handed male patient was selected. He has right hemisphere cerebral infarction. He showed a left homonymous hemianopia by confrontation. There was no limitation of eye movement. Severe left hemiparesis and a left-sided sensory disturbance were presented. His score of the regular task of Behavioural Inattention Test [8] is 125/146. Brain CT scan showed a lesion involving right caudate nucleus and internal capsule. He provided written informed consent before testing and was examined with local ethical committee approval.

Table 1
Specifications of the developed system

Image presentation	Horizontal visual field angle	45°
	Vertical visual field angle	35°
	Distance from eyes	1.4 m
Eye measurement	Horizontal resolution	0.1°
	Vertical resolution	0.2°
	Time resolution	60 Hz
Human factors	Inter pupil distance	58.0–68.0 mm
	Eye relief	15.0 mm

M0 (subjective midpoint of the straight line) → R0 (right; 20.0 deg) → R1 (right 10.3 deg) → C0
(center; 0.0 deg) → L0 (left; 10.3 deg) → L1 (left 20.0 deg) →
  M1 (subjective midpoint of the straight line) → R2 (right; 20.0 deg) → R3 (right 10.3 deg) → C1
(center; 0.0 deg) → L2 (left; 10.3 deg) → L3 (left 20.0 deg)

Fig. 2. The sequence procedure of the gaze point to the target instructed to the subject to gaze at.

2.2. Apparatus

The authors have developed a new measurement system in which a head set can not only detect eye movement, but also simultaneously present visual video images. The appearance of the whole system and the schematic of the optics in the head set are shown in Fig. 1A and B, respectively. A subject can only view the virtual image generated by the embedded liquid crystal displays in the head set. Concerning detection of eye movement, a CMOS image sensor was utilized in infrared band area. Two coordinate systems of eye movement measurement and visual presentation are always fixed inside the head set, the wearer is not forced to fix his/her head without movement, which feature made the measurement more reliable. As shown in Table 1, the subject can view the virtual image for 45° in the horizontal field at the distance of 1.4 m. A sample of the obtained eye image, as shown in Fig. 1C, can be automatically processed to calculate eye movement data at sampling rate of 60 Hz.

2.3. Procedure

The subject was instructed to gaze at the subjective midpoint of a horizontal straight-line (M0 shown in Fig. 2) which length ranges from 20.0° right to the same degree left. Next, after the straight-line was turned off, a target appeared in the specific direction as the following sequence shown in Fig. 2 (R0, R1, C0, L0, L1). Such sequence was repeated twice. Only one target was displayed at any time.

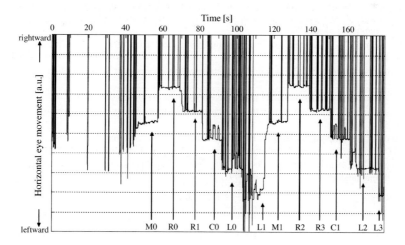

Fig. 3. The right eye movement of the patient while gazing at the targets.

3. Results

Fig. 3 shows the result of the subject's right eye movement while gazing at the targets. In the figure, a lot of sudden rises indicate occurrence of eye blinks. The stops of fixations corresponding to each target shown in Fig. 2 can be easily seen. However, fixations leftward such as L0 and L1 are more unstable than those rightward such as R0 and R1. This instability indicates the presence of UN. In addition, though M0, M1 C0, C1 are located at the same position geometrically in the visual field, the points of fixation corresponding to the subjective midpoint of the straight line (M0, M1) are deviated from the center (C0, C1) to the right direction. The degree of this deviation represents the severity of the patient's sensory neglect.

4. Discussion

In this study, we attempted to develop a new device that minimises motor and other kind of bias and that enable us to asses sensory neglect.

Past studies reported that sensory and motor neglect are dissociable [9,10]. However the studies attempting to demonstrate sensory bias are few. In the presented method, directional and intentional motor bias is minimized in reaction. Therefore, it is considered that the rightward deviation of gaze represents sensory bias that was eliminated from other bias.

As an additional advantage of the method, the test can be easily carried out. It is physically and intellectually much less demanding on the patients than the conventional pencil- and paper type description test. Therefore it may be applicable even to the patient for whom a normal standard description test is not suitable.

References

[1] E. Bisiach, V. Giuseppe, Unilateral neglect in humans, 2nd edition. In Handbook of neuropsychology, Laird S. Cermak, Elsevier 2000, pp. 459–502.
[2] E. Bisiach, C. Luzzatti, Unilateral neglect of representational space, Cortex 14 (1978) 129–133.
[3] A.D. Milner, M. Harvey, C.L. Pritchard, Visual size processing in spatial neglect, Exp. Brain Res. 123 (1–2) (1998) 192–200.
[4] K.M. Heilman, E. Valenstein, Mechanisms underlying hemispatial neglect, Ann. Neurol. 5 (2) (1979) 166–170.
[5] A. Colombo, E. De Renzi, P. Faglioni, The occurrence of visual neglect in patients with unilateral cerebral disease, Cortex 12 (3) (1976) 221–231.
[6] M.L. Albert, A simple test of visual neglect, Neurology 23 (6) (1973) 658–664.
[7] E. Bisiach, et al., Brain and conscious representation of outside reality, Neuropsychologia 19 (4) (1981) 543–551.
[8] B. Wilson, J. Cockburn, P. Halligan, Behavioural inattention test, Thames Valley Test, Amsterdam, 1987.
[9] E. Bisiach, et al., Perceptual and premotor factors of unilateral neglect, Neurology 40 (8) (1990) 1278–1281.
[10] R. Tegner, M. Levander, Through a looking glass, A new technique to demonstrate directional hypokinesia in unilateral neglect, Brain 114 (PT 4) (1991) 1943–1951.

International Congress Series 1270 (2004) 345–347

www.ics-elsevier.com

EEG source gravity center location changes after a single dose of atypical antipsychotics in healthy volunteers

Toshiaki Isotani[a,*], Keizo Yamada[a], Satoshi Irisawa[a],
Masafumi Yoshimura[a], Aran Tajika[b], Naomi Saito[c],
Takami Yagyu[a], Akemi Saito[a], Toshihiko Kinoshita[a]

[a] Department of Neuropsychiatry, Kansai Medical University, 10-15 Fumizono-cho, Moriguchi,
Osaka 570-8506, Japan
[b] Department of Public Health, Kansai Medical University, Osaka, Japan
[c] Saito Neuropsychiatric Clinic, Osaka, Japan

Abstract. EEG source localization effects of 4 different novel atypical antipsychotics were compared with 2 conventional typical antipsychotics and a placebo in 14 male, right-handed normals (24.1 ± 4.1 years). All subjects went through seven sessions. In each session, a subject received orally either 0.5-mg risperidone, 4-mg perospirone, 33-mg quetiapine, 1.25-mg olanzapine, 50-mg chlorpromazine, 1-mg haloperidol or placebo according to a single-blind, crossover, Latin-square design. EEG was recorded from 19 scalp-electrodes prior to as well as 2, 4 and 6 h after drug administration. Twenty-second artifact-free/subject/drug/time-point EEG were analyzed into FFT dipole approximation source models for seven frequency bands. Assuming the maximal effect would correspond to serum-concentration, 2 h after perospirone and quetiapine, 4 h after risperidone, olanzapine and chlorpromazine, and 6 h after haloperidol were chosen. Differences from pre-drug source gravity center locations (3D values) were compared using one-way repeated measures ANOVAs, then post-hoc LSD multiple comparisons were applied. The source gravity center of excitatory β3 frequency band (21.5–30 Hz) after perospirone was more right than after risperidone, olanzapine, chlorpromazine and placebo, while after quetiapine and haloperidol were more right than after olanzapine ($p < 0.05$). Our results suggest that the seven test drugs including placebo acted differently on neural populations after a single administration. © 2004 Elsevier B.V. All rights reserved.

Keywords: Human multi-channel EEG; Quantitative pharmaco-EEG; EEG source localization; FFT dipole approximation; Risperidone; Perospirone; Quetiapine; Olanzapine

* Corresponding author. Tel.: +81-6-6992-1001; fax: +81-6-6995-2669.
E-mail address: isotani@takii.kmu.ac.jp (T. Isotani).

1. Introduction

Are there differences, demonstrable effects on EEG source localization among atypical antipsychotic agents? We compared source gravity center locations of brain electric activity after a single dose of four atypical antipsychotics or two conventional antipsychotics with placebo in healthy subjects using FFT dipole approximation.

2. Materials and methods

Fourteen right-handed healthy male volunteers (mean age $\pm$ S.D. = 24.1 $\pm$ 4.1 years) who participated in this study gave their written consent after being fully informed about the study. The study was approved by the institutional review board of Osaka Pharmacology Research Clinic.

The study was designed to be single-blind, crossover, two-fold Latin square. All subjects went through 7 session days. On each session day, each subject received either 0.5-mg risperidone, 4-mg perospirone, 33-mg quetiapine, 1.25-mg olanzapine, 50-mg chlorpromazine, 1-mg haloperidol or placebo. The doses were decided to be equivalent to 1-mg haloperidol. EEGs were recorded from 19 scalp electrodes (band-pass: 0.3–60 Hz, A/D sampling time: 128 Hz) prior to as well as 2, 4 and 6 h after each drug administration.

A sample of the 20-s EEG/subject/drug/time-point was analyzed into FFT dipole approximation (modeling by a single generator process) [1] for seven independent frequency bands (δ: 1.5–6 Hz, θ: 6.5–8 Hz, $\alpha 1$: 8.5–10 Hz, $\alpha 2$: 10.5–12 Hz, $\beta 1$: 12.5–18 Hz, $\beta 2$: 18.5–21 Hz, $\beta 3$: 21.5–30 Hz) [2].

Assuming the maximal effect of each drug would correspond to its serum concentration, 2 h after perospirone and quetiapine, 4 h after risperidone, olanzapine and chlorpromazine, and 6 h after haloperidol were chosen.

For placebo as a control, the arithmetic means of 2, 4 and 6 h were calculated. Differences from pre-drug source gravity center locations: i.e., each of 3D (anterior–posterior (A-P), left–right (L-R) and superior–inferior (S-I)) values were compared using

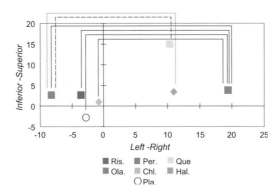

Fig. 1. Source location for beta3 frequency band after drug administration. Differences (subtraction values) from baseline (= 0) are shown on L-R × S-I axis. Repeated measures ANOVAs and post-hoc multiple comparisons of LSD indicated significant differences on L-R axis for the beta3 band. Red lines indicate significant differences at p < 0.05; Ris.: risperidone, Per.: perospirone, Que.: quetiapine, Ola.: olanzapine, Chl.: chlorpromazine, Hal.: haloperidol, Pla.: placebo.

one-way repeated measures ANOVAs, then post-hoc multiple comparisons using LSD method were applied.

3. Results

The source gravity center of β3 frequency band after perospirone was more right than after risperidone, olanzapine, chlorpromazine and placebo, while after quetiapine and haloperidol deviated to more right than after olanzapine ($p < 0.05$) (Fig. 1).

4. Discussion

Our results suggest that the seven test drugs including placebo acted differently on neural populations after a single administration. Only the source gravity center of β3 frequency band differed among the six antipsychotics tested.

References

[1] D. Lehmann, C.M. Michel, Intracerebral dipole source localization for FFT power maps, Electroencephalogr. Clin. Neurophysiol. 76 (1990) 271–276.
[2] S. Kubicki, et al., Reflections on the topics: EEG frequency bands and regulation of vigilance, Pharmakopsychiatr. Neuro-Psychopharmakol. 12 (1979) 237–245.

International Congress Series 1270 (2004) 348–351

ELSEVIER

www.ics-elsevier.com

Combined LORETA and fMRI study of recognition of eyes and eye movement in schizophrenia

Akihiko Suzuki, Eiji Kirino*

Department of Psychiatry, Juntendo University School of Medicine, Juntendo Izunagaoka Hospital, 1129 Nagaoka Izunagaokacho Tagatagun, Shizuoka 4102211, Japan

Abstract. Schizophrenics and controls participated in functional MRI (fMRI) and event-related potential (ERP) experiments, in which they viewed a face, eyes and moving eyes. Low-resolution brain electromagnetic tomography (LORETA) was reconstructed using ERPs. In fRMI, controls exhibited more eminent activations for the face in the fusiform gyrus and superior temporal gyrus bilaterally than did schizophrenics. For eyes, controls exhibited more prominent activations in the left inferior temporal gyrus and fusiform gyrus than did schizophrenics. In controls, moving eyes activated the posterior portion of the superior temporal region and transverse temporal gyrus right-dominantly or the middle and inferior occipital gyrus bilaterally. In contrast, schizophrenics tended to have greater activation in the left amygdala than controls. In LORETA, controls exhibited greater current density for the static face in the right middle temporal gyrus than did patients. In contrast, patients showed greater current density for the static eyes in the left insula. Furthermore, patients showed greater current density for moving eyes to the left in the left insula. Overactivation for eyes or moving eyes in the amygdala, insula, or extrastriate cortex observed in patients might indicate their hypersensitivity in the processing of feature details before processing the gestalt of the face or facial expression as a whole, which might be implicated in their deficits in interpersonal skills or in the formation of a variety of their clinical manifestations. © 2004 Elsevier B.V. All rights reserved.

Keywords: fMRI; LORETA; ERP; Schizophrenia; Face; Eye movement; Extrastriate; Fusiform gyrus

1. Introduction

The ventral occipitotemporal cortex and, in particular, the fusiform gyrus respond preferentially to faces [4,9,10,11]. Further, there exist neuronal systems sensitive to face parts in the lateral occipitotemporal cortex [1,14,15]. Neuroimaging findings [10,14,15] demonstrated that a region of the superior temporal cortex, located primarily in the superior temporal sulcus, is activated preferentially by moving eyes and mouths. It has been demonstrated that schizophrenic patients show deficits in facial–affect recognition [6,7], to which the deficits in interpersonal skills of the disease might be attributed. It might be plausible that their distorted interpersonal skills are due to impaired recognition of eyes or eye movement.

---

* Corresponding author. Tel.: +81-55-948-3111; fax: +81-55-948-5088.
E-mail address: ekirino@med.juntendo.ac.jp (E. Kirino).

0531-5131/ © 2004 Elsevier B.V. All rights reserved.
doi:10.1016/j.ics.2004.05.043

The goal of the present study is to explore the schizophrenics' deteriorations of face, eye, and eye movement recognition. Functional MRI (fMRI) and low-resolution brain electromagnetic tomography (LORETA) complemented time/spatial resolution of each of the measures.

2. Subjects and methods

A total of 10 schizophrenics and 10 healthy controls participated in the fMRI sessions, and 15 patients and 12 controls were in ERP sessions. After a complete description of the study to the subjects, all gave informed consent for the protocol. In fMRI, a blocked design was used. Experimental tasks had two sessions: ① static face and eyes, ② moving eyes (Fig. 1). ①-1 a static colored face superimposed on a radial pattern;①-2 static, colored, check patterns with the same background as ①-1; ①-3 static eyes cropped from ①-1; ①-4 same size static check patterns as ①-3.2-1, 2 the same static face as ①-1, initially gazed at the subject (S1), and then suddenly the eyes deviated to the right (②-1) or left (②-2) (S2); ②-3 simulated eye movement, in which the same check patterns as ①-2 moved in the same part of the visual field as in eyes, and with the same timing as ②-1; ②-4 face with eyes gazing unchanged, but the background rings changed between S1 and S2 with the same timing as ②-1, producing a perception consisting of an inwardly moving radial stimuli. The stimulus durations of S1 and S2 were 800 ms each and the onset-to-onset interval was 2100 ms. The imaging session of each task consisted of 24 blocks with a duration of 21 s (7 TR) with six cycles in four categories (168 TR/504 s in total). MRI data were acquired using the 1.5-T Toshiba VISART Ex system (gradient–echo echoplanar sequence: $TR = 3000$ ms $TE = 45$ ms, matrix $= 96 \times 96$, slice thickness $= 8$ mm, gap $= 1.0$ mm, Slice no. $= 13$, FOV $= 260$ mm, flip angle $= 70°$). Functional image analysis relied on the SPM99 software package (Wellcome Institute of Cognitive Neuroscience, London, UK). ERP experiments were conducted using the identical stimulus categories used in the fMRI studies, except for stimulus duration of ① (250 ms) and timing of the onset-to-onset interval of ① ② (1800–2300 ms). Each stimulus in a given category was pseudo-randomly distributed with equal probability over a session. Each stimulus category was presented 100 times. The electroencephalogram was recorded from 10 to 20 standard sites (Fp_1, Fp_2, F_7, F_3, Fz, F_4, F_8, T_3, C_3, Cz, C_4, T_4, T_5, P_3, Pz, P_4, T_6, O_1, O_2). LORETA was used to estimate the three-dimensional, intracerebral, and current density distribution. LORETA was reconstructed with ERPs using the LORETA program (LORETA-KEY; The Key Institute for Brain–Mind Research).

3. Results

3.1. fMRI

In task ①, controls exhibited more eminent activations for the face in the fusiform gyrus (BA 37) and superior temporal gyrus (BA 40) bilaterally than did schizophrenics (Fig. 2A).

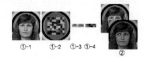

Fig. 1. Stimuli.

In contrast, for eyes, schizophrenics exhibited more prominent activations in the left inferior temporal gyrus (BAs 20 and 37) and fusiform gyrus (BA 37) than did controls (Fig. 2B). In task ②, controls showed greater activation for moving eyes (averaged activation of both directions) in the posterior portion of the superior temporal region and transverse temporal gyrus (BAs 41 and 42) right-dominantly (contrasting moving eyes with moving background) or the middle and inferior occipital gyrus (BAs 18 and 19) bilaterally (contrasting moving eyes with simulated moving eyes) (Fig. 2C,D). In contrast, schizophrenics tended to have greater activation in the left amygdala than did controls (Fig. 2E).

3.2. LORETA

In comparing patients and controls at each time frame in task ①, at a latency of 166–174 ms, controls exhibited greater current density for the face in the right middle temporal gyrus (BA 21) than did patients (Fig. 3) (Fig. 3A). In contrast, at a latency of 202 ms, patients showed greater current density for eyes in the left insula (BA 13) (Fig. 3B). Furthermore, at a latency of 238–240 ms in task ②, patients showed greater current density for moving eyes to the left in the left insula, as well as for eyes (Fig. 3C).

4. Discussion

Schizophrenics have been reported to be associated with more efficient processing of feature details than the gestalt [16], resulting in their segmented perception that the patients process stimulus fragments first and at the expense of the stimulus as a whole [12]. This type of processing leads to an overemphasis on non-critical features and to a depletion of available attention recourse before processing the critical features or interpreting wholes as meaningful gestalts. This might be implicated in their deficient facial–affect recognition [6] or impaired capacity to differentiate between relevant and irrelevant stimulus fragments [2]. The present finding revealed patients' attenuated activation for the static face in the temporal regions either in fMRI or LORETA. In contrast, patients exhibited more prominent activation for static eyes or moving eyes in the left amygdala, insula, or extrastriate cortex. Amygdala activation has been observed in response to fearful facial expressions [5], and anterior insula activation has been evoked by facial expressions of disgust [8]. The

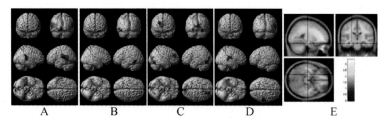

Fig. 2. Voxel-wise *t* test results for fMRI activation; (A) contrasting static face with checker pattern (controls>schizophrenics, $P_{uncorrected} < 0.01$ at voxel level, $P_{corrected} < 0.05$ at cluster level), (B) contrasting static eyes with checker pattern (schizophrenics>controls, $P_{uncorrected} < 0.01$ at voxel level, $P_{uncorrected} < 0.05$ at cluster level), (C) contrasting moving eyes with simulated moving eyes (controls>schizophrenics $P_{uncorrected} < 0.01$ at voxel level, $P_{uncorrected} < 0.05$ at cluster level), (D) contrasting moving eyes with moving background (controls>schizophrenics, $P_{uncorrected} < 0.01$ at voxel level, $P_{corrected} < 0.05$ at cluster level), (E) contrasting moving eyes with simulated moving eyes (schizophrenics>controls, $P_{uncorrected} < 0.05$ at voxel level).

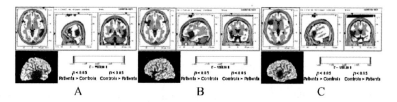

A   B   C

Fig. 3. Voxel-wise t test results for LORETA values of current density for static face (A) (controls>schizophrenics, $P < 0.05$), (B) static eyes (schizophrenics>controls $P < 0.05$), moving eyes to the left (C) (schizophrenics>controls $P < 0.05$).

extrastriate cortex, including face-specific regions of the fusiform gyrus [4,11], is activated more extensively by emotional facial expressions than emotionally neutral faces [3,13]. Overactivation for eyes or moving eyes in the amygdala, insula, or extrastriate cortex observed in schizophrenics might indicate their hypersensitivity in processing feature details before processing the face or facial expression as a whole, which might be implicated in their deficits in interpersonal skills or the formation of a variety of their clinical manifestations, such as fear of eye-to-eye confrontation or delusion of reference.

References

[1] S. Bentin, et al., Electrophysiological studies of face perception in humans, J. Cogn. Neurosci. 8 (6) (1996) 551–565.
[2] A.H. Buss, P.J. Lang, Psychological deficit in schizophrenia: I. Affect, reinforcement, and concept attainment, J. Abnorm. Psychology 70 (1965) 2–24.
[3] P.J. Lang, et al., Emotional arousal and activation of the visual cortex: an fMRI analysis, Psychophysiology 35 (2) (1998) 199–210.
[4] G. McCarthy, A. Puce, J.C. Gore, T. Allison, Face-specific processing in the human fusiform gyrus, J. Cogn. Neurosci. 9 (5) (1997) 605–610.
[5] J.S. Morris, et al., A differential neural response in the human amygdala to fearful and happy facial expressions, Nature 383 (6603) (1996) 812–815.
[6] R.L. Morrison, A.S. Bellack, K.T. Mueser, Deficits in facial–affect recognition and schizophrenia, Schizophr. Bull. 14 (1) (1988) 67–83.
[7] M.L. Phillips, A.S. David, Facial processing in schizophrenia and delusional misidentification: cognitive neuropsychiatric approaches, Schizophr. Res. 17 (1) (1995) 109–114.
[8] M.L. Phillips, et al., A specific neural substrate for perceiving facial expressions of disgust, Nature 389 (6650) (1997) 495–498.
[9] A. Puce, et al., Differential sensitivity of human visual cortex to faces, letterstrings, and textures: a functional magnetic resonance imaging study, J. Neurosci. 16 (16) (1996) 5205–5215.
[10] A. Puce, et al., Temporal cortex activation in humans viewing eye and mouth movements, J. Neurosci. 18 (6) (1998) 2188–2199.
[11] A. Puce, et al., Face-sensitive regions in human extrastriate cortex studied by functional MRI, J. Neurophysiol. 74 (3) (1995) 1192–1199.
[12] D. Shakow, Segmental set, Arch. Gen. Psychiatry 6 (1962) 1–17.
[13] R. Sprengelmeyer, et al., Neural structures associated with recognition of facial expressions of basic emotions, Proc. R. Soc. Lond., B Biol. Sci. 265 (1409) (1998) 1927–1931.
[14] S. Watanabe, et al., Human face perception traced by magneto- and electro-encephalography, Brain Res. Cogn. Brain Res. 8 (2) (1999) 125–142.
[15] S. Watanabe, et al., It takes longer to recognize the eyes than the whole face in humans, NeuroReport 10 (10) (1999) 2193–2198.
[16] D.S. Wells, D. Leventhal, Perceptual grouping in schizophrenia: replication of Place and Gilmore, J. Abnorm. Psychology 93 (2) (1984) 231–234.

International Congress Series 1270 (2004) 352–355

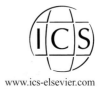

www.ics-elsevier.com

Combined LORETA and fMRI study of global–local processing in schizophrenia

Rie Inami, Eiji Kirino*

*Department of Psychiatry, Juntendo University School of Medicine, Juntendo Izunagaoka Hospital,
1129 Nagaoka, 4102211 Izunagaokachu, Tagatagun, Shizuoka, Japan*

Abstract. The goal of the present study is to explore schizophrenic patients' deteriorations of global–local (hierarchical stimulus) processing. Schizophrenics and healthy controls participated in functional MRI (fMRI) and event-related potentials (ERP) experiments. Low-resolution brain electromagnetic tomography (LORETA) was reconstructed using ERPs. In fMRI, global attention in controls exhibited more prominent activations for incongruent stimuli in the posterior portion of the superior temporal region and bilaterally transverse temporal gyrus than did schizophrenics. In global/local attention, controls exhibited more prominent activations for incongruent stimuli in the middle and inferior occipital gyrus right-dominantly than did schizophrenics. In local attention, schizophrenics showed greater activation in the left precuneus than did controls. Further, even in global attention, schizophrenics showed greater activation in the left middle occipital gyrus than did controls. In LORETA, global attention in controls showed greater current density in the posterior portion of the superior/middle temporal region and transverse temporal gyrus right-dominantly than did patients. In contrast, patients exhibited greater current density in the middle frontal gyrus and inferior frontal gyrus left-dominantly than did controls. The present results support the concept of left hemisphere overactive-right hemisphere underactive in schizophrenic patients. Schizophrenics' processing of hierarchical visual stimuli might be deficient in perceptual integration during processing in the occipitemporal cortex or be interfered with by the to-be-ignored local level, which might consequently increase the loads needed in higher processing in the prefrontal cortex reflected by enhanced activation in the left inferior frontal gyrus. © 2004 Elsevier B.V. All rights reserved.

Keywords: fMRI; LORETA; ERP; Schizophrenia; Global–local processing

1. Introduction

Natural visual processing involves the analysis of global and local form within hierarchically organized visual stimuli [4]. Loci within the temporal, parietal, or extrastriate cortex, and hemispheric asymmetry associated with human perception of hierarchical stimuli [4,11] have been documented. Most reports supported hemispheric specialization of the right for global forms and the left for local forms. Schizophrenics have been reported to be more associated with efficient processing of feature details than the gestalt [10,13],

---
* Corresponding author. Tel.: +81-55-948-3111; fax: +81-55-948-5088.
E-mail address: ekirino@med.juntendo.ac.jp (E. Kirino).

0531-5131/ © 2004 Elsevier B.V. All rights reserved.
doi:10.1016/j.ics.2004.05.044

resulting in their segmented perception that the patients process stimulus fragments first, at the expense of the stimulus as a whole [12]. This type of processing leads to an overemphasis on non-critical features and to a depletion of available attention recourse before processing the critical features or interpreting wholes as meaningful gestalts. This might be implicated in their deficient facial-affect recognition [8] or impaired capacity to differentiate between relevant and irrelevant stimulus fragments [1,6]. The global–local paradigm, using hierarchical visual stimuli composed of small local forms arranged into a large global form, is a useful tool for investigating hemispheric asymmetry, as well as aberrant attention and visual perception with schizophrenic patients [3,7,9]. Schizophrenic patients exhibited asymmetry in global–local perceptions, however, advantaged hemisphere is not consistent [2,3]. It still remains to be elucidated which hemisphere was responsible for the schizophrenics' deterioration in perception of hierarchical visual stimuli. The goal of the present study is to explore the schizophrenics' deteriorations of global–local processing employing functional MRI (fMRI) and low-resolution brain electromagnetic tomography (LORETA).

2. Subjects and methods

A total of 11 schizophrenics and 11 healthy controls participated in the fMRI sessions, and 12 patients and 10 controls were in event-related potentials (ERP) sessions. After a complete description of the study to the subjects, all gave informed consent for the protocol. In *fMRI*, a blocked design was used. Experimental tasks consisted of three tasks (Fig. 1): ① global-attention task, ② local-attention task, and ③ global/local-attention task. ①-1 usual, large capital letters (A, E, H, S); ①-2 global letters constructed from congruent local capital letters (A/A, E/E, H/H, S/S); ①-3 global letters constructed from incongruent local capital letters (A/H, E/S, H/A, S/E). Subjects were instructed to pay attention to the global level and press a button whenever targets (A or E) appeared at the global level. ②-1 usual, small capital letters constructing squares with the same height as ①-1 (A, E, H, S); ②-2 identical to ①-2; ②-3 identical to ①-3. Subjects were instructed to pay attention to the local level and press a button whenever targets (A or E) appeared at the local level. In ① ②, stimulus in each category was pseudo-random with an equal probability. ③. All stimuli are global letters constructed from incongruent, local capital letters (A/H, E/S, H/A, S/E. A/S, E/H, H/S, S/A). Subjects were instructed to pay attention to both the global and local levels and press a button whenever target (A) appeared at any level; ③-1 targets appear only on the local level with probability of 50%; ②-2 targets appear only on the global level with a probability of 50%; ③-3 targets appear on both levels with a probability of 50%. Each stimulus, other than the target in a given category, was pseudo-randomly distributed such that they each comprised equal probability (12.5%) in a block. The stimulus duration was 500 ms and the onset-to-onset interval was 750 ms. The imaging session of each task consisted of 288 stimuli. Each session included 18

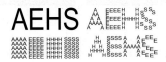

Fig. 1. Stimuli; large capital letters, small capital letters, congruent hierarchical stimuli (A/$_A$, E/$_E$, H/$_H$, S/$_S$), incongruent hierarchical stimuli (A/$_H$, E/$_S$, H/$_A$, S/$_E$).

blocks with 6 cycles by three categories. To exclude influence of expectation, the block duration varied from 14 to 18 stimuli. MRI Data were acquired using the 1.5-T Toshiba VISART Ex system (gradient-echo echoplanar sequence: TR = 3000 ms TE = 45 ms, Matrix = 96 × 96, Slice Thickness = 8 mm, Gap = 1.0 mm, Slice # = 13, FOV = 260 mm, Flip angle = 70°). Image analysis relied on the SPM99 software package (Wellcome Institute of Cognitive Neuroscience, London, UK). ERP experiments were conducted using the identical stimulus categories used in fMRI studies, except for the onset-to-onset interval of 1250–1750 ms. In each experiment, each stimulus category was presented 100 times. One button was used to respond to targets A and E in , A in ③) and another for all non-targets. The electroencephalogram was recorded from 10 to 20 standard sites (Fp$_1$, Fp$_2$, F$_7$, F$_3$, Fz, F$_4$, F$_8$, T$_3$, C$_3$, Cz, C$_4$, T$_4$, T$_5$, P$_3$, Pz, P$_4$, T$_6$, O$_1$, Oz, O$_2$), in addition to PO$_3$, PO$_4$, PO$_7$, PO$_8$, and POz. LORETA was reconstructed with ERPs using the LORETA-KEY program (The Key Institute for Brain–Mind Research).

3. Results

3.1. fMRI

In global attention, controls exhibited more prominent activations for incongruent stimuli in the posterior portion of the superior temporal region and transverse temporal gyrus (BA41, 42) bilaterally than did schizophrenics (contrasting global attention with local-attention). In global/local-attention, controls exhibited more prominent activations for incongruent stimuli in the middle and inferior occipital gyrus (BA18, 19) right-dominantly than did schizophrenics (contrasting global/local-attention with local-attention). In local-attention, schizophrenics showed greater activation in the left precuneus (BA19) than did controls (contrasting incongruent stimuli with congruent ones). Further, even in global attention, schizophrenics showed greater activation in the left middle occipital gyrus (BA18) than did controls (contrasting incongruent with congruent) (Figs. 2 and 3).

3.2. LORETA

In comparison to LORETA values of ERPs for incongruent stimuli at each time frame during global attention between patients and controls, at a latency of 168 ms, controls showed greater current density in the posterior portion of the superior/middle temporal

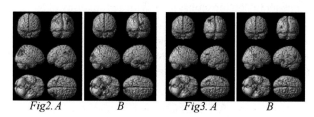

Fig2. A   B   Fig3. A   B

Fig. 2. Voxel-wise t-test results (controls>schizophrenics) for fMRI activation contrasting incongruent stimuli during global attention (A) and global/local (B) attention with those during local attention ($P_{uncorrected}$ < 0.05 at voxel level, $P_{uncorrected}$ < 0.05 at cluster level). Fig. 3. Voxel-wise t-test results (schizophrenics>controls) for fMRI activation contrasting incongruent stimuli with congruent stimuli during local attention (A) and global attention (B) ($P_{uncorrected}$ < 0.01 at voxel level, $P_{uncorrected}$ < 0.05 at cluster level).

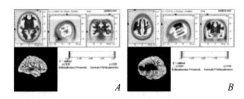

Fig. 4. Voxel-wise t-test results for current density for incongruent stimuli at each time frame during global attention (A controls>schizophrenics $P < 0.1$, B; schizophrenics>controls $P < 0.05$).

region and transverse temporal gyrus (BA 21, 22) right-dominantly than did patients. During 220–226 ms, patients exhibited greater current density in the middle frontal gyrus and inferior frontal gyrus (BA 9, 46) left-dominantly than did controls (Fig. 4).

4. Discussion

Schizophrenics exhibited attenuated activation of the right hemisphere in global attention; however, they showed more prominent activation in local attention predominantly in the left hemisphere. As revealed in greater activation of the left occipital middle gyrus even in global attention, patients' global processing of hierarchical visual stimuli is likely to be interfered with by the to-be-ignored local level, which supports the concept of left hemisphere overactive-right hemisphere underactive in schizophrenic patients [3]. Furthermore, patients exhibited greater current density in the middle frontal gyrus and the inferior frontal gyrus left-dominantly than did controls during global attention. These findings are compatible with the previous reports of aberrant prefrontal cortex activation, especially in the left inferior frontal gyrus during a visual oddball paradigm containing task-irrelevant distracters in schizophrenia [5]. Schizophrenics' processing of hierarchical visual stimuli might be deficient in perceptual integration during processing in the occipitemporal cortex or be interfered with by the to-be-ignored local level, which might consequently increase the loads needed in higher processing in PFC reflected by enhanced activation in the left inferior frontal gyrus.

References

[1] A.H. Buss, P.J. Lang, J. Abnorm. Psychology 70 (1965) 2–24.
[2] C.S. Carter, et al., Psychiatry Res. 62 (2) (1996) 111–119.
[3] T.J. Ferman, et al., J. Int. Neuropsychol. Soc. 5 (5) (1999) 442–451.
[4] H.J. Heinze, et al., J. Cogn. Neurosci. 10 (4) (1998) 485–498.
[5] E. Kirino, A. Belger, in: K. Hirata, Y. Koga, K. Nagata, K. Yamazaki (Eds.), Recent Advances in Human Brain Mapping, Elsevier, Amsterdam, 2002, pp. 691–696.
[6] P.J. Lang, A.H. Buss, J. Abnorm. Psychology 70 (1965) 77–106.
[7] J. Miller, D. Navon, Q. J. Exp. Psychol., A 55 (1) (2002) 289–310.
[8] R.L. Morrison, A.S. Bellack, K.T. Mueser, Schizophr. Bull. 14 (1) (1988) 67–83.
[9] D. Navon, Perception 12 (3) (1983) 239–254.
[10] E.J. Place, G.C. Gilmore, J. Abnorm. Psychology 89 (3) (1980) 409–418.
[11] L.C. Robertson, et al., J. Exp. Psychol. Hum. Percept. Perform. 19 (3) (1993) 471–487.
[12] D. Shakow, Arch. Gen. Psychiatry 6 (1962) 1–17.
[13] D.S. Wells, D. Leventhal, J. Abnorm. Psychology 93 (2) (1984) 231–234.

International Congress Series 1270 (2004) 356–360

ELSEVIER

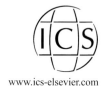

www.ics-elsevier.com

Combined fMRI and LORETA study of illusory contour perception in schizophrenia

Chisako Ikeda, Eiji Kirino*

Department of Psychiatry, Juntendo University School of Medicine, Juntendo Izunagaoka Hospital, 1129 Nagaoka, Izunagaokacho Tagatagun, Shizuoka 4102211, Japan

Abstract. Schizophrenic patients and healthy controls participated in functional MRI (fMRI) experiments with blocked design using Echo Planner Imaging, in which illusory contour (IC) (Kanizsa's square) and control objects (no contour: NC; real contour: RC) were passively presented. Subjects underwent ERP (event-related potentials) sessions using identical stimuli with fMRI studies, and then LORETA (low resolution brain electromagnetic tomography) was reconstructed using ERPs. Controls exhibited more eminent activations for IC in the extrastriate cortex encompassing the V2 area than did schizophrenics. In contrast, schizophrenics demonstrated more prominent activations for IC in the right anterior cingulate gyrus (ACC) and bilateral middle frontal gyrus than those of controls. Comparing LORETA values of ERPs for IC at each time frame between patients and controls, patients showed greater current density in the left insula than that of controls. Schizophrenics might be deficient in perceptual integration during processing in the extrastriate cortex, which might consequently increase the loads needed for higher processing in the prefrontal cortex reflected by the enhanced fMRI activation in ACC. Otherwise, an ambiguous object like IC, unless processed optimally at the pre-attentive level, might be perceived as disgusting stimuli and evoke activation in the insula of schizophrenic patients. © 2004 Elsevier B.V. All rights reserved.

Keywords: LORETA; fMRI; ERP; Extrastriate; Schizophrenia; Illusory contour

1. Introduction

Object recognition occurs despite ambiguous or incomplete information in the retinal images, as in situations of partial occlusion and poor lighting. The brain can therefore reconstruct absent from visual images [3,10]. Examples are provided by the Kanizsa figures/ illusory contours (IC), where the arrangement of a simple component induces the perception of contours and shapes, which are more than the sum of the parts in the stimuli themselves [6]. Neuroimaging studies have shown IC sensitivity in the lower-tier of area V2, and to a lesser extent of V1 [4,5,7,12]. Ffytche and Zeki [4] demonstrated that IC perception was associated with significant activity only in the early visual area, in particular in area V2,

---

* Corresponding author. Tel.: +81-55-948-3111; fax: +81-55-948-5088.
E-mail address: ekirino@med.juntendo.ac.jp (E. Kirino).

0531-5131/ © 2004 Elsevier B.V. All rights reserved.
doi:10.1016/j.ics.2004.04.101

without higher order cognitive influences. Others propose that IC sensitivity occurs at higher processing stages in the lateral-occipital cortex (LOC) areas [9].

Schizophrenic patients experience a loss of perceptual stability, fragmentation of percepts, and inability to interpret wholes as meaningful gestalts [1,2]. Given the feature integration theory [14], at the first or pre-attentive level in visual perception, separate sensory features are coded automatically, in parallel and without focused attention—an automatic, effortless or "bottom-up" processing. This level leads to the formation of the "feature maps," which are organized into groups, textures or homogeneous areas. These "maps" provide a preliminary organization of the stimulus fields and prepare stimulus input for optimal serial processing. The second level is the feature integration stage in which focused attention is used in serially scanning the stimulus fields—a controlled, effortful, or "top-down" processing. It still remains to be elucidated whether schizophrenic patients' fragmented perception or deficit in feature integration is attributed to bottom-up/parallel/automatic process or top-down/serial/controlled process or both. To investigate these issues, functional MRI (fMRI), event-related potentials (ERPs), and low-resolution brain electromagnetic tomography (LORETA) during IC perception were employed to complement time/spatial resolution of each of the other measures.

2. Subjects and methods

Fifteen schizophrenics and fifteen healthy controls participated in the fMRI sessions, and nineteen patients and fifteen controls in ERP sessions. After complete description of the study to the subjects, all gave informed consent for the protocol. In fMRI, a blocked design was used. There were these stimulus categories: illusory contour (IC); Kanizsa's square [6], no contour (NC); four inducers positioned misangled such that no illusory contour was generated, and real contour (RC); a real square, filling the same field of IC, with inducers (Fig. 1). The imaging session consisted of six blocks with a duration of 42 s (21 TR), each of which consisted of a specific stimulus category presentation (126 TR/252 s in total). Every category was presented totally for 126 s in a given session. Images were acquired using a 1.5 Tesla Toshiba VISART Ex system and functional images were acquired using a gradient-echo echoplanar sequence (TR = 2000 ms TE = 45 ms, Matrix = 96 × 96, Slice Thickness = 8 mm, Gap = 1.0 mm, Slice # = 13, FOV = 260 mm, Flip angle = 70°). Functional image analysis relied on the SPM99 software package (Wellcome Institute of Cognitive Neuroscience, London, UK). ERP experiments were conducted using the identical stimulus categories used in the fMRI studies, except for stimulus duration (250

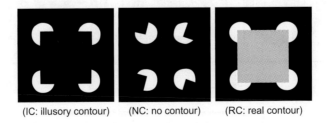

(IC: illusory contour)   (NC: no contour)   (RC: real contour)

Fig. 1. Stimuli.

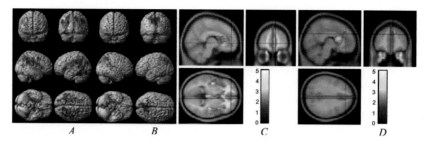

Fig. 2. Voxel-wise t-test results for fMRI activation contrasting the IC (A, C) with NC (B, D) (A; controls> schizophrenics, $P_{uncorrected} < 0.05$ at voxel level, $P_{corrected} < 0.05$ at cluster level) and RC (B; controls> schizophrenics, $P_{uncorrected} < 0.05$ at voxel level, $P_{uncorrected} < 0.05$ at cluster level). (C, D; schizophrenics> controls, $P_{uncorrected} < 0.05$ at voxel level, $P_{uncorrected} < 0.05$ at cluster level).

ms) and timing of the onset-to-onset interval (1800–2300 ms). Each of three stimulus categories was pseudo-randomly distributed with equal probability over a single session. In each experiment, each stimulus category was presented 100 times. The electroencephalogram (EEG) was recorded from 10 to 20 standard sites (Fp1, Fp2, F7, F3, Fz, F4, F8, T3, C3, Cz, C4, T4, T5, P3, Pz, P4, T6, O1, O2). LORETA was used to estimate the three-dimensional intracerebral current density distribution. LORETA was reconstructed with ERPs using the LORETA program (LORETA-KEY; The Key Institute for Brain-Mind Research).

3. Results

3.1. fMRI

In contrast both between IC and NC and between IC and RC, controls exhibited more eminent activations for IC in the extrastriate cortex encompassing the V2 area (BA18) than did schizophrenics (Fig. 2A,B). In contrast, schizophrenics demonstrated more prominent activations for IC in the right anterior cingulate gyrus (ACC) (BA 9, 24, 32) and bilateral middle frontal gyrus (BA 9) those of controls (Fig. 2C,D).

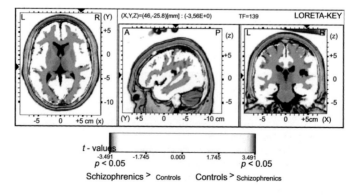

Fig. 3. Voxel-wise t-test results (schizophrenics> controls) for current density for IC ($P < 0.05$).

3.2. LORETA

Comparing LORETA values of ERPs for IC at each time frame between patients and controls, at the latency of 276, patients showed greater current density in the left insula (BA 13) than that of controls (Fig. 3).

4. Discussion

The present findings revealed that IC processing in schizophrenia might be underactive in the occipital visual fields, but overactive in ACC and the insula. The previous reports have been trying to model IC processing. Murray et al. [10] proposed that IC sensitivity described in V2 and V1 may predominantly reflect feedback modulation from a higher-tier LOC area, where IC sensitivity first occurs. They suggested a model of IC processing wherein dorsal stream regions, which are initially insensitive to an IC presence, coarsely demarcate the spatial extent of a given stimulus array and then input to ventral stream structures as LOC. Namely, IC effects observed previously in lower-tier areas are likely to be driven by feedback inputs from higher-tier areas. Given that IC processing was modelled as feedback loops between bottom-up/lower tier/process and top-down/higher tier process, schizophrenic patients' impaired IC processing might be attributed to their deterioration of feedback loops between the hierarchical subsystems during visual processing. Although speculative, a higher tier system might be implicated in the frontal cortex containing the prefrontal cortex including ACC, as well as the occipital visual fields.

The processing of affective/emotional stimuli has been studied using both PET and fMRI. Anterior insula activation has been evoked by facial expressions of disgust [11]. Processing of stimuli evoking fear, anger, disgust or other emotions may be based on separate neural systems, and the output of these systems may converge on frontal regions for further information processing [13].

The present findings and the previous reports reviewed above might support the views that dysfunction in the pre-attentive, automatic stage of processing necessitates the use of consciously controlled serial processing for perceptual assembly operations that would normally be conducted automatically and in parallel [1,2,8]. Schizophrenics might be deficient in perceptual integration during processing in the extrastriate cortex, which might consequently increase the loads needed in later processing in the prefrontal cortex as reflected by the enhanced fMRI activation in the ACC. Otherwise, an ambiguous object like IC, unless processed optimatically in the pre-attentive level, might be perceived as disgusting stimuli and evoke activation in the insula of schizophrenic patients.

References

[1] V.J. Carr, S.A. Dewis, T.J. Lewin, Preattentive visual search and perceptual grouping in schizophrenia, Psychiatry Res. 79 (2) (1998) 151–162.
[2] J. Chapman, The early symptoms of schizophrenia, Br. J. Psychiatry 112 (484) (1966) 225–251.
[3] G.M. Doniger, et al., Visual perceptual learning in human object recognition areas: a repetition priming study using high-density electrical mapping, NeuroImage 13 (2) (2001) 305–313.
[4] D.H. Ffytche, S. Zeki, Brain activity related to the perception of illusory contours, NeuroImage 3 (2) (1996) 104–108.

[5] J. Hirsch, et al., Illusory contours activate specific regions in human visual cortex: evidence from functional magnetic resonance imaging, Proc. Natl. Acad. Sci. U. S. A. 92 (14) (1995) 6469–6473.

[6] G. Kanizsa, Subjective contours, Sci. Am. 234 (4) (1976) 48–52.

[7] J. Larsson, et al., Neuronal correlates of real and illusory contour perception: functional anatomy with PET, Eur. J. Neurosci. 11 (11) (1999) 4024–4036.

[8] A. McGhie, J. Chapman, Disorders of attention and perception in early schizophrenia, Br. J. Med. Psychol. 34 (1961) 103–116.

[9] J.D. Mendola, et al., The representation of illusory and real contours in human cortical visual areas revealed by functional magnetic resonance imaging, J. Neurosci. 19 (19) (1999) 8560–8572.

[10] M.M. Murray, et al., The spatiotemporal dynamics of illusory contour processing: combined high-density electrical mapping, source analysis, and functional magnetic resonance imaging, J. Neurosci. 22 (12) (2002) 5055–5073.

[11] M.L. Phillips, et al., A specific neural substrate for perceiving facial expressions of disgust, Nature 389 (6650) (1997) 495–498.

[12] M. Seghier, et al., Moving illusory contours activate primary visual cortex: an fMRI study, Cereb. Cortex 10 (7) (2000) 663–670.

[13] R. Sprengelmeyer, et al., Neural structures associated with recognition of facial expressions of basic emotions, Proc. R. Soc. Lond., B Biol. Sci. 265 (1409) (1998) 1927–1931.

[14] A.M. Treisman, G. Gelade, A feature-integration theory of attention, Cogn. Psychol. 12 (1) (1980) 97–136.

International Congress Series 1270 (2004) 361–364

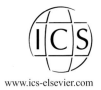

www.ics-elsevier.com

Neuroimaging of the information processing flow in schizophrenia during the Stroop task using a spatially filtered MEG analysis

Shunsuke Kawaguchi[a,*], Satoshi Ukai[a], Kazuhiro Shinosaki[b],
Masakiyo Yamamoto[a], Ryouhei Ishii[a], Asao Ogawa[a],
Yuko Mizuno-Matsumoto[a], Norihiko Fujita[c],
Toshiki Yoshimine[d], Masatoshi Takeda[a]

[a] Department of Psychiatry and Behavioral Science, Osaka University Graduate School of Medicine D-3,
2-2, Yamada-oka, Suita, Osaka 565-0871, Japan
[b] Department of Neuropsychiatry, Wakayama Medical University, Wakayama, Japan
[c] Department of Radiology, Osaka University Graduate School of Medicine, Osaka, Japan
[d] Department of Neurosurgery, Osaka University Graduate School of Medicine, Osaka, Japan

Abstract. We examined transient neural activations from the input of a stimulus to the output of a response during the Stroop task for schizophrenic subjects with/without auditory hallucinations using a spatial filtered technique, synthetic aperture magnetometry (SAM), which provides high temporal and spatial resolution. MEG signals from the presentation of incongruent stimuli to responses were analyzed with a time window of 200 ms in steps of 50 ms. According to our previous studies with healthy subjects, regions showing significant decrease of current source density (CSD) in the 25–60-Hz band, corresponding to event-related desynchronization, were regarded to be activated. The non-hallucinators showed neural activations in the inferior parietal or temporal regions in the early stage of information processing, and successive and temporally overlapping neural activations in the left dorsolateral prefrontal cortex (DLPFC) and primary motor area (M1). The hallucinators showed neural activations in the right DLPFC and M1. Our preliminary results suggest that the schizophrenic subjects showed transient neural activations along the fundamental information flow (sensory input system–executive control system–motor output system), and that lateralization of DLPFC might be related with auditory hallucinations in schizophrenia. © 2004 Elsevier B.V. All rights reserved.

Keywords: Spatial filter; Synthetic aperture magnetometry (SAM); Magnetoencephalography; Information processing flow; Schizophrenia; Stroop task

* Corresponding author. Tel.: +81-6-6879-3051; fax: +81-6-6879-3059.
E-mail address: kawaguch@psy.med.osaka-u.ac.jp (S. Kawaguchi).

0531-5131/ © 2004 Elsevier B.V. All rights reserved.
doi:10.1016/j.ics.2004.05.050

1. Introduction

The information processing flow of the brain neural network in schizophrenia is still unknown, although neuroimaging approaches, such as PET and fMRI, have focused on it. These techniques have poor temporal resolution and merely examine the information processing flow by estimating functional connectivity of the pre-specified regions of interest using correlation analysis of the hemodynamics.

Previously, using a spatial filtered technique, synthetic aperture magnetometry (SAM) [1,2] of MEG with high temporal and spatial resolution, we successfully visualized the information processing flow during the Stroop task from the input of a stimulus to the output of a response in nearly real time for the healthy subjects [3]. In this study, using SAM, we examined the information processing flow for the schizophrenic patients with/ without auditory hallucinations.

2. Materials and methods

2.1. Subjects

Six schizophrenic patients were studied. All subjects provided written informed consent after the explanation of this study. According to the scores of the hallucinatory behavior item on the Brief Psychiatric Rating Scale, the patients were subdivided into the hallucinators (three patients) and the non-hallucinators (three patients).

2.2. Stroop task

Using red, blue, yellow and green, the stimuli of the task consisted of 12 incongruent and 4 congruent stimuli. Each name of a color was displayed in a Japanese kanji character, which was written in a color of ink different from that of the word for the incongruent stimuli or the same as that of the word for the congruent stimuli. Each stimulus set consisted of an eye fixation cross of 500 ms and an incongruent/congruent stimulus of 1250 ms. The stimulus sets of the incongruent and congruent stimuli were pseudo-randomly presented on a 15-in. TFT display placed 2 m away from the subjects. The subjects were asked to name the color quickly and accurately in a very small voice.

2.3. Synthetic aperture magnetometry: SAM

SAM can produce three-dimensional current source density (CSD) mapping from band-limited MEG signals. A statistical parametric map can be produced using voxel-to-voxel comparison by the Student's t-test of the CSD mappings taken in active (task) and control (rest) states. A statistical parametric map image is fused with a subject's MRI, and examined for regions showing statistically significant differences in CSD in the prescribed frequency bands.

2.4. MEG acquisition and data analysis

MEG recordings were performed using a helmet-shaped, 64-channel SQUID sensor array (CTF Systems). The data acquisition rate was 250 Hz. MEG data were digitally filtered using an online, combined 80-Hz low pass filter and 60-Hz notch filter and were recorded on disks for the offline analysis.

One hundred unaveraged, incongruent stimulus sets were analyzed for each subject. The 200-ms period, just before the presentation of incongruent stimuli for the control state (− 200–0 ms), and the 200-ms post-stimulus period (0–200 ms) and a moving step of 50 ms (50–250,..., 650–850 ms), for a total of 14 active states, were analyzed.

According to our previous study [3], we estimated the statistical parametric map images for the 25–60-Hz band with a 5-mm voxel resolution, and examined regions showing significantly decreased CSD corresponding to event-related desynchronization (ERD), considered to be neural activation.

3. Results

Fig. 1 shows the SAM statistical imaging of significant ERD for a non-hallucinator and a hallucinator. Fig. 2 shows the time course maps of significant ERD during the Stroop task for all subjects. The non-hallucinators showed significant ERD in the inferior parietal or temporal regions in the early stage of information processing, while the hallucinators did not. They also showed significant ERD in the left prefrontal polar area, left dorsolateral prefrontal cortex (DLPFC), left inferior frontal gyrus and mid- to lower-primary motor area (M1). The hallucinators showed significant ERD in the right DLPFC and the M1. All subjects showed significant ERD in the DLPFC. The non-hallucinators showed ERD in the left DLPFC, hallucinators in the right DLPFC.

4. Discussion

The schizophrenic subjects showed the successive and temporally overlapping transient neural activations from the input of a stimulus to output of a response during the Stroop task. The left inferior parietal or temporal regions might subserve the processing of words

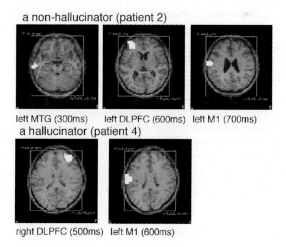

a non-hallucinator (patient 2)

left MTG (300ms)   left DLPFC (600ms)   left M1 (700ms)

a hallucinator (patient 4)

right DLPFC (500ms)   left M1 (600ms)

Fig. 1. The SAM statistical imaging in the 25–60-Hz band for a non-hallucinator (patient 2) and a hallucinator (patient 4) showing significant neural activation with its maximum t value. The time given is the median of each time window. MTG: middle temporal gyrus; DLPFC: dorsolateral prefrontal cortex; M1: mid- to lower-primary motor area.

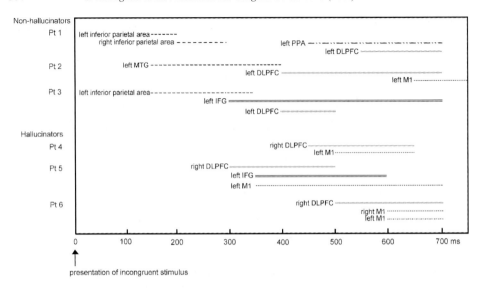

Fig. 2. The time course maps of significantly activated regions for all subjects. The thick line indicates periods of significant neural activations. The time given is the median of each time window. DLPFC: dorsolateral prefrontal cortex; MTG: middle temporal cortex; IFG: inferior frontal gyrus; M1: mid- to lower-primary motor area.

in the early stage of information processing in order to maintain a good performance of the Stroop task. The DLPFC and M1 are thought to be associated with executive control functions and vocalization, respectively. The schizophrenic subjects showed spatial and temporal patterns of neural activations along the fundamental information flow (sensory input system–executive control system–motor output system). In addition, the neural activations in the DLPFC were left-lateralized for the non-hallucinators, while right-lateralized for the hallucinators, suggesting that lateralization of the DLPFC activation might be related to auditory hallucinations in schizophrenia.

References

[1] S.E. Robinson, D.F. Rose, Current source image estimation by spatially filtered MEG, in: M. Hoke, S.N. Eme, Y.C. Okada (Eds.), Biomagnetism: Clinical Aspects, Proceedings of the 8th International Conference on Biomagnetism, Elsevier, New York, 1992, pp. 761–765.

[2] R. Ishii, et al., Theta rhythm increases in left superior temporal cortex during auditory hallucinations in schizophrenia: a case report, Neuroreport, (2000) 3283–3287.

[3] S. Ukai, et al., Parallel distributed processing neuroimaging in the Stroop task using spatially filtered magnetoencephalography analysis, Neurosci. Lett. 334 (2002) 9–12.

International Congress Series 1270 (2004) 365–369

ELSEVIER

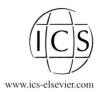

www.ics-elsevier.com

Event-related fMRI study of prefrontal and anterior cingulate cortex during response competition in schizophrenia

Mayuko Fukuta, Eiji Kirino*

Department of Psychiatry, Juntendo University School of Medicine, Juntendo Izunagaoka Hospital, 1129 Nagaoka, Izunagaokacho Tagatagun, Shizuoka 4102211, Japan

Abstract. Carter et al. [Science 280 (1998) 747] demonstrated that anterior cingulate cortex (ACC) detects conditions in which errors are likely to occur. Kirino and Belger [E. Kirino, A. Belger, fMRI and ERP evidence of prefrontal cortex mediation of novelty bias and distractibility in schizophrenia, in: K. Hirata, Y. Koga, K. Nagata, K. Yamazaki (Eds.), Recent Advances in Human Brain Mapping, Elsevier, Amsterdam, 2002, pp. 691–696.] further observed aberrant prefrontal cortex (PFC) activation during a visual oddball paradigm containing task-irrelevant distracters in schizophrenia. We hypothesized that schizophrenics show distorted PFC and ACC activation during response competition. We imaged patients and controls performing variants of Continuous Performance Test (CPT) that were designed to increase error rates and manipulate response competition. Subjects made a response whenever the probe was an X proceeded by a cue A, and to make a nontarget response to all other stimuli (AY, BX and BY). When targets (AX) occurred with 70% frequency, AY and BX were previously reported to elicit higher levels of response competition than BY (1998). Event-related design for the functional MRI (fMRI) experiment was employed with AX ($p = 86\%$) as baseline response and AY, BX, and BY ($p = 4.7\%$ for each) as event stimuli. Echo Planner images were acquired on a 1.5-T MR system. Schizophrenics showed attenuated activation in PFC and ACC under condition that elicits response competition. These findings might indicate that they are less sensitive to override prepotent responses. Schizophrenics' deficits in working memory might be attributed to the deteriorated central executive system, which involved response competition, rather than slave systems in the working memory model of Baddeley [Science 255 (1992) 556]. © 2004 Elsevier B.V. All rights reserved.

Keywords: fMRI; Schizophrenia; Prefrontal; Anterior cingulate cortex

1. Introduction

Physiological studies in monkeys have demonstrated dorsolateral prefrontal cortex (dPFC) involvement in processes underlying working memory [10]. Neuroimaging studies in humans have supported this assertion by demonstrating dPFC activation during varieties of working memory tasks [2,7,17,19,21]. Baddeley [1] divided working memory system

* Corresponding author. Tel.: +81-55-948-3111; fax: +81-55-948-5088.
 E-mail address: ekirino@med.juntendo.ac.jp (E. Kirino).

into three subcomponents: the central executive, which is assumed to be an attention-controlling system, and two slave systems, namely the visuospatial sketchpad and phonological loop. McCarthy et al. [18] and Kirino et al. [14] demonstrated activation of prefrontal cortex (PFC), primarily middle frontal gyrus (MFG) and ACC, in response to infrequently and irregularly presented visual target stimuli during target detection tasks. Anterior cingulate cortex (ACC) detects conditions in which errors are likely to occur [4,11]. These findings might be interpreted as that dPFC and ACC are critically involved in the central executive system.

Schizophrenic patients have demonstrated working memory deficits as revealed by psychophysiological studies or P300 or MMN abnormality in ERP studies [3,12,15,16]. However, these findings leave unsettled whether working memory deficits observed in schizophrenic patients are attributed predominantly to impairment of the central executive or that of the slave systems. To investigate this issue, employing event-related functional MRI (fMRI) during Continuous Performance Test (CPT), we explored activation PFC and ACC for response competition in schizophrenic patients.

2. Subjects and methods

2.1. Subjects

Schizophrenics (9) and healthy controls (13) participated in fMRI sessions. After complete description of the study to the subjects, all gave informed consent.

2.2. fMRI

2.2.1. Experimental task

CPT was modified such that error rates increased to manipulate response competition. Subjects made a target response whenever the probe was an X proceeded by a cue that was A, and no overt or covert response was required to all other type of cue–probe (AY, BX and BY). When targets (AX) occurred with 70% frequency, AY and BX are previously reported to elicit higher levels of response competition than BY [6]. Each stimulus was presented for 500 ms against a white background that subtended a visual angle of $5.4 \times 5.4°$. The onset-to-onset interval was 1500 ms including 1 S of interstimulus interval, i.e. cue–cue interval was 3000 ms (1 TR). AX type of cue–probe pair was designed as baseline/reference response and AY, BX and BY as events of interests. Each imaging session consisted of three blocks with duration of 450 s (150 of cue–probe/150 TRs). Each pair of cue–probe was pseudo-randomly distributed such that AX, AY, BX and BY comprised, respectively, 86%, 4.7%, 4.7%, 4.7% of the stimulus in a given session. Subsequent events (AY, BX, BY) were separated by a minimum of 7 AXs. Every event was presented a total of 21 times in a given session.

2.2.2. Acquisition of MRI data

1.5 Tesla Toshiba EXELART system (gradient-echo echoplanar sequence: $TR = 3000$ ms $TE = 45$ ms, Matrix $= 96 \times 96$, Slice Thickness $= 8$ mm, Gap $= 1.0$ mm, Slice $\# = 13$, FOV $= 260$ mm, Flip angle $= 70°$).

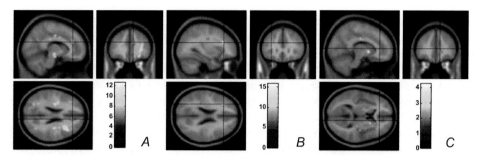

Fig. 1. Grand-average of 13 Controls (A) ($P_{uncorrected} < 0.00001$ at voxel level, $P_{corrected} < 0.05$ at cluster level) and 9 Schizophrenics (B) ($P_{uncorrected} < 0.0001$ at voxel level, $P_{corrected} < 0.05$ at cluster level) of fMRI activation for AY and BX. Voxel-wise t-test results (controls > schizophrenics) of fMRI activation for AX and BY ($P_{uncorrected} < 0.01$ at voxel level, $P_{uncorrected} < 0.05$ at cluster level) (C).

2.2.3. Functional image analysis

SPM99 software package (Wellcome Institute Cognitive Neuroscience, London, UK).

3. Results

Controls exhibited prominent activations in right ACC (BA 32) and right MFG (BA 9,10) (Fig. 1A). Schizophrenics exhibited limited activations in left MFG for AY and BX (BA 9) nonetheless no activation was observed in ACC (Fig. 1B). Voxel-wise t-test results revealed that controls exhibited more eminent activation in right ACC (BA 32) than that of schizophrenics (Fig. 1C).

4. Discussion

Referring to previous findings concerning memory of schizophrenic patients, McKenna et al. [20] reported a distinctive pattern of memory impairment in schizophrenia with sparing of short-term/primary memory coupled with clear impairment in long-term/secondary memory. In their findings, schizophrenics showed preservation on short-term memory tasks such as the forward digit span test although they showed ubiquitous impairment on long-term memory tasks. Goldberg et al. [9] assessed memory in monozygotic pairs of individuals discordant for schizophrenia and normal pairs of monozygotic twins. Forward short-term memory for digit did not differ significantly between groups. However, in the performance of digits span in backward order, the affected groups did worse. Further, the affected group had relatively preserved recognition memory for faces and words on the Warrington test, and did not show profoundly accelerated rates of forgetting on the Wechsler Memory Scale. Frame and Oltmanns [8] assessed schizophrenics' performance on serial-recall of six nouns shortly after hospitalization and again after their symptoms had improved. Schizophrenics' performance continued to be impaired particularly on the word presented in the first serial position, despite an overall improvement in their accuracy as they recover from an acute psychotic episode. They also reported that schizophrenics' performance deteriorated in the presence of distraction at both point of assessment and suggested their tendency toward greater distractibility. They accounted that the schizophrenics problems involve active, organizational processes rather than passive or automatic functions. Goldberg et al. [9] accounted the characterized memory impairment of schizophrenics as the inability to acquire new information rapidly, access old information propitiously, and divide attention between important environmental stimuli. Internal information processing might be difficult in even the most routine mental operations of everyday life. These findings concerning schizophrenics' memory suggest that their memory is preserved when they do not need to employ the attention-controlling system such as the central executive system, which coordinates information from the slave systems in working memory model of Baddeley [1] referred above. They might be intact as concerns the slave system. Further, Kirino and Belger [13] observed less PFC activation during a visual oddball paradigm containing task-irrelevant distracters in schizophrenia. Carter et al. [5] also reported less positron emission tomography (PET) activation of ACC during stroop task, and which has been related to cingulated morphology [22].

In conjunction with data from studies of schizophrenic patients' memory, the present findings might indicate that they are less sensitive to override prepotent responses. Schizophrenics' deficits in working memory might be attributed to the deteriorated central executive system, which involved response competition, rather than slave systems in the working memory model of Baddeley [1].

References

[1] A. Baddeley, Working memory, Science 255 (5044) (1992) 556–559.
[2] A. Belger, et al., Dissociation of mnemonic and perceptual processes during spatial and nonspatial working memory using fMRI, Hum. Brain Mapp. 6 (1) (1998) 14–32.
[3] D.H. Blackwood, et al., Changes in auditory P3 event-related potential in schizophrenia and depression, Br. J. Psychiatry 150 (1987) 154–160.
[4] C.S. Carter, et al., Anterior cingulate cortex, error detection, and the online monitoring of performance, Science 280 (5364) (1998) 747–749.
[5] C.S. Carter, et al., Anterior cingulate gyrus dysfunction and selective attention deficits in schizophrenia: [15O]H$_2$O PET study during single-trial Stroop task performance, Am. J. Psychiatry 154 (12) (1997) 1670–1675.
[6] J.D. Cohen, T.S. Braver, R.C. O'Reilly, A computational approach to prefrontal cortex, cognitive control and schizophrenia: recent developments and current challenges, Philos. Trans. R. Soc. Lond., B Biol. Sci. 351 (1346) (1996) 1515–1527.
[7] J.D. Cohen, et al., Activation of prefrontal cortex in a non-spatial working memory task with functional MRI, Hum. Brain Mapp. 1 (1994) 293–304.
[8] C.L. Frame, T.F. Oltmanns, Serial recall by schizophrenic and affective patients during and after psychotic episodes, J. Abnorm. Psychology 91 (5) (1982) 311–318.
[9] T.E. Goldberg, et al., Learning and memory in monozygotic twins discordant for schizophrenia, Psychol. Med. 23 (1) (1993) 71–85.
[10] P.S. Goldman-Rakic, Circuitry of primate prefrontal cortex and regulation of behavior by representational memory, in: F. Plum (Ed.), Handbook of Physiology, The Nervous System, Higher Functions of the Brain, American Physiological Society, Bethesda, 1987, pp. 373–417.
[11] K.A. Kiehl, P.F. Liddle, J.B. Hopfinger, Error processing and the rostral anterior cingulate: an event-related fMRI study, Psychophysiology 37 (2) (2000) 216–223.
[12] E. Kirino, Correlation between P300 and EEG Rhythm in schizophrenia, Clin. Electroencephalogr. 35 (4) (2004) (in press).
[13] E. Kirino, A. Belger, fMRI and ERP evidence of prefrontal cortex mediation of novelty bias and distractibility in Schizophrenia, in: K. Hirata, Y. Koga, K. Nagata, K. Yamazaki (Eds.), Recent Advances in Human Brain Mapping, Elsevier, Amsterdam, 2002, pp. 691–696.

[14] E. Kirino, et al., Prefrontal activation evoked by infrequent target and novel stimuli in a visual target detection task: an event-related functional magnetic resonance imaging study, J. Neurosci. 20 (17) (2000) 6612–6618.

[15] E. Kirino, R. Inoue, Relationship of mismatch negativity to background EEG and morphological findings in schizophrenia, Neuropsychobiology 40 (1) (1999) 14–20.

[16] E. Kirino, R. Inoue, The relationship of mismatch negativity to quantitative EEG and morphological findings in schizophrenia, J. Psychiatr. Res. 33 (5) (1999) 445–456.

[17] G. McCarthy, et al., Functional magnetic resonance imaging of human prefrontal cortex activation during a spatial working memory task, Proc. Natl. Acad. Sci. U. S. A. 91 (18) (1994) 8690–8694.

[18] G. McCarthy, et al., Infrequent events transiently activate human prefrontal and parietal cortex as measured by functional MRI, J. Neurophysiol. 77 (3) (1997) 1630–1634.

[19] G. McCarthy, et al., Activation of human prefrontal cortex during spatial and nonspatial working memory tasks measured by functional MRI, Cereb. Cortex 6 (4) (1996) 600–611.

[20] P.J. McKenna, et al., Amnesic syndrome in schizophrenia, Psychol. Med. 20 (4) (1990) 967–972.

[21] E.E. Smith, et al., Spatial versus object working memory: PET investigations, J. Cogn. Neurosci. 7 (1995) 337–356.

[22] M. Yucel, et al., Anterior cingulate activation during Stroop task performance: a PET to MRI coregistration study of individual patients with schizophrenia, Am. J. Psychiatry 159 (2) (2002) 251–254.

International Congress Series 1270 (2004) 370–373

ELSEVIER

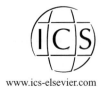

www.ics-elsevier.com

Evaluation of missing fundamental phenomenon with auditory selective attention in the human auditory cortex

Tetsushi Ookushi[a], Yoshinori Matsuwaki[b], Tsuneya Nakajima[b,*],
Jirou Iimura[a], Masafumi Nakagawa[c], Masuro Shintani[d],
Hiroshi Moriyama[a], Tatsuya Ishikawa[d]

[a] Department of Otorhinolaryngology, JIKEI University School of Medicine, Japan
[b] Department of Otorhinolaryngology, Tokyo Dental College Ichikawa General Hospital, 5-11-13 Sugano, Ichikawa, Chiba 272-0824, Japan
[c] Department of Otorhinolaryngology, Juntendo University School of Medicine, Japan
[d] Department of Oral Health Science Center, Tokyo Dental College, Japan

Abstract. When complex tones consisting of four or more continuous harmonic tones of a certain fundamental frequency are perceived as the pitch of the fundamental frequency, it is referred to as the missing fundamental phenomenon (MFP) or the virtual pitch. We reported that MFP occurred in the human transverse and superior temporal gyri, namely, the primary auditory cortex, between P50 and N100 by 306 ch magnetoencephalography (MEG). It is also reported that auditory selective attention probably occurs in the human auditory cortex. The purpose of this study was to investigate whether MFP was produced in the same process even during auditory selective attention. We measured MFP by 306 ch MEG. The subjects had two tasks. One task was listening to some complex tones while counting the total numbers of the target tone (attention task), and the other task was accomplished while ignoring the target tone (no attention task). MFP also occurred in the transverse and superior temporal gyri between P50 and N100 even in the case of auditory selective attention, the same as in that of the without attention atmosphere. MFP and auditory selective attention occurred in the human auditory cortex at adjoining locations. © 2004 Elsevier B.V. All rights reserved.

Keywords: Missing fundamental phenomenon (MFP); Human auditory cortex; Harmonic complex tones; Magnetoencephalography (MEG); Auditory selective attention; Transverse temporal gyrus; Superior temporal gyrus

1. Introduction

Circumstances can be perceived by hearing sensation based on the perception of complex tones. When complex tones consisting of four or more continuous harmonic tones of a

---

* Corresponding author. Tel.: +81-47-322-0151; fax: +81-47-325-4456.
E-mail address: nakajima@tdc.ac.jp (T. Nakajima).

0531-5131/ © 2004 Elsevier B.V. All rights reserved.
doi:10.1016/j.ics.2004.05.148

certain fundamental frequency are perceived as the pitch of the fundamental frequency, it is referred to as the missing fundamental phenomenon (MFP) or the virtual pitch [1–5].

MFP is thought to be produced in the auditory center, not in the periphery, because of the following reasons: (1) MFP was observed in the primary auditory area at a single unit level when one ear was stimulated in a monkey [6,7]; (2) this phenomenon was not masked by low frequency noises [6]; (3) the pitch of a fundamental frequency was perceived even when both ears were independently stimulated with complex tones consisting of two continuous harmonic tones of the fundamental frequency (dichotic listening) [8,9]; and (4) this phenomenon was not observed when part of the temporal lobe was surgically removed to treat epilepsy [10]. We reported that MFP occurs in the transverse and superior temporal gyri, the primary auditory cortex between P50 and N100, by using 306 ch magnetoencephalography (MEG) [11].

By the way, we can hear clearly even in a noisy environment by concentrating on a selected sound or voice. It is also reported that auditory selective attention probably occurs in the human auditory cortex [12,13]. But the relation between attention effect and MFP is uncertain. We investigated whether MFP was observed in the same process even during auditory selective attention by using 306 ch MEG.

2. Subjects and method

We examined the right hemisphere of five subjects who were healthy right-handed adult volunteers with normal auditory sensation in the following experiment.

We measured MFP by 306 ch MEG, as previously described [11]. Briefly, each ear was stimulated with a pure tone burst at a duration of 20 ms (rise/fall: 1 ms). Sound pressure was established at the most comfortable level for each subject. Ears were randomly stimulated with six different complex tones (STIM1-6) at intervals of 500 ± 50 ms, up to 300 times, respectively. STIM1-5 were connected with MFP, while STIM6 had no connection with MFP and was the target tone. The subjects had two tasks. One task was listening to STIM1-6 and counting the total numbers of the target tone (STIM 6) (attention task), and the other task was accomplished while ignoring the target tone (no attention task). Following left ear stimulation with STIM1 (fundamental frequency tone, 330 Hz) and STIM 2 (four harmonic complex tones, $660 + 990 + 1320 + 1650$ Hz), the location and direction of ECD were evaluated at P50 and N100 in the right temporal lobe.

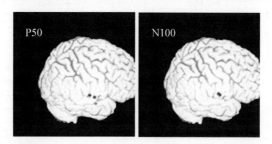

Fig. 1. Localization of ECD evoked by STIM1-5 on the 3-dimensionally constructed brain surface. Green point: STIM1; yellow point: STIM2; turquoise point: STIM3; red point: STIM4; and blue point: STIM5. (For interpretation of the references to colour in this figure legend, the reader is referred to the web version of this article.)

STIM3 and STIM4 (each of those consisting of two harmonic complex tones, $660 + 1650$ Hz, $990 + 1320$ Hz) were used for dichotic listening, and the results were compared with those of bilateral stimulation with STIM5 (fundamental frequency tone, 330 Hz). Similarly, the location and direction of ECD were evaluated at P50 and N100 after auditory stimulation with STIM3–STIM5. Using source modeling (Neuromag), single dipole analysis was performed in the right hemisphere (153 ch), based solely on data showing 80% or higher GOF. Dispersion of the source of ECD at P50 and N100 was respectively evaluated by comparing the distance of the source of ECD evoked by STIM1–STIM5 (between STIM1 and STIM2, as well as between STIM3 + STIM4 and STIM5) and comparing the difference with and without attention task.

Paired *t*-test was used to compare the two variables. Differences with *P* value were considered statistically significant.

3. Results and discussion

We have already reported that the MFP occurred in the human transverse and superior temporal gyri, which constitute the primary auditory cortex between P50 and N100 in the no attention task when using 306 ch MEG [11]. The purpose of this study was to investigate whether MFP was produced in the same process even during auditory selective attention. The location and direction of ECD evoked by STIM1–STIM5 varied at P50 depending on the direction of the gyrus in the transverse temporal and superior temporal gyrus. However, the location and direction of ECD at N100 evoked by STIM1–STIM5 were almost identical in the transverse temporal gyrus. These results were observed in both tasks (Fig. 1). When the distance was compared between each location of ECD evoked by STIM1 and STIM2, it was significantly shorter (nearer) at N100 than at P50 in both tasks (Fig. 2A). These phenomena were similarly observed, even when STIM3–STIM5 (dichotic and bilateral listening) were stimulated in both tasks (Fig. 2B). These findings suggest that the MFP is processed at the transverse temporal gyri and superior temporal, the primary auditory cortex between P50 and N100 (about 40–120 ms after auditory stimulation), even during auditory selective attention. MFP was observed not only by one side listening but also by dichotic listening even in the attention task; it may be produced in the central auditory system, but not by peripheral tone differences.

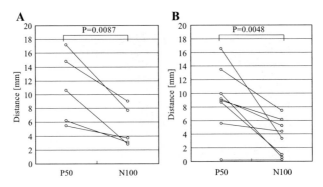

Fig. 2. Comparison of distance between several sources of ECD at P50 and N100 in the attention task. (A) STIM1 vs. STIM2. (B) STIM3 and STIM4 vs. STIM5.

Table 1
Lag of ECD location in the attention task compared with each ECD location in the no attention task (mm, mean ± standard deviation)

		STIM1	STIM2	STIM3	STIM4	STIM5
P50	X	− 0.48 ± 6.27	− 3.8 ± 3.49	5.05 ± 5.09	− 0.48 ± 2.91	10.15 ± 17.86
	Y	− 2.8 ± 4.35	0 ± 3.84	− 5.15 ± 9.71	2.25 ± 8.54	5.6 ± 14.16
	Z	0.93 ± 12.41	− 4.63 ± 7.61	− 0.86 ± 6.61	− 0.83 ± 5.14	− 7.35 ± 13.17
N100	X	− 0.45 ± 5.54	− 0.9 ± 4.16	− 0.7 ± 2.01	− 2.83 ± 2.9	− 0.36 ± 3.15
	Y	2.33 ± 5.42	− 2.1 ± 5.73	1.53 ± 5.23	1.58 ± 6.77	0.33 ± 4.23
	Z	− 0.9 ± 1.85	− 3.55 ± 4.71	− 2.85 ± 5.39	− 1.83 ± 3.01	0.48 ± 5.08

X corresponds to anterodorsal direction, Y to bilateral direction, and Z to superoinferior direction.

We also investigated the lag of ECD location in the attention task in relation to each location of ECD in the no attention task. There was no characteristic trend of P50 in either task. On the other hand, at N100, the ECD in the attention task tended to locate in front from that of the no attention task, although it was within the error range of MEG measuring (Table 1). Arthur et al. [12] reported that ECD for auditory attention were localized anterior to ECD for the no attention task in the human posterior regions of the sylvian fissure. If there is a component of auditory selective attention ECD in the front of primary auditory cortex, ECD of MFP would be falsely transferred to the front in the attention task. Because single dipole analysis shows just center of the target, brain activity was performed in this study. A recent study showed that the location of auditory selective attention ECD and those of no attention ECD did not differ significantly [13]. These data show that MFP and auditory selective attention occur in the human auditory cortex, locations probably adjoining each other. We reported that MFP was observed in the same process even during auditory selective attention.

References

[1] J.L. Goldstein, An optimum processor theory for the central formation of the pitch of complex tones, J. Acoust. Soc. Am. 54 (1973) 1496–1516.
[2] J.C.R. Licklider, A duplex theory of pitch perception, Experientia 7 (1951) 128.
[3] R.J. Risma, Frequencies dominant in the perception of the pitch of complex sounds, J. Acoust. Soc. Am. 42 (1967) 191–198.
[4] E. Terhardt, Pitch, consonance and harmony, J. Acoust. Soc. Am. 55 (1974) 1061–1069.
[5] F.L. Wightman, The pattern-transformation model of pitch, J. Acoust. Soc. Am. 54 (1973) 407–416.
[6] D.W. Schwarz, R.W. Tomlinson, Spectral response patterns of auditory cortex neurons to harmonic complex tones in alert monkey (Macaca mulatta), J. Neurophysiol. 64 (1990) 282–298.
[7] Y.I. Fishman, et al., Pitch vs. spectral encoding of harmonic complex tones in primary auditory cortex of the awake monkey, Brain Res. 786 (1998) 18–30.
[8] C. Pantev, et al., Binaural fusion and the representation of virtual pitch in the human auditory cortex, Hear Res. 100 (1996) 164–170.
[9] A.J.M. Houtsma, et al., The central origin of the pitch of complex tones: evidence from musical interval recognition, J. Acoust. Soc. Am. 51 (1972) 520–529.
[10] R.J. Zatorre, Pitch perception of complex tones and human temporal-lobe function, J. Acoust. Soc. Am. 84 (1988) 566–572.
[11] Y. Matsuwaki, et al., Evaluation of missing fundamental phenomenon in the human auditory cortex, ANL (in press).
[12] D.L. Arthur, et al., A neuromagnetic study of selective auditory attention, Electro. Clin. Neuro. 78 (1991) 348–360.
[13] N. Fujiwara, T. Nagamine, M. Imai, Role of the primary auditory cortex in auditory selective attention studied by whole-head neuromagnetometer, Brain Res. Cogn. Brain Res. 7 (1998) 99–109.

Author index

Keyword index